DETOX
KITCHEN
VEGETABLES

DETOX KITCHEN VEGETABLES

LILY SIMPSON

BLOOMSBURY PUBLISHING
LONDON · OXFORD · NEW YORK · NEW DELHI · SYDNEY

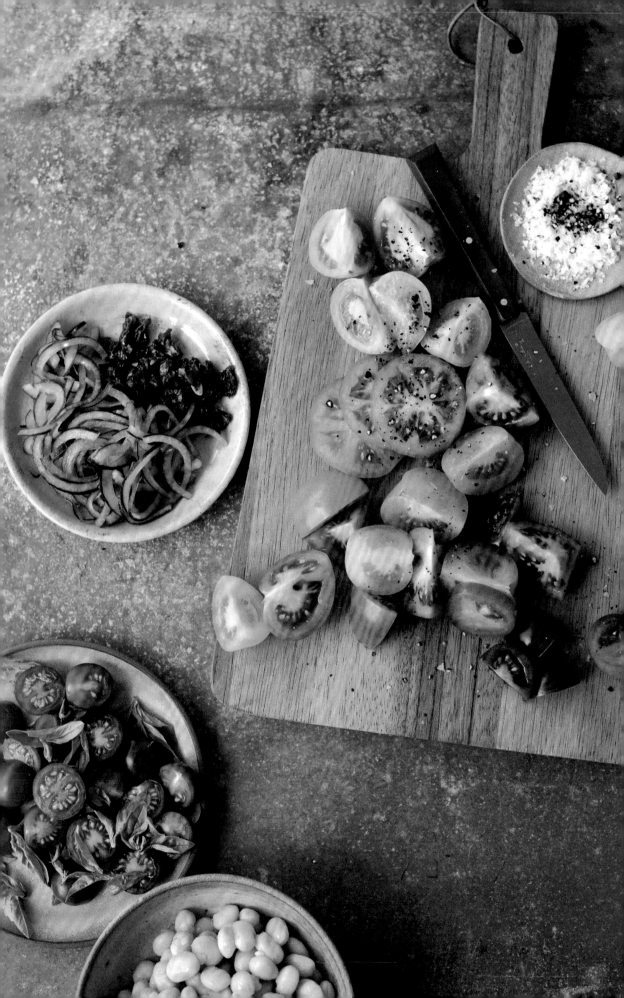

Contents

Joyfulness and good health 7

Cooking with vegetables 8

Stocking your larder 9

Broad beans 12

Peas 20

Asparagus 30

Globe artichoke 40

Fennel 48

Rhubarb 58

Radish 66

Cucumber 76

Spinach 84

Kale 90

Watercress 98

Pak choi 104

Cabbage 112

Brussels sprouts 118

Broccoli 124

Cauliflower 134

Okra 148

Butternut squash 154

Pumpkin 166

Sweet potato 176

Jerusalem artichoke 186

Carrot 192

Parsnip 202

Beetroot 208

Leek 218

Onion 224

Mushroom 232

Aubergine 240

Pepper 252

Tomato 260

Courgette 272

Marrow 282

Sweetcorn 288

Index 296

Acknowledgements 303

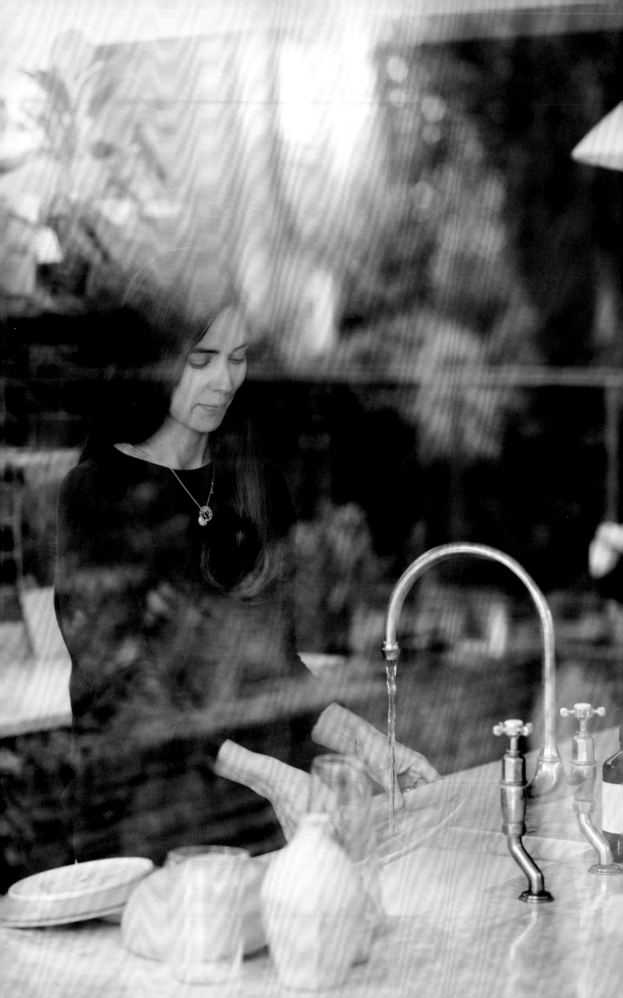

Joyfulness and good health

First and foremost, I want to clarify that this book is not just for vegetarians. It is a book about vegetables, to show how versatile and delicious they can be.

In 2012 I launched Detox Kitchen, a food business with natural ingredients at its core. Since then, I have had the pleasure of creating and sharing hundreds of vegetable-based dishes with thousands of customers and have seen first-hand how moving towards a diet that is abundant in good-quality, predominantly plant-based foods can have a truly beneficial impact on your health and well-being.

Over the years I have also mastered the art of cooking without wheat, dairy or refined sugar. While these are not necessarily foods that we all should avoid or completely eliminate – I believe that there is a place for every type of food in a well-balanced diet – I do think that we tend to over-consume them. Through the recipes in this book, I hope to show you how easy it can be to eat in a more balanced way.

At home and at work I want to create food that makes you feel good and that makes you feel nurtured; I also want to celebrate the fact that we are able to enjoy three meals a day. From breakfast-time, sitting on the rug with my kids – a hot cup of tea carefully placed out of their reach – to the dinner I rush home to prepare (at home even chefs have to wing it sometimes!), it all culminates in total calmness once I am settled at the table with the people I love most.

My way of cooking and eating is guided by two clear principles: everyday joyfulness and good health. When both of them are in balance you'll find that you're enjoying a nutritious diet that can make you feel truly happy.

Cooking with vegetables

The food that we put into our bodies has a huge effect on our overall health and well-being. Ultimately, we all know that fresh, 'real' food is much better for us than food that has been over-sprayed with chemicals and industrially processed. Eating well can be very easy and inexpensive as well as entirely delicious. Enjoying an abundance of vegetables will ensure that you consume a wide variety of the nutrients that play such an important role in your body's health. This is because vegetables contain a huge array of essential vitamins and minerals.

When I started to write this book I was not a vegetarian. I was raised in a meat-eating household where no main meal was complete if chicken, lamb, beef or pork didn't feature. But over the past few years, because of a growing concern for animal welfare and the environmental impact of rearing animals for meat, I have taken the personal decision that I don't want to make the problem worse and would stop eating meat. I believe that anyone can cook their way to a delicious diet by eating less meat generally, even without becoming a full-time vegetarian.

The thirty-three vegetables in this book are the ones that are always in my kitchen, that I like to grow in my garden and that I look forward to when they are about to come into season. But what is a vegetable, when you get right down to it? The general rule, botanically speaking, is that an edible plant is a fruit if it has seeds; if it is seedless, then it is a vegetable. The culinary classifications, however, sometimes differ. I have followed the basic principle that if you use something like a vegetable, then that's what it is – so tomato, cucumber and squash, for example, have made the cut. I have snuck rhubarb in because technically it is a vegetable that just happens to be treated like a fruit.

In this book you'll see that the only frozen vegetables I use are peas, broad beans and sweetcorn. These often contain as many nutrients as freshly picked peas, broad beans or sweetcorn as they will have been prepared and frozen within a few hours of being harvested. As a general rule, however, fresh vegetables in season have the best flavour and texture, and are likely to be the most nutritious.

Stocking your larder

Today we are lucky enough to have a fabulous variety of vegetables to cook with, from beautifully coloured heirloom tomatoes and heritage carrots to knobbly little Jerusalem artichokes, architectural 'Romanesco' cauliflowers and perfect podded peas. With this cornucopia comes a great opportunity to play with flavours and textures.

By pairing vegetables with carefully chosen grains, herbs and spices, I hope to encourage you in a bolder approach to cooking with them. My recipes can be adapted and developed to suit your own palate (and store cupboard or fridge contents). If you don't have all the ingredients for a recipe, don't be afraid to experiment and throw other things in – you might end up creating a new dish!

Herbs

Finding confidence in your herb selection will open up wonderful ways of cooking vegetables. Pairing a vegetable with its perfect herb can transform its flavour. Below I have listed my most used herbs and indicated how best to cook with them, but my advice is simply to experiment and work out the flavour combinations you prefer.

Coriander
You either love it or hate it. For me, the complex flavour of coriander – fresh and citrussy with nutty notes – can really bring a dish to life. Used widely in Asian and South American cuisine, the leaves of this herb work well in fresh, crunchy salads, as well as to garnish curries, soups and stews. Using the stalks in curries will add a deep, floral flavour.

Dill
This delicate, feathery leaf adds a light aniseed flavour to salads, soups and stews. Its fragrant taste is similar to fresh coriander, with a sweet undertone. Dill is best used as a finishing touch or garnish, as the flavour decreases when cooked.

Parsley
Parsley is the hardiest soft-leaved herb, so can be cooked in a dish for a long period or added raw as a garnish. When cooked, it develops a woody, savoury flavour, which is why it works so well in stocks and stews. Widely used in Middle Eastern cooking, parsley adds a grassy, fresh flavour to contrast deep, smoky notes of other ingredients. I prefer flat-leaf parsley for its more robust taste.

Basil
Basil is found in many cuisines but it is most frequently used in Mediterranean cooking, in particular Italian. This sweet, strongly aromatic, soft-leaved herb is the perfect garnish for tomato salads; it is delicious as the base of a pesto, and it will bring many classic pasta dishes to life.

Chives
Chives will give a fresh, oniony kick to any dish, and can always be on hand if you grow a pot of them on a windowsill. This herb is particularly good in dressings, where it adds a subtle savoury flavour and a flash of bright green colour.

Mint

I use mint often in salads, especially one that will accompany a spicy dish. I love the combination of mint and coriander – they complement each other to give a complex, lingering flavour. I also love fresh mint tea and have a cup every day, which means that mint is always in my fridge or growing on the windowsill.

Rosemary

Rosemary is a hardy herb that works amazingly well with root vegetables. It's easy to grow and should take up residence in every garden. It's best to cook this herb, as the sweet, nutty, floral notes will develop more and the texture of the rosemary spikes will become softer and more palatable.

Thyme

With its pungent aroma and flavour, thyme is perfect for slow-cooked dishes. It works well in savoury recipes and, teamed with citrus flavours, it creates an aromatic Middle Eastern twist.

Spices

When cooking vegetables, a bit of spice can open up a new world of exciting flavours and aromas. The following are my favourite spices, always on hand in my store cupboard.

Cardamom

Cardamom has a unique sweet and floral flavour. The complex citrussy, earthy and aromatic taste works just as well in curries as it does in sweet dishes. I use it often in baking to bring a more savoury twist to a cake or bread.

Cinnamon

Cinnamon will bring out the sweetness in most vegetables, which is why I use it often in tagines and curries to balance earthier spices. It is also the perfect companion to porridge – a sprinkle is all you need to bring the creamy oats to life.

Cloves

These dried flowerbuds have a wonderfully strong, aromatic flavour. Widely used in Asian and African cooking, they add a floral, sweet taste with citrus notes. Cloves work well in curries and stews, as well as in sweet dishes.

Fennel seeds

The aniseed flavour of fennel seeds brings out sweetness in root vegetables. Used in stews and curries, it adds an aromatic, floral taste, which works especially well with the heat of chilli.

Cumin

Cumin's flavour – earthy, nutty and bitter – is distinctive and powerful. Just a teaspoon of ground cumin makes its presence felt in a bold curry sauce, and sprinkled over vegetables before roasting, it gives them a rich, smoky flavour.

Turmeric

This bright yellow spice will transform the dullest dish. I use ground turmeric in curries to add an earthy, mustardy flavour. I also like to add it when roasting cauliflower to give a deep colour, as well as a peppery, slightly bitter flavour that works well with a sweeter ingredient, such as sultanas.

Grains

These are the staple foods of a healthy, nutritious vegetable-based diet. I keep a good stock of them.

Rice

I use a variety of different rices. I love the texture and nuttiness of black, red and wild rices. Their dark colour also gives a touch of theatre to a dish. Brown rice, with its good firm texture and lovely earthy flavour, is the whole rice grain, so is more nutritious than white rice. The cooking times for brown, black, red and wild rices tend to be longer than that of white rice, but it is worth it for the delicious flavour and texture that they offer.

Quinoa

Quinoa has long been part of the staple diet in South America – the Incas called it the 'Mother Grain' – and it provides a complete source of protein. I use it in salads as well as to accompany curries and stews in place of rice. Quinoa is also great added to soups to give them more substance.

Buckwheat

Seasoned well, buckwheat has a deep, nutty flavour that is a great backdrop for salads, as well as providing a good accompaniment to rich, saucy stews. It's easy to prepare and inexpensive too.

Flour

I tend to use three types of flour, depending on what I am cooking. For sauces and baking I like Doves Farm gluten-free flour, which is made up of rice and buckwheat flour. I use chickpea (gram) flour for flatbreads, as its rich, nutty flavour gives the breads a wonderful earthiness. And for the fluffiest gluten-free pancakes, my choice is buckwheat flour.

Nuts and seeds

A sprinkle of nuts or seeds on a vegetable dish provides a delightful contrast in flavour and texture as well as a boost of protein. I couldn't be without these nuts and seeds in my kitchen.

Cashews
These creamy, crunchy nuts are widely used in my cooking. They form the base of my pesto (see page 36), giving it a good coarse texture; I add the nuts whole to curries for an extra crunch; and toasted, they top many of my salads.

Pecans
Sweet, softly crunchy pecans work well with root vegetables, as well as in sweet dishes.

Almonds
I often use flaked almonds to garnish Middle Eastern-style stews. The sweet almond flavour also lends itself to use in cakes and other treats. Ground almonds can make a great alternative to wheat flour in many breads and pastry.

Pumpkin and sunflower seeds
These are an absolute staple in my kitchen cupboard. I toast them to add crunch and nuttiness to salads, soups and stews.

Eggs

I will always buy organic eggs. For an ingredient that forms one of the main protein sources in a vegetarian diet, I think it's worth spending the extra amount for really good-quality eggs that taste delicious.

Dairy alternatives

I use a number of dairy alternatives, such as oat milk, brown rice milk and soya yoghurt. If you do not consume any dairy in your diet, it's important to ensure that you choose the varieties of these that are unsweetened and fortified with calcium, where possible.

Salt and pepper

I always cook with Maldon sea salt flakes because of the fresh, light flavour. Unlike table salts, which are processed and contain an additive to prevent clumping, Maldon salt is simply salt crystals produced by the evaporation of filtered sea water.

I splash out on good-quality cracked black pepper because I think it is such a key ingredient – it will enhance all the herbs and spices that you cook with. Pepper also adds a touch of heat to a dish, to awaken your tastebuds and make them more open to the other flavourings.

Vegetable stock

I make my own stock, using onion, celery, fennel and bay leaves, and keep it in the freezer, usually in ice cube trays, ready to use. If I have run out of home-made stock, I use a good-quality vegetable bouillon powder.

Broad beans

Broad beans (also known as fava beans) are legumes. They generally come in two varieties – 'Windsor', which has four large beans in each pod, and 'Longpod', with about eight smaller beans per pod. They are hardy little things that can grow in most climates, and are at their best during the months of June to September in the UK.

The floury, nutty flavour of a broad bean packs a real punch for its small size and it is a very versatile vegetable. When you tear open a broad bean pod, you'll find each of the beans inside covered in a light green skin. If the beans are very young, you can use them straight away. The skin of older beans can be tough so you might want to remove it (this is sometimes called 'double podding') to reveal the tender, bright green bean beneath. This colour will bring the dullest of dishes to life.

Frozen broad beans normally have the thick skin left on, though you can track down the double-podded kind too. Beans with skin on work well in stews, adding a good firm texture. They are also delicious simply boiled for a few minutes, then tipped into a food processor with a drizzle of oil and some fresh mint to make a dip for slathering over toast or serving with crudités.

Nutritional bonus

Broad beans are an excellent source of **protein** and **fibre**, perfect for a vegetarian diet. The beans are also rich in both **folate** and **B vitamins**, which we need for healthy nerves and peak energy levels.

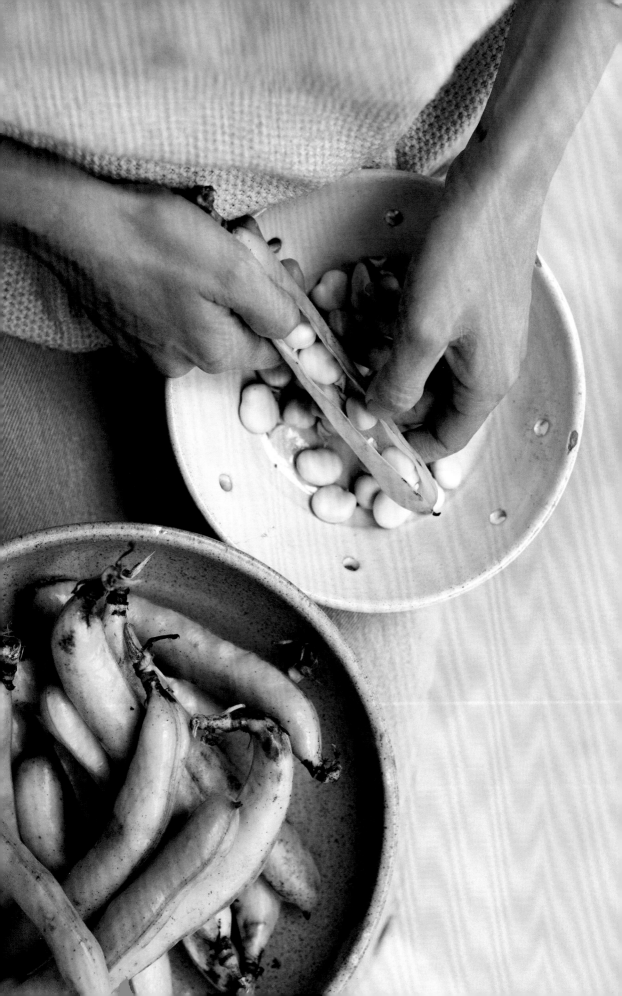

Broad bean bruschetta

Serves 2
331 calories per serving

Skinning broad beans is a perfect way to block out the rest of the world while you focus on the repetitive action of gently squeezing thumb to forefinger to make each bright green bean burst out of its skin. These bruschette are great for brunch and a good way to enjoy fresh beans.

1 cucumber
A handful of fresh mint, leaves picked
1 garlic clove
2 tbsp soya yoghurt
Zest of 1 lemon
600–800g fresh broad beans in their pods
2 fresh tarragon sprigs, roughly chopped
A handful of sunflower seeds

For the bruschette
1 garlic clove, crushed
1 small loaf rye bread, preferably thick crust,
    cut into 4 slices lengthways
Olive oil for drizzling
Flaked sea salt and cracked black pepper

1 Cut the cucumber across in half. Peel one half, then cut in half lengthways and scoop out the seeds. Finely chop the peeled cucumber, mint and garlic together and mix with the yoghurt. Add the lemon zest and season with salt and pepper. Reserve the other cucumber half.

2 Pod the broad beans (you want about 200g podded weight). Bring a pan of water to the boil. Drop in the beans and cook for 1 minute, then drain and rinse under cold water. Pop the beans out of their skins by gently squeezing. Place in a bowl and add the tarragon. Crush the beans coarsely with a fork.

3 Toast the sunflower seeds in a small dry frying pan until golden.

4 Run the prongs of a fork down the sides of the reserved cucumber half. Cut it in half lengthways and scoop out the seeds, then cut across into half-moons.

5 Set a ridged griddle/grill pan on a high heat. For the bruschette, rub the garlic over the rye bread and drizzle with oil. Place the slices in the hot pan and toast/char on both sides.

6 Remove the bruschette from the pan and immediately top with the cucumber and yoghurt mixture followed by the broad beans. Garnish with the cucumber half-moons and sprinkle over the toasted sunflower seeds.

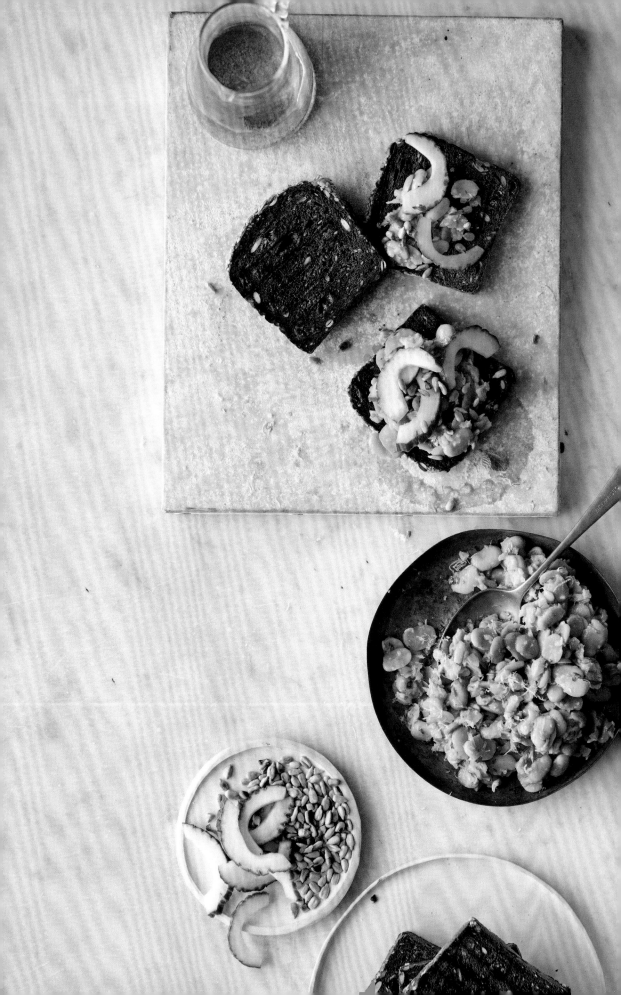

Broad bean and herb frittata

Serves 4
290 calories per serving
Here's a perfect go-to supper when you are short
of time and want to cook up something both tasty
and satisfying. Eggs are a good source of protein,
so they fill you up, and fresh herbs and broad
beans are delicious flavourings. If it's broad bean
season (between June and September), the skin
of the beans should be tender, so there will be no
need to peel them for this recipe.

200g podded fresh broad beans
Rapeseed oil for frying
150g new potatoes, diced
50ml water
6 eggs
1 tbsp chopped fresh flat-leaf parsley,
    plus extra to garnish
1 tbsp chopped fresh tarragon
1 tbsp chopped fresh chives
100ml oat milk
2 tbsp sunflower seeds

For the salad
1 tbsp Dijon mustard
1 tbsp rapeseed oil
Juice of 1 lemon
100g cherry tomatoes, cut in half
100g rocket
Flaked sea salt and cracked black pepper

1   Bring a pan of water to the boil. Drop in the
    broad beans and cook for 1 minute, then drain
    and rinse under cold water. If the beans are not
    young and tender, pop them out of their skins
    by gently squeezing. Tip the broad beans on to
    a chopping board and roughly chop them.
2   Preheat the grill to high.
3   Heat a little oil in a large, ovenproof, non-stick
    frying pan and add the diced potatoes with
    a pinch each of salt and pepper. Sauté until
    golden. Add the water and continue cooking
    until the potatoes are soft, adding a little more
    water if needed to prevent sticking. Add the
    broad beans and cook for a few more minutes.
    Spread out the bean mixture evenly.
4   Whisk the eggs with the herbs, oat milk and
    some salt and pepper in a bowl. Tip the egg
    mixture into the frying pan and cook for a few
    minutes until the base of the frittata has set.
    Sprinkle over the sunflower seeds. Place the
    frying pan under the grill and grill until the top
    of the frittata is golden and set. Remove from
    the grill and cut into four wedges.
5   To make the salad, simply combine the
    mustard, oil and lemon juice with some
    seasoning and use to dress the tomatoes
    and rocket. Serve with the frittata.

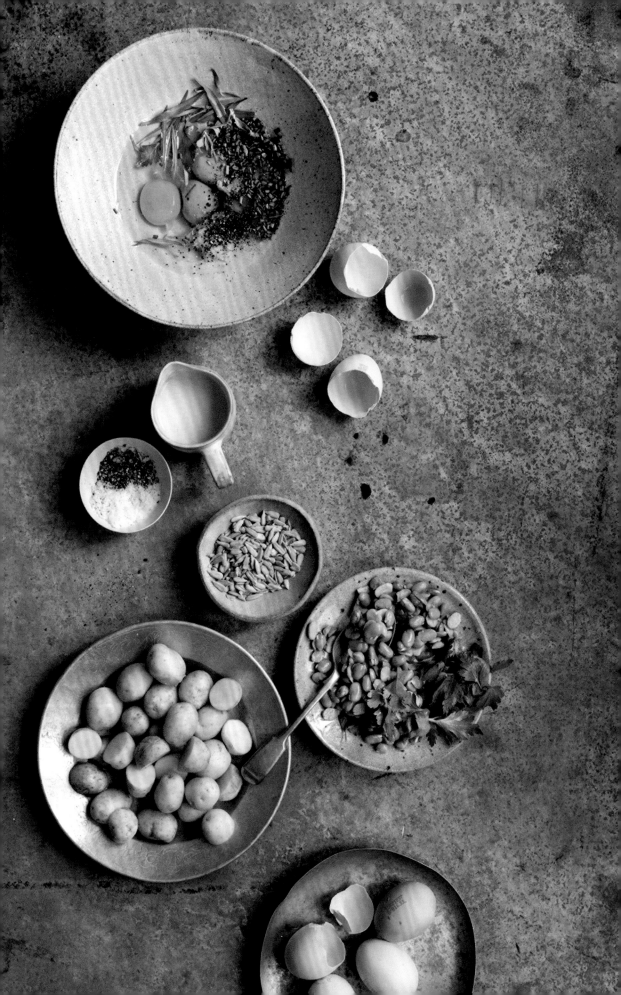

Broad bean and
buckwheat salad

Serves 2
588 calories per serving

Pull up a chair and let the minutes float by while
you skin the broad beans for this salad. If you don't
have time, or fresh beans aren't in season, frozen
broad beans will do the job too, although they
won't give you such an intensely fresh, sweet
flavour. To my mind, hazelnut and buckwheat are
perfect companions for broad beans, and they
give this salad a background of earthy nuttiness,
punctuated with sweet cherry tomatoes.

600–800g fresh broad beans in their pods
1 tbsp olive oil
5 fresh mint sprigs, leaves picked
A big handful of spinach
50g hazelnuts
150g buckwheat
Zest of 1 lemon
100g cherry tomatoes, cut in half
A handful of watercress, roughly chopped
Flaked sea salt and cracked black pepper

1   Pod the broad beans (you want about 150g
    podded weight). Bring a pan of water to the
    boil, add the beans and simmer for 1 minute.
    Drain and tip into a bowl of cold water. Pop the
    beans out of their skins – I do this by pinching
    the top so that the skin breaks. Put half of the
    broad beans in a food processor and set the
    rest aside.

2   Add the olive oil, mint leaves, spinach, half
    of the hazelnuts and 1 teaspoon salt to the
    food processor. Blitz to a coarse pesto-like
    texture. Set aside.

3   Put the buckwheat in a pan with a pinch of
    salt and cover with three times the amount
    of water. Bring to the boil, then simmer for
    15–20 minutes until the buckwheat is tender
    and has become a lighter shade of green. Drain
    in a sieve and rinse under cold water, then tip
    into a large mixing bowl.

4   Add the broad bean paste as well as the
    remaining broad beans, the lemon zest, cherry
    tomatoes and watercress. Season to taste with
    salt and pepper and toss together.

5   Toast the remaining hazelnuts in a dry frying pan.
    Put them in a pestle and gently crush with the
    mortar. Sprinkle over the salad before serving.

Broad bean and broccoli hummus

Serves 2
214 calories per serving

The best dips are those that can be made quickly because – let's be honest – there are many more important things to be getting on with if you have friends coming over for dinner. This easy, fresh green broad bean and broccoli hummus is a guaranteed crowd-pleaser – especially for the chef, as it takes only 10 minutes to make!

100g frozen broad beans
250g broccoli, roughly chopped
200g jarred chickpeas, drained
1 tsp tahini
2 fresh mint sprigs
Flaked sea salt and cracked black pepper

1   Bring a pan of water to the boil. Add the broad beans and broccoli and cook for just a few minutes, then drain in a colander and rinse under cold water to stop the cooking.
2   Tip the vegetables into a food processor and add the chickpeas, tahini, mint, and a pinch each of salt and pepper. Blitz until completely smooth (this may take a few minutes – to ensure that all the flavour from the broccoli and broad beans has been evenly distributed).
3   Serve the hummus with crudités or smother over slices of rye bread.

Peas

Few things in life are certain, but one thing's for sure: there will always be a packet of peas in my freezer. Normally I am not that keen on the idea of frozen vegetables but peas are different because they're put on ice so soon after being picked, usually within three hours. At moments when the cupboards seem bare and I simply cannot muster enough energy to go out and buy supplies, I know that I can always whip something up with those trusty frozen peas (this is why the pea soup with black rice on page 26 appears so regularly on the Sunday night dinner table at our house).

Having said that, I must admit that there is nothing quite like the delicate crunch of a freshly plucked pea straight from the pod – if you are ever lucky enough to find yourself in front of a pea plant.

When I was growing up, peas were always served on the side of a main dish but I've come to realise that they can and should sometimes be the centre of attention. Peas were the first real food I gave my daughter Eva, blitzed up with some fresh mint and a dollop of yoghurt. Ever since then she has loved anything with peas in it, including the lemony pea and broad bean pasta on page 24, which is as satisfying for grown-ups as it is for children.

Nutritional bonus
Considering their small size, peas pack a surprising nutritional punch – they are a significant source of **vitamin C,** which supports your immune system, and are also a good source of **folate**, needed for heart health.

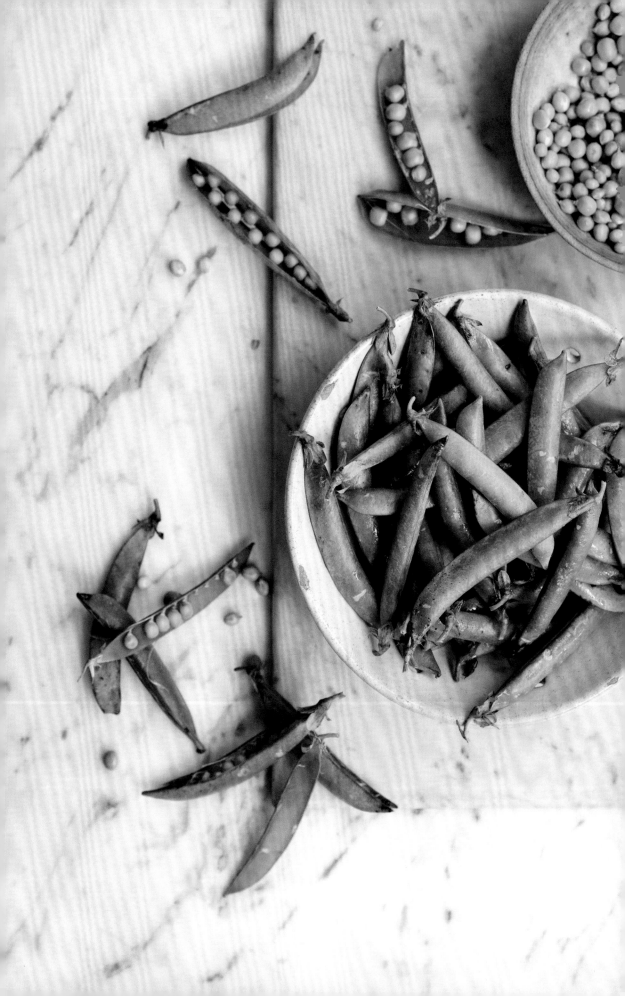

Pea, leek and tarragon omelette

Serves 1

311 calories per serving

Peas and tarragon make a great combination, the aniseed flavour of the tarragon enhancing the sweetness of the peas. Teamed with softly fried sliced leeks, they make an indulgent omelette for weekend breakfasts.

1 tsp rapeseed oil
1 leek, finely sliced
150g podded fresh peas (or thawed frozen peas)
A few fresh tarragon sprigs
4 eggs
50ml water
Flaked sea salt and cracked black pepper

1   Heat the oil in a frying pan, add the leek and cook on a low heat until soft but not browned. Add the peas and tarragon and cook for a few more minutes until the peas are tender.

2   Meanwhile, whisk the eggs in a bowl with the water and a pinch each of salt and pepper. Pour the egg mixture into the frying pan. Once browned on the base, fold the omelette in half and cook for a few more minutes until cooked throughout. Slide out of the pan to serve.

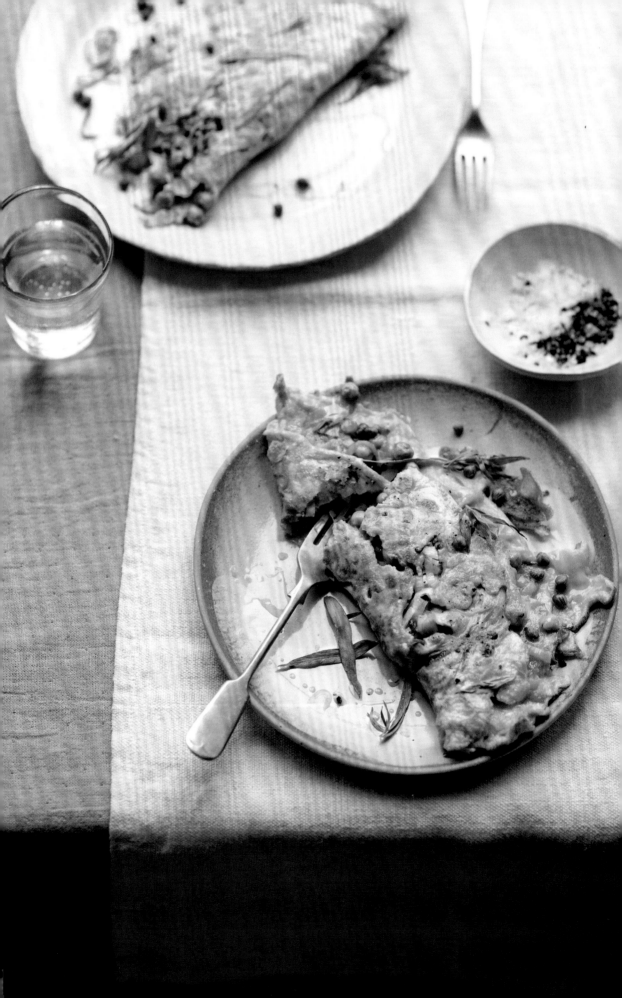

Pea and broad bean pasta with lemon

Serves 2
546 calories per serving

Penne pasta dressed with lemony peas and broad beans, spiked with fried capers, is a great family dish. Frying capers until they turn golden gives them a deliciously deep flavour that works well with the vegetables. If I'm feeding the kids I tend to leave out the chilli, or add it as a fresh garnish just to the adults' bowls.

150g podded fresh broad beans
200g gluten-free penne pasta
1 tbsp olive oil
2 garlic cloves, finely chopped
3 fresh thyme sprigs
4 tbsp capers
150g podded fresh peas (or thawed frozen peas)
1 green chilli, sliced
Zest and juice of 2 lemons
Flaked sea salt and cracked black pepper
Cherry tomatoes, cut in half (optional)

1   Bring a large saucepan of water to the boil. Drop in the broad beans and cook for 1 minute, then scoop them out with a spider or slotted spoon and tip into a bowl of cold water. Keep the pan of water boiling.

2   Season the boiling water with a good pinch of salt, then add the pasta and cook until it is al dente. While the pasta is cooking, pop the broad beans out of their skins.

3   Put the olive oil, garlic and thyme into a frying pan, set it over a medium heat and add the capers. Fry until they are slightly golden. Add the peas and cook until they are a deep green. Add the broad beans, chilli, lemon zest and a pinch each of salt and pepper. Cook for a few minutes, then remove the thyme sprigs.

4   Drain the pasta, keeping a few spoonfuls of the water in the pan. Tip the pasta back into the pan and add the pea and broad bean mixture along with the lemon juice. Mix through and serve, topped with the cherry tomatoes, if using.

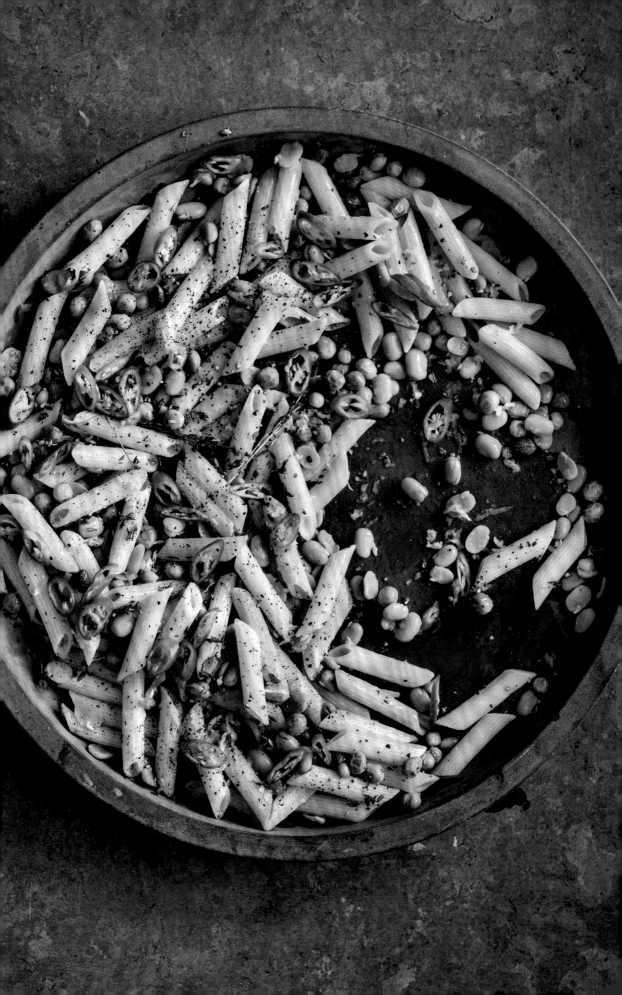

Pea soup with black rice

Serves 4
472 calories per serving

A simple and classic pea soup is a thing of beauty.
All you really need is sweet peas and a good stock,
but here I've added a few extras to make a more
substantial soup. The black rice offers a bit of
extra texture and the flecks of black against the
bright green soup look stunning.

100g black rice
500ml vegetable stock
4 celery sticks, diced
½ tsp celery salt
150g frozen peas
100g spinach
50g pistachios, roughly chopped
A small handful of fresh chives, roughly chopped

1   Put the black rice in a pan with a pinch of salt
    and cover with three times the amount of water.
    Bring to the boil, then leave to simmer gently for
    30–35 minutes until the rice is tender and fluffy.
    Drain and set aside.

2   Put the vegetable stock in a pan with the celery
    and bring to a simmer. Add the celery salt and
    peas and bring to the boil. Remove from the
    heat. Add the spinach to the pan and, using
    a hand blender, blitz until smooth.

3   Ladle the soup into bowls and top with the
    black rice, chopped pistachios and chives.

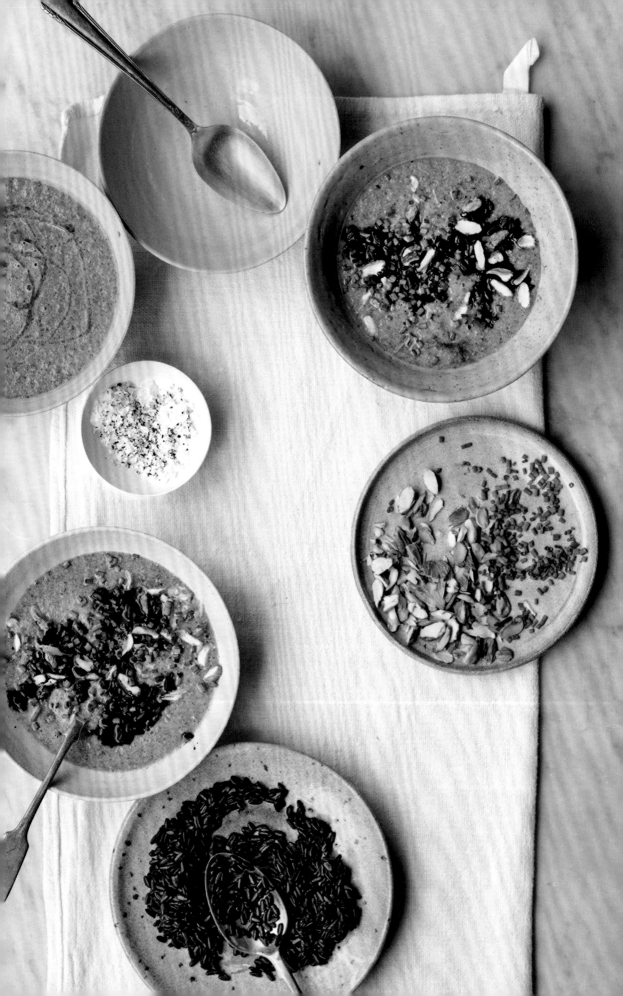

Pea and cashew pesto with quinoa and pickled beetroot

Serves 4
625 calories per serving

Preparing the beetroot for this recipe takes time but it's a pleasing task, perfect for a Saturday morning if you are pottering around. Roasting the beetroot before pickling it will help it to absorb the pickling liquor and results in a sweet yet sharp flavour. You could very easily eat the beetroot just as it is – dipped in the accompanying creamy, nutty pea pesto – but tossed with some quinoa and chopped spinach, it makes a colourful salad.

500g raw beetroots (unpeeled)
300ml water
1 tbsp honey
3 tbsp brown rice vinegar
200g quinoa
2 tbsp pumpkin seeds
100g baby spinach, roughly chopped
Zest and juice of 1 lemon

For the pesto
200g podded fresh peas (or frozen peas)
150g cashew nuts
2 tbsp olive oil
A small handful of fresh basil, leaves picked
100ml water
Flaked sea salt and cracked black pepper

1   Preheat the oven to 200°C/Fan 180°C/Gas 6.
2   Wrap each beetroot in foil and place on a baking tray. Roast for 40–60 minutes until the beetroots are cooked through. Leave to cool, then peel off the skin and cut each beetroot into quarters.
3   Pour the water into a saucepan and add the honey and rice vinegar. Bring to the boil. Add the beetroots and simmer for about 5 minutes. Remove from the heat and leave the beetroots to soak in the pickling liquid for at least 1 hour.
4   To make the pesto, cook the peas in a pan of boiling water for a few minutes, then drain and rinse under cold running water until completely cooled. Put the cashews and oil in a blender or food processor and blitz to a paste. Add the basil, peas, water and ½ teaspoon salt. Blitz again until smooth. Set aside until you are ready to serve.
5   Put the quinoa in a saucepan with a pinch of salt and cover with three times the amount of water. Bring to the boil, then leave to simmer for 10–12 minutes until the quinoa is cooked and the tail has separated from the seed. Drain in a sieve and rinse under cold water to cool.
6   Toast the pumpkin seeds in a hot dry frying pan until golden. Set aside.
7   Gently mix the quinoa with the drained pickled beetroot, spinach, and lemon zest and juice. Season with salt and pepper. Serve with the pesto, either mixed through or dolloped on top, and sprinkled with the pumpkin seeds.

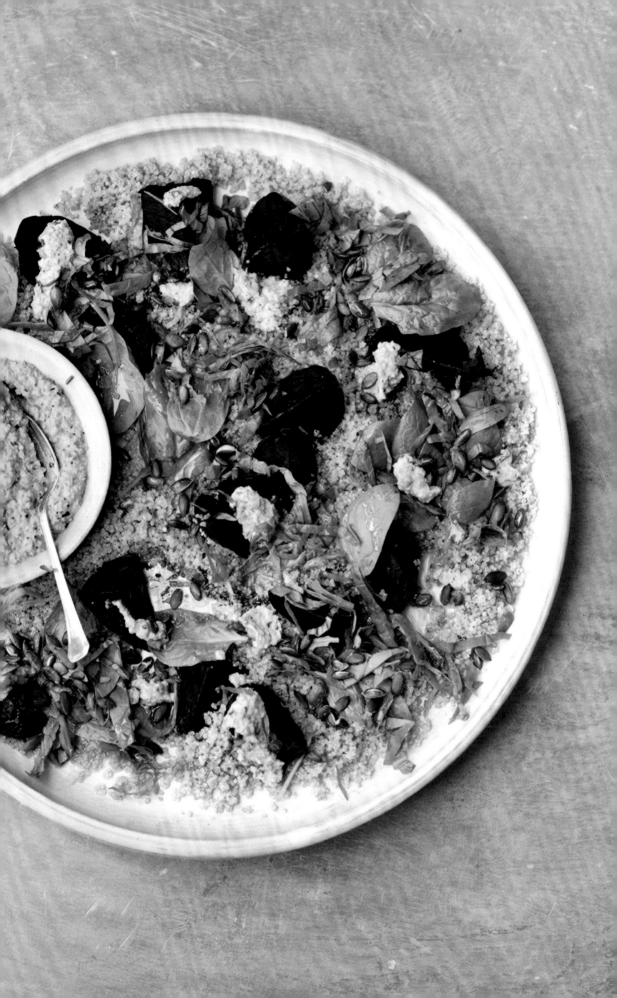

Asparagus

There are several varieties of asparagus out there. In France, for example, they tend to like the white variety, which has a milder and slightly sweeter taste than the usual green. I actually prefer that bright green type, which we produce here in the UK. British asparagus tastes divine when it's in season, and eating it is a real treat. Pretty much any dish you add asparagus to is immediately catapulted into 'special occasion' status – even if it's just breakfast for one, it will feel like the queen of breakfasts (see the breakfast stack recipe on page 32 for an example of this).

Asparagus does not lend itself to long, slow cooking methods as it becomes mushy and loses its flavour and brilliant colour. Instead it's best to steam, flash-fry, grill, griddle or just blanch it. The less you mess around with asparagus the better: griddled asparagus with a good drizzle of olive oil, a sprinkle of Maldon salt and some cracked black pepper is one of life's simplest yet most wonderful pleasures. It is just as good loaded on to a big platter with a selection of lovely dips, or eaten on its own in blissful, solitary silence.

Nutritional bonus
Asparagus provides **vitamins A and C** and it is high in **folate**, which is important for making red blood cells. In addition, asparagus is fat-free and low in calories.

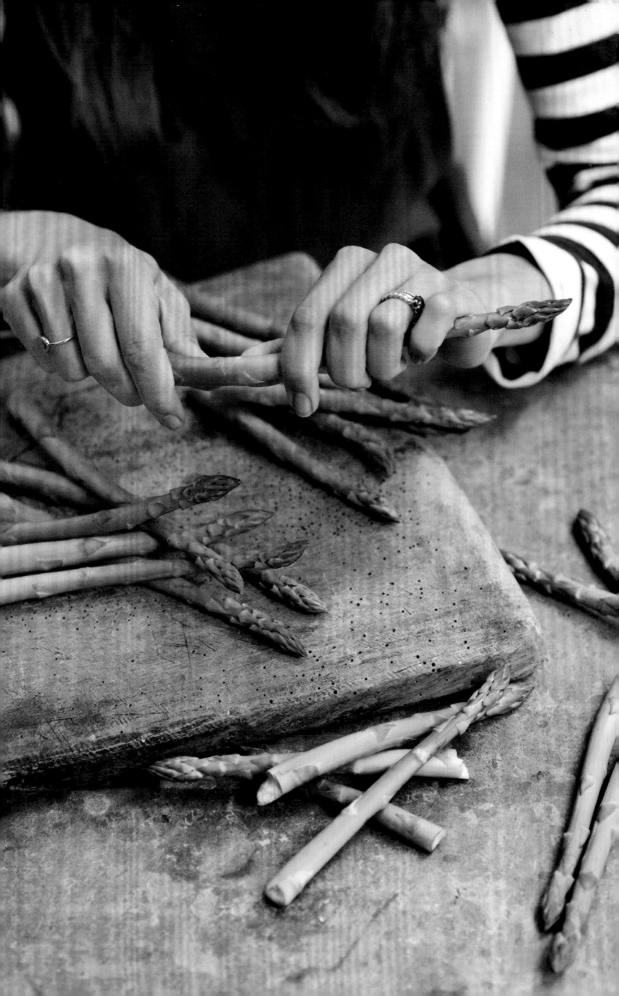

Asparagus and sweet potato frittata

Serves 4

174 calories per serving

Frittata is perfect as a weekday supper, as it's so easy and quick. Sweet potatoes are a good replacement for normal spuds, and their softer texture and sweeter flavour work well with the crunchy, earthy asparagus here.

1 sweet potato (unpeeled), cut into small wedges
1 tsp fennel seeds
1 fresh rosemary sprig, leaves picked and roughly chopped
3 tsp rapeseed oil
8 asparagus spears (tough ends broken off)
8 large eggs
1 tbsp sunflower seeds
1 tbsp Dijon mustard
1 tbsp lemon juice
Baby Gem lettuce leaves
Flaked sea salt and cracked black pepper

1 Preheat the oven to 200°C/Fan 180°C/Gas 6. Line a baking tray with greaseproof paper.
2 Spread the sweet potato wedges on the tray and scatter over the fennel seeds, rosemary, 1 teaspoon of the oil and a pinch each of salt and pepper. Roast for 20–25 minutes until the wedges are tender.
3 Heat 1 teaspoon of the oil in a heavy-based ovenproof frying pan and sauté the asparagus until slightly browned. Tip in the roasted sweet potato and spread out evenly.
4 Whisk the eggs together in a bowl with a pinch each of salt and pepper. Pour the eggs into the frying pan and sprinkle the sunflower seeds over the surface. Transfer the pan to the oven and cook for 5–10 minutes until the frittata is set and the top is golden.
5 Quickly whisk together the remaining teaspoon of oil, the mustard, lemon juice and some salt and pepper. Use to dress the lettuce leaves to serve with the frittata.

Asparagus and mushroom breakfast stack

Serves 4

324 calories per serving

The addition of sautéed asparagus takes this breakfast of eggy bread and mushrooms to a new level of sophistication. I love cooking all the individual parts of the recipe and bringing them together in a neat tower, only to demolish it at the first forkful.

4 Portobello mushrooms
200g cherry tomatoes on the vine
Olive oil for drizzling and frying
4 eggs
50ml oat milk
8 slices gluten-free bread
200g asparagus spears (tough ends broken off)
A handful of pumpkin seeds
Flaked sea salt and cracked black pepper

1 Preheat the oven to 200°C/Fan 180°C/Gas 6. Line a baking tray with greaseproof paper.
2 Place the Portobello mushrooms and cherry tomatoes (still on the vine) on the lined tray, drizzle over a teaspoon of oil and season with salt and pepper. Roast for 20 minutes.
3 Meanwhile, make the eggy bread. Whisk the eggs with the oat milk and some salt and pepper in a shallow dish. Place the slices of bread in the dish. Leave to soak, rearranging the slices as necessary so they all become evenly moistened.
4 Place a non-stick frying pan on a high heat and add a little oil. Fry the eggy bread, in batches if necessary, for 5 minutes on each side until golden. Remove and keep hot.
5 Add the asparagus and pumpkin seeds to the hot pan, season and sauté until the asparagus is lightly browned but still crunchy.
6 Place a slice of eggy bread on each plate and stack up on top a mushroom, four tomatoes, three asparagus spears and a good sprinkle of pumpkin seeds.

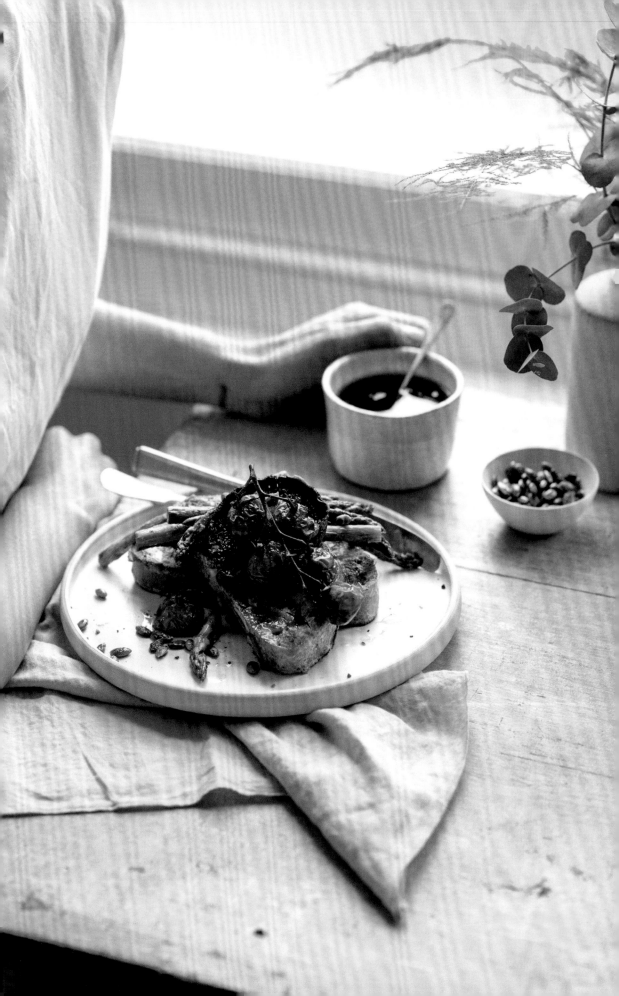

Asparagus and spinach soup

Serves 4
393 calories per serving
This super-green, super-tasty springtime soup is made using a few simple ingredients that would very likely grow next to each other in a vegetable garden. I add the spinach at the very end, whizzing it up with the asparagus in the hot soup to create a deep shade of green.

Rapeseed oil for frying
2 spring onions, finely chopped
2 garlic cloves, finely chopped
250g new potatoes
2 celery sticks, diced
500ml vegetable stock
8 asparagus spears (tough ends broken off)
250g spinach
Flaked sea salt and cracked black pepper
Toasted sunflower seeds, to garnish

1   Heat a little oil in a saucepan, add the spring onions and garlic, and cook until soft. Add the potatoes, celery and vegetable stock. Bring to the boil, then simmer until the potatoes are softened.

2   Cut the asparagus tips from the stalks, then cut the tips lengthways in half. Chop the stalks. Add all the asparagus to the pan and cook it for 2–3 minutes until almost tender. Add the spinach and cook for 1 minute.

3   Transfer half of the mixture to a blender or food processor and blitz until smooth. Pour this back into the pan. Add a good pinch each of salt and pepper. Reheat, if necessary, before serving hot, sprinkled with sunflower seeds.

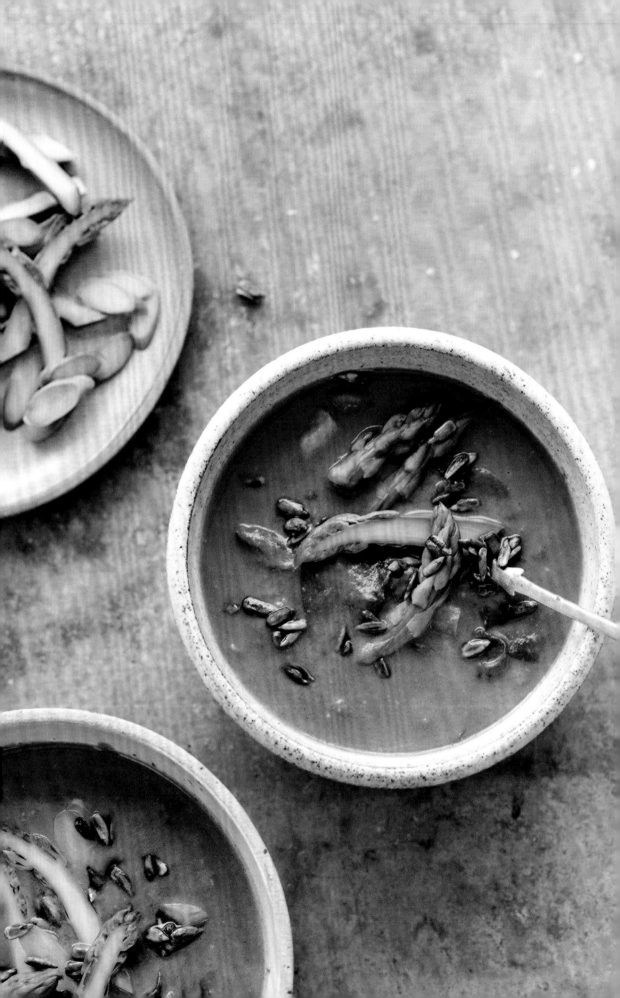

Asparagus and wild rice salad with tarragon pesto

Serves 4
604 calories per serving

This is a classic 'throw lots of delicious ingredients together in a bowl and smother them with a really punchy pesto' kind of a dish. It looks as good as it tastes: the asparagus and broad beans are richly green against the deep, dark colours of the rice, – woodland shades with a flash of bright green.

200g mixed red and wild rice
600–800g fresh broad beans in their pods
Rapeseed oil for frying
6–8 asparagus spears (tough ends broken off),
    sliced in half lengthways
1 tbsp pumpkin seeds
1 tbsp sunflower seeds

For the pesto
A handful of cashew nuts
A handful of sunflower seeds
A small handful of fresh tarragon, leaves picked
    (keep a few sprigs to garnish)
Zest of 1 lemon
A handful of spinach leaves
2 tbsp rapeseed oil
150ml water
Flaked sea salt and cracked black pepper

1. Put the rice in a pan with a pinch of salt and cover with three times the amount of water. Bring to the boil, then leave to simmer gently for 30–35 minutes until the rice is tender and fluffy. Drain in a sieve, rinse under cold water and tip into a large mixing bowl.

2. Pod the broad beans (you want about 150g podded weight). Bring a small pan of water to the boil. Drop in the beans and cook for 3 minutes. Drain and rinse under cold water, then cover with cold water. Skin the beans – you should be able to pop out each bean by gently squeezing it. This is a fairly laborious task but well worth it as the skinned beans add a lively green colour to the dish. Add the beans to the cooked rice.

3. Place a non-stick frying pan over a medium heat and add a few drops of rapeseed oil. Fry the asparagus with the pumpkin seeds, sunflower seeds and some salt and pepper until the asparagus is slightly charred and the seeds are golden. Add all this to the rice and toss gently together.

4. To make the pesto, toast the cashew nuts and sunflower seeds in a small dry frying pan until golden. Tip into a small food processor, add the remaining pesto ingredients and blitz to a coarse texture.

5. Serve the salad on a large platter or plates, garnished with tarragon sprigs. Offer the pesto separately, in a small bowl, for spooning over.

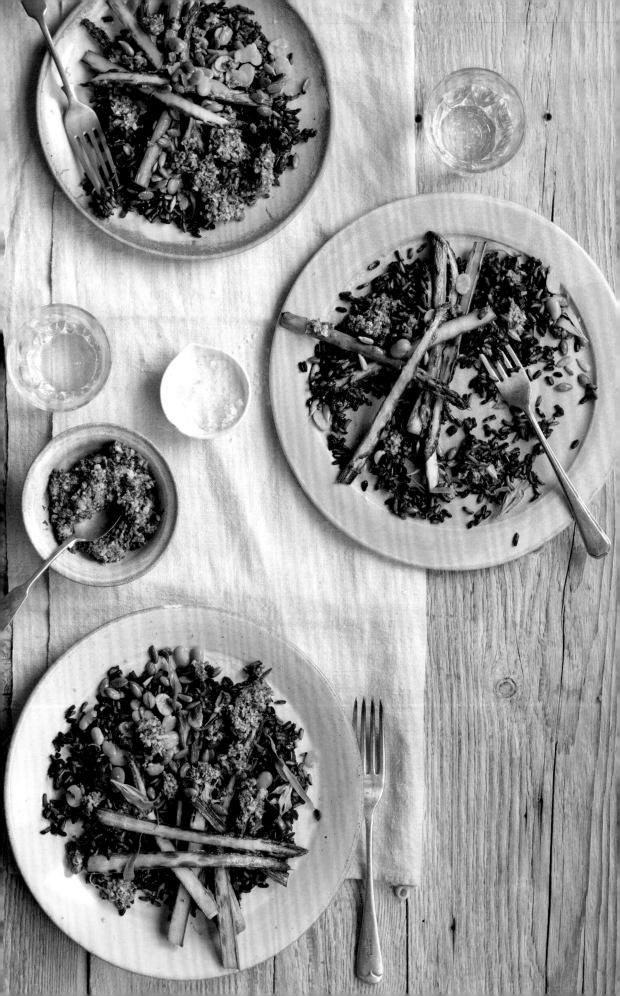

Asparagus and shallot tart

Serves 4

379 calories per serving

Slow-cooking the shallots for this asparagus tart is essential. They need to be sweet, sticky and oozing with deep savouriness to offer the perfect foil for the baby asparagus. The dough for the tart base is very easy to make and holds together well for a gluten-free pastry. It can be kept in the fridge, well wrapped in cling film, for three days, so you can prepare it in advance.

Rapeseed oil for frying
6 shallots, sliced
2 garlic cloves, chopped
1 tsp honey
6 eggs
100ml brown rice milk
200g baby asparagus spears
A handful of sunflower seeds
Flaked sea salt and cracked black pepper

For the pastry
2 eggs
2 fresh rosemary sprigs, leaves picked and
    finely chopped
2 tbsp rapeseed oil
1 tsp flaked sea salt
100g porridge oats
50g gluten-free flour, plus extra for dusting

1   Preheat the oven to 190°C/Fan 170°C/Gas 5. Lightly flour a 24cm loose-bottomed flan tin.

2   To make the pastry, beat the eggs together, then add the rest of the ingredients and bring together into a ball of dough. Wrap in cling film and leave to rest in the fridge for 20 minutes.

3   Roll out the dough on a lightly floured surface. This is quite a dry dough, so don't worry too much if it crumbles. Once you have a large round that is about 5mm thick, place it in the tin and mould it with your fingers to line the bottom and sides. You can fill in any holes with the trimmings.

4   Line the pastry case with baking paper and fill with baking beans. Blind bake for 15 minutes. Remove from the oven and take out the baking paper and beans. Set the tart case aside while you make the filling. Leave the oven on.

5   Place a small frying pan on a medium heat and add a drizzle of oil, followed by the shallots, garlic and honey. Cook over a low heat, stirring occasionally, until the shallots have become sticky, slightly browned and soft. This will take about 20 minutes. Evenly spread the shallots over the bottom of the tart case.

6   Mix the eggs with the milk and some salt and pepper. Pour this over the shallots. Top with the asparagus and sunflower seeds. Bake for 15–20 minutes until the filling has set. Remove the tart from the tin to serve.

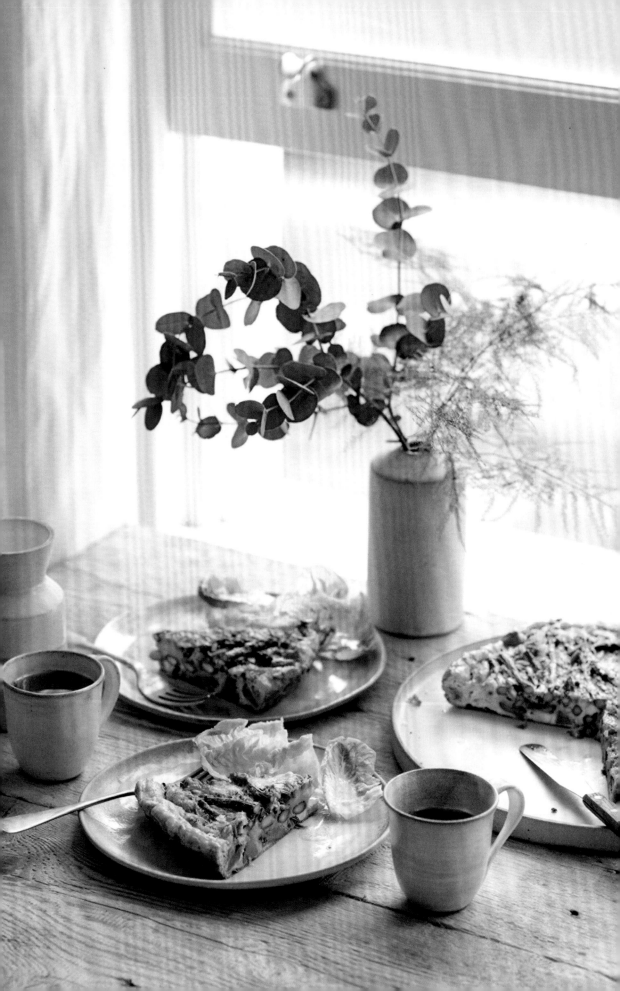

Globe artichoke

'A woman is like an artichoke: you must work hard to get to her heart.' So said Jacques Clouseau, detective and protagonist of *The Pink Panther* films. Artichokes do look rather intimidating with their thick, armour-like petals. However, there are impressive rewards on offer for the undaunted cook because as well as being uniquely delicious, globe artichokes are good for you.

The Italian vegetable stew called vignole sings to me of spring and early summer, and the recipe on page 46 is one of my absolute favourites. The preparation of fresh artichoke hearts may be slightly time-consuming – there's the trimming, the simmering, the gentle peeling back of each petal until you reach the heart, and the delicate job of removing the 'choke' – but for vignole it is worth it.

I always keep a jar of artichoke hearts in my cupboard as they make so many dishes taste just that bit more special with minimal culinary effort. It's very easy to preserve your own artichoke hearts – if you are preparing them fresh for vignole or another recipe, you might as well do double the amount and keep some for later. Put the artichoke hearts in a spotlessly clean jar, add lemon zest and dried chilli flakes, cover with rapeseed oil and seal. The hearts should keep in the fridge for 4–6 weeks.

Artichokes are best during the summer and autumn months. When you're choosing which ones to buy, look for artichokes with tightly closed, undamaged leaves or petals. Smaller 'baby' artichokes tend to have more tender leaves, but larger ones will have a bigger heart.

Nutritional bonus

Globe artichokes are a good source of **fibre** and **folate**, as well as providing **potassium**, which helps to regulate blood pressure and heart-beat.

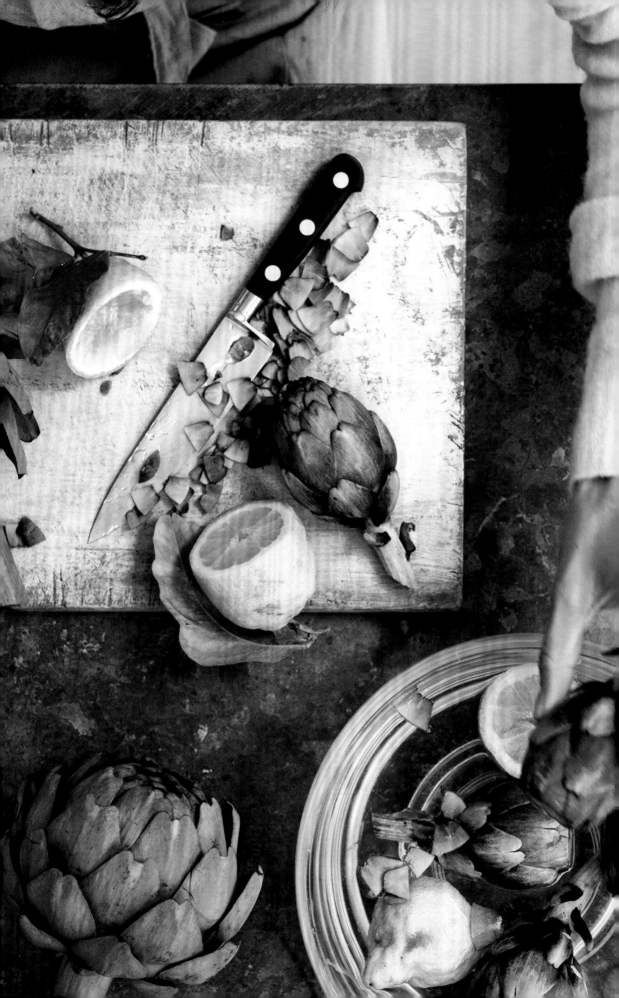

Artichoke heart and pomegranate salad

Serves 2
545 calories per serving

Pomegranate seeds are one of my favourite fruity additions to a salad. Not only do they have a lovely sweet-and-sour flavour and a crunchy 'pop' when you bite into them, they also add a burst of deep pink prettiness to your plate. The salad here is the perfect example of how, with just a jar of artichoke hearts and a few other ingredients, you can create something that is utterly satisfying and delicious in a matter of minutes.

200g jarred artichoke hearts packed in oil
1 courgette, shaved into ribbons
1 Baby Gem lettuce, separated into leaves
A handful of spinach
1 avocado, peeled and diced
2 tbsp pomegranate seeds
50g sunflower seeds

For the dressing
1 tbsp English mustard powder
Juice of 2 lemons
Zest of 1 lemon
1 tbsp honey
1 tbsp rapeseed oil
Flaked sea salt and cracked black pepper

1   First make the dressing. Whisk the mustard powder with the lemon juice until the powder has dissolved, then add the zest, honey and oil and whisk to combine. Season to taste with salt and pepper, then set aside.

2   Drain the artichoke hearts and cut each one into quarters. Put them into a mixing bowl with the courgette, lettuce, spinach, avocado and pomegranate seeds. Pour over the dressing and toss together gently.

3   Toast the sunflower seeds in a dry frying pan until golden.

4   Divide the salad into bowls and sprinkle over the toasted sunflower seeds. Season with salt and pepper.

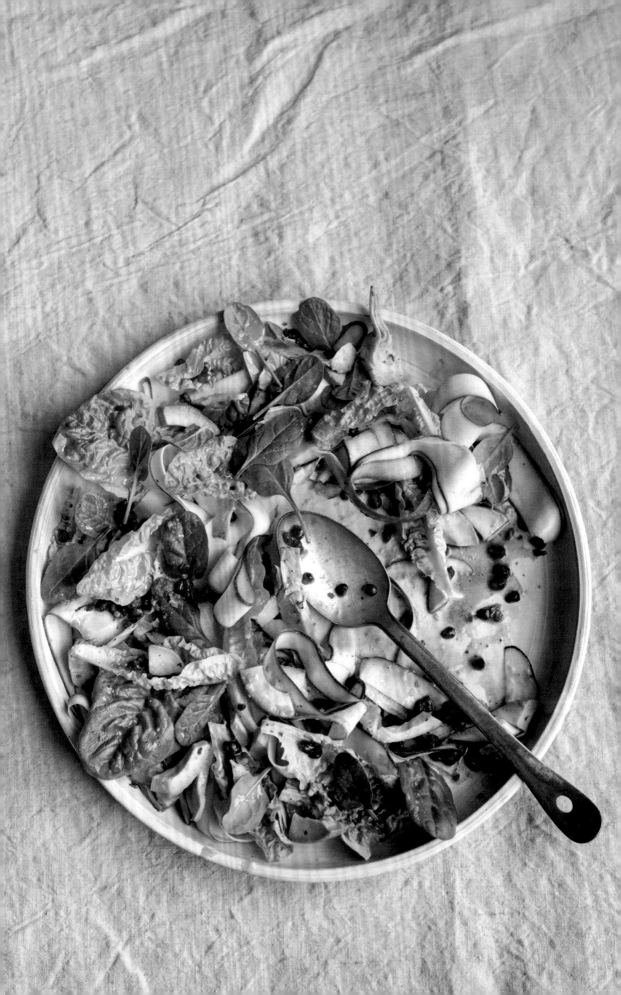

Artichoke and borlotti bean salad

Serves 2
441 calories per serving
This salad is a weekday-dinner-party kind of dish: simple yet delicious and very pretty. The quality of the ingredients you use will be the making of the dish, so buy good, ripe cherry tomatoes and try to find borlotti beans in jars, which don't have the metallic taste of tinned beans. I like to use jarred artichoke hearts that have been packed in a flavoured oil – you can find a good choice in larger supermarkets or delis these days. Artichoke hearts in oil flavoured with Provençal herbs and chilli would work really well here.

400g jarred borlotti beans
200g jarred artichoke hearts packed in oil
200g cherry tomatoes, cut in half
A handful of fresh basil leaves, to garnish

For the dressing
A big handful of fresh basil, leaves picked
    and chopped
A handful of fresh flat-leaf parsley, leaves picked
1 garlic clove
2 tbsp capers
4 sun-dried tomatoes
1 tbsp olive oil
Flaked sea salt and cracked black pepper

1   Drain the borlotti beans and rinse under cold water, then tip them into a mixing bowl. Drain the artichoke hearts and add them to the bowl.
2   To make the dressing, place all the ingredients on a board and chop them together to create a well-mixed, coarse-textured dressing. Add to the beans and artichokes and mix together gently but thoroughly. Season with salt and pepper to taste.
3   Tip the salad on to a serving platter. Arrange the cherry tomatoes on top along with the basil leaves.

Artichoke fritters with caraway

Serves 2
552 calories per serving
Artichoke fritters make a fantastic canapé for a dinner party. You can prepare the artichokes ahead of time and have all the ingredients for the batter ready to whizz together. The fritters look and taste sensational. All you need to serve with them is sea salt and cracked black pepper.

300g jarred artichoke hearts packed in oil
140g gluten-free flour
¼ tsp gluten-free bicarbonate of soda
3 eggs, beaten
100ml oat milk
100ml sparkling water
1 tbsp caraway seeds
1 tsp flaked sea salt, plus extra for seasoning
Rapeseed oil for frying
Cracked black pepper

1   Drain the artichoke hearts and cut each one in half. Lay them on some kitchen paper and pat dry. Sift over some of the flour to cover them completely, then set aside until you are ready to fry them.
2   To make the batter, sift the remaining flour and the bicarbonate of soda into a bowl. Gradually add the eggs to the flour, mixing with a spatula or spoon. Whisk in the oat milk and water. The consistency of this batter should be fairly thin and able to drip off a spoon. It is similar to a tempura batter.
3   Toast the caraway seeds in a small dry frying pan for a few minutes until fragrant. Add them to the batter along with the salt, then leave the batter in the fridge until you are ready to fry.
4   Place a non-stick frying pan on a high heat and add some oil. When the oil is hot, dip a few of the artichoke halves into the batter, then place straight into the pan. Add as many artichokes as will fit, making sure you have enough space to flip them over. Cook until they are golden on both sides. Remove and drain on kitchen paper. Repeat with the rest of the artichokes.
5   Sprinkle the fritters with a pinch each of salt and pepper before serving hot.

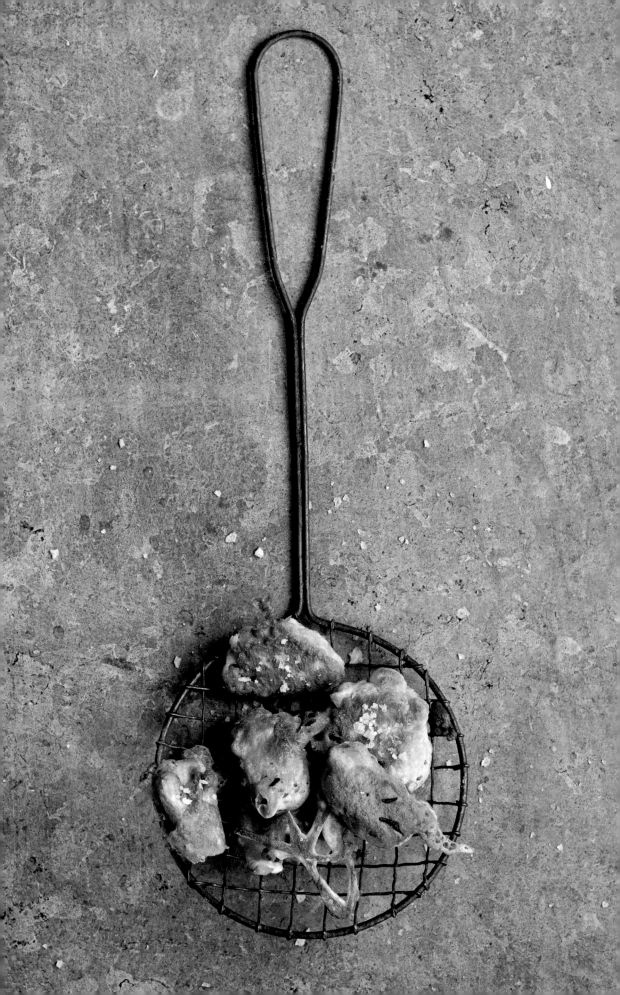

Italian vignole

Serves 4
486 calories per serving

If you haven't cooked fresh artichoke hearts from scratch before, I suggest you head straight to your local greengrocer when artichokes are in season and buy some. Don't get me wrong – there is a time and a place for jarred artichoke hearts, but nothing beats preparing your own fresh ones, peeling back each petal until you reveal the vegetable's soft centre or heart. Artichokes and fresh peas are the joint stars of the show in this dish, which is traditionally made with the early crop of baby artichokes.

2 lemons
6 baby/small globe artichokes
600–800g fresh peas in their pods
1 tbsp olive oil
1 red onion, diced
100g kale (tough stalks trimmed), shredded
300ml vegetable stock
3 fresh mint sprigs, leaves picked and finely
    chopped, plus extra to garnish
1 slice dark rye bread
Flaked sea salt and cracked black pepper

1   Cut one of the lemons in half and squeeze the juice of one half into a large bowl of water; add the squeezed half too. Trim each artichoke stalk, leaving about 5cm, then cut off the very thick top part of the leaves. As each artichoke is prepared, rub all the cut surfaces with the other lemon half, then drop into the bowl of lemon water.

2   Bring a pan of water to the boil. Add the (drained) artichokes and simmer for about 20 minutes until they are tender (test by inserting the tip of a knife into the top: there should be no resistance). Drain and leave to cool. Pull off the outer leaves until you reach the lighter, softer centre, or heart. Using a teaspoon, scrape out the hairy choke and discard it. Cut each artichoke heart into quarters and set aside.

3   Pod the peas (you want about 150g podded weight) and place them in a small bowl. Zest and juice the second lemon.

4   Heat some of the olive oil in a frying pan over a medium heat and fry the diced onion until translucent. Add the peas and kale and cook until the kale has wilted and the peas are a bright green. Pour in the vegetable stock and add the lemon zest and juice along with the artichokes. Simmer for about 10 minutes. Remove from the heat, stir in the mint and season to taste.

5   In a small frying pan heat the rest of the olive oil. Crumble the rye bread into the pan and fry until crisp. Scatter the rye breadcrumbs and extra mint over the artichoke stew and serve.

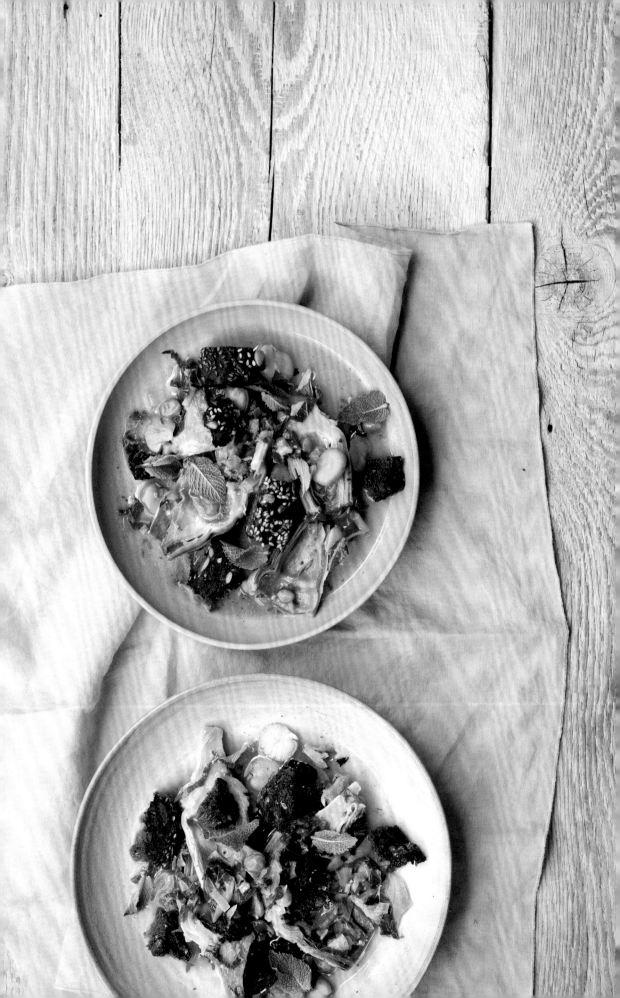

Fennel

Fennel is at its best in summer. Young fennel will be tender then, so look out for white bulbs with bright green feathery tops when you're shopping. The flowers, leaves and seeds of the plant can all be eaten, not just the bulb.

With its fresh aniseed-like flavour and bright lemony aftertaste, raw fennel is a great addition to salads: cut thinly on a mandoline, it adds a crisp texture, and its white and pale green tones look beautiful.

When fennel is cooked, its flavour becomes mellow and rounded, with sweet caramelised notes. It works well in soups and stews, as well as being absolutely delicious simply roasted with some fresh chilli, salt and pepper. I also like to use fennel in vegetable stock, first braising the fennel with onion, celery and bay leaves before adding water and simmering for a few hours to release all of the sweetness and rich aniseedy flavour.

Fennel works surprisingly well in sweet recipes too. The fennel and chocolate cake on page 56 was inspired by a brilliant chef named Steve Groves, who introduced me to this wonderful flavour combination.

Nutritional bonus

Fennel is a good source of **fibre** and **potassium**. It is also thought to reduce bloating. Try making some fennel tea with a teaspoon of fennel seeds, plus lemon juice and honey. Not only is this tea refreshing, it could settle your stomach.

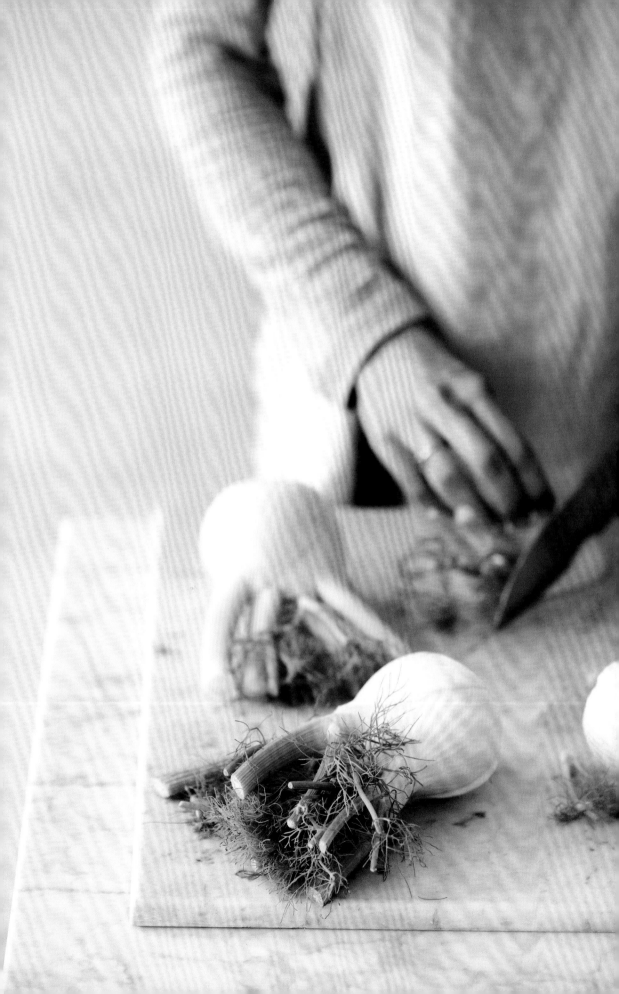

Spiced fennel, Puy lentil and apple salad

Serves 2
423 calories per serving

Thinly slicing fennel on a mandoline is one of the best ways to prepare it, as it keeps its freshness and crispness. Here it is paired with soft, earthy lentils. When using raw fennel in a recipe, I would always recommend you select a small bulb, as it will be younger and thus more tender with a more delicate aniseedy flavour.

150g Puy lentils
1 tsp rapeseed oil
2 red onions, sliced
A pinch of ground cinnamon
1 tsp ground cumin
1 tsp smoked paprika
50g sultanas
Zest and juice of 1 lemon
A handful of fresh coriander, chopped
A handful of fresh dill, chopped
1 small fennel bulb
1 Braeburn apple
Flaked sea salt and cracked black pepper

1 Put the lentils in a medium saucepan and cover with three times the amount of water. Place on a high heat and bring to the boil, then simmer for 15–20 minutes until the lentils are cooked but still have a bite to them. Drain and place in a large mixing bowl.

2 Heat the oil in a small frying pan, add the red onions and sauté for 10 minutes until soft. Stir in the cinnamon, cumin and smoked paprika and cook for a few minutes until the spices are fragrant. Remove from the heat and add the sultanas, lemon juice and a pinch each of salt and pepper. The lemon juice should turn the onions a brighter shade of pink.

3 Mix the onions into the lentils along with half of the chopped coriander and dill.

4 Remove the core and outer layer of the fennel. Slice the fennel and apple very thinly using a mandoline or a microplane shaver. Place them in a bowl and mix with the lemon zest and a pinch of salt.

5 To assemble the dish, place the lentil mixture in a serving bowl and top with the fennel and apple slices. Garnish with the remaining dill and coriander.

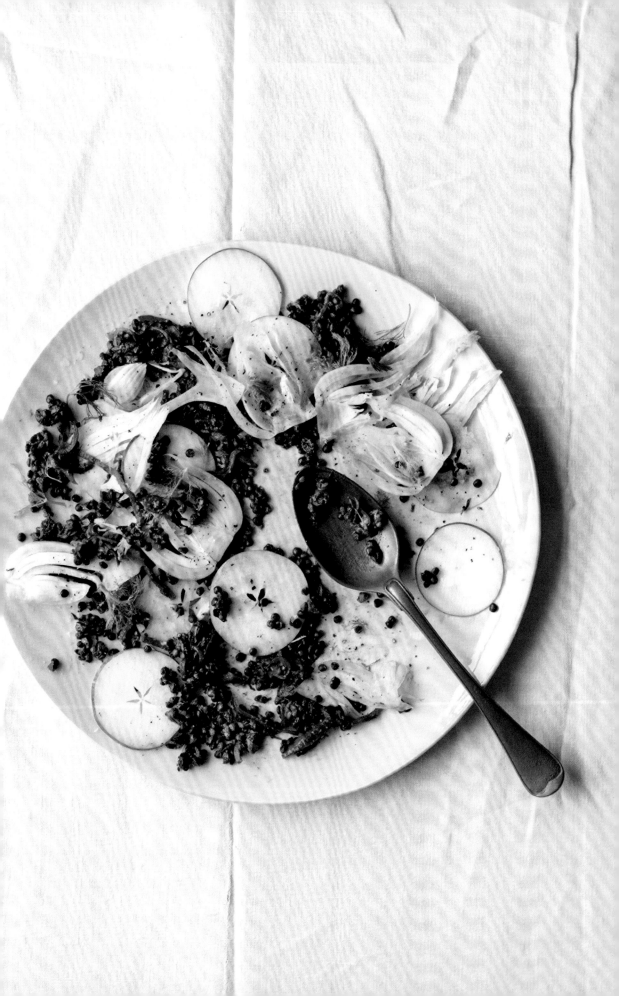

Honey and tamari-roasted fennel salad

Serves 2
227 calories per serving
Sticky, sweet, salty and spicy, roasted fennel is a thing of deliciousness. You can enjoy this salad as a side dish or combine it with rice or lentils to make a more substantial main-dish version.

4 fennel bulbs
2 tbsp honey
1 tbsp rapeseed oil
2 tbsp tamari
1 tsp dried chilli flakes
3 tbsp coconut yoghurt
A small handful of fresh dill, finely chopped
A small handful of fresh mint, leaves picked
    and finely chopped
100g baby spinach
Flaked sea salt and cracked black pepper

1   Preheat the oven to 200°C/Fan 180°C/Gas 6. Line a baking tray with greaseproof paper.
2   Remove the core and outer layer of the fennel bulbs as well as any leafy tops (keep these to garnish, if you like). Cut lengthways into 1cm slices, through the root. Place the slices on the baking tray. Whisk together the honey, oil, tamari, chilli flakes, and a pinch each of salt and pepper. Pour evenly over the fennel. Roast for about 20 minutes until the fennel is tender and the sauce has crisped in places.
3   While the fennel is cooking, mix together the yoghurt and herbs.
4   To serve, place the spinach leaves on plates, add the roasted fennel and top with the herbed yoghurt. Garnish with the reserved fennel leaves, if you wish.

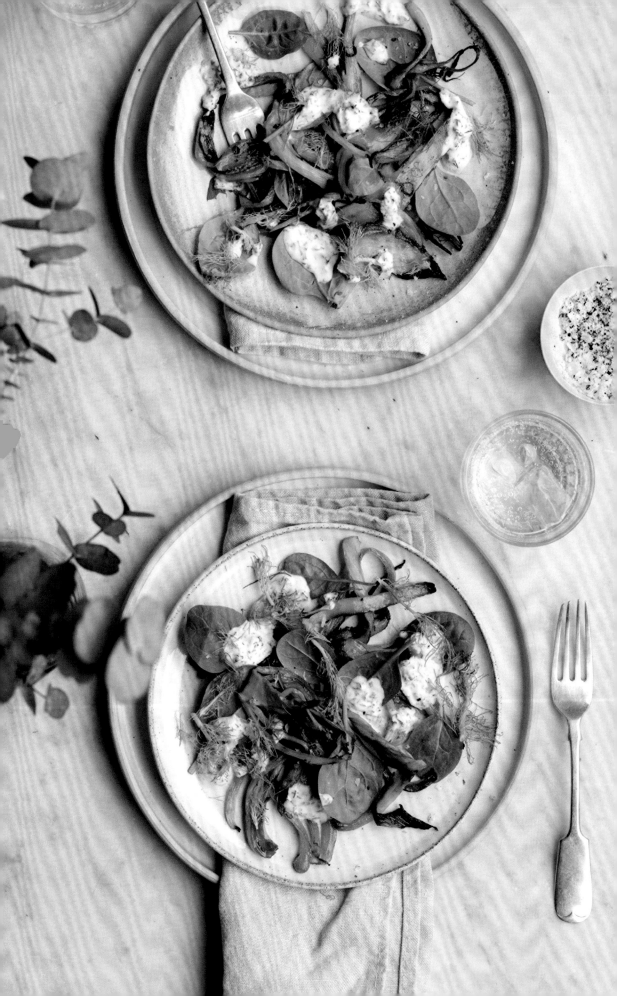

Fennel and date balls

Makes 12
166 calories per ball
The fennel in these sweet date balls has a lovely
fresh flavour that cuts through the rich cacao.
The balls are a good snack – they offer a sweet
hit, but are full of fibre, which will help to prevent
spikes in your blood sugar levels.

300g pitted dates
150g ground almonds
4½ tbsp cacao powder, plus extra for dusting
A good pinch of flaked sea salt
1½ tsp fennel seeds
12 hazelnuts

1 Put the dates into a bowl and cover with
boiling water. Leave to soften for 20 minutes.
Drain the dates and place them in a food
processor with the ground almonds, cacao
powder and sea salt.

2 Toast the fennel seeds in a small dry frying pan
until they are fragrant. Tip into a mortar and
crush to a powder using the pestle. Add to the
mixture in the food processor and blitz until
you have a soft paste.

3 Remove the paste from the food processor
and divide into 12 equal pieces. One at a time,
flatten each piece in your hand, put a hazelnut
in the middle and roll the paste around the nut
to form a small ball. Place extra cacao powder
on a plate and roll the balls in it to give them
a fine coating.

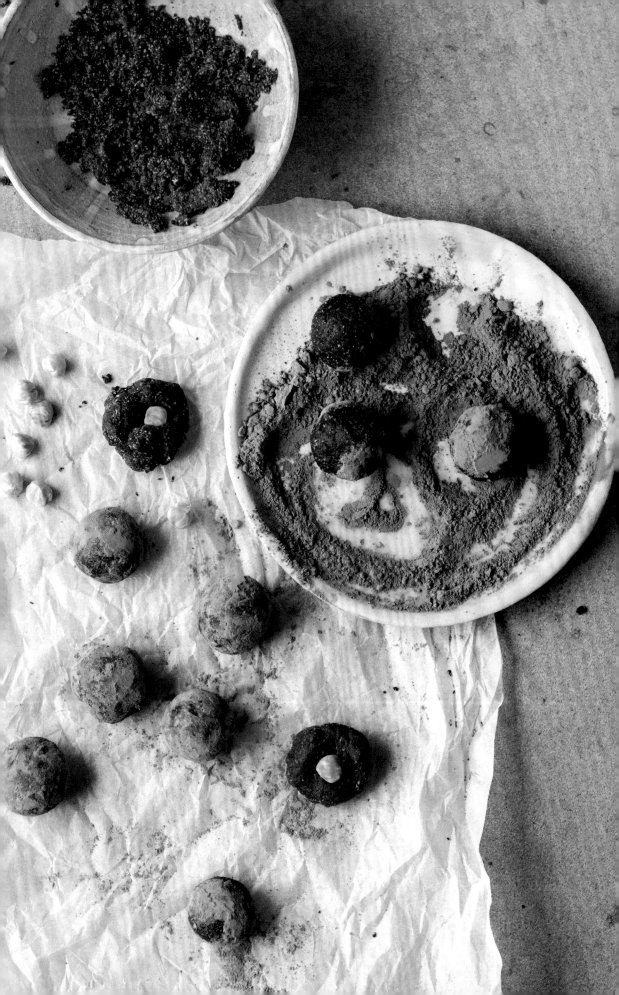

Fennel and chocolate cake

Serves 8

415 calories per serving (with ice cream)

Fennel works surprisingly well with chocolate in desserts, the aniseed flavour cutting through the sweetness of chocolate. Here this pairing creates a rich and intensely flavoured cake. The dairy-free ice cream to accompany is utterly luxurious.

1 tsp fennel seeds

100g cacao powder, plus extra for sprinkling

200ml honey

60ml boiling water

1 vanilla pod, split open and seeds scraped out

3 eggs

130ml olive oil

120g ground almonds

½ tsp gluten-free bicarbonate of soda

A pinch of flaked sea salt

For the ice cream

3 very over-ripe bananas (with brown skin), peeled

1 vanilla pod, split open and seeds scraped out

2 tbsp coconut yoghurt

100ml almond or coconut milk

1 To make the ice cream, put all the ingredients in a bullet or high-speed blender and blend until smooth. Pour into a small tray and leave to set in the freezer.

2 Preheat the oven to 190°C/Fan 170°C/Gas 5. Line a 20–22cm loose-bottomed cake tin with baking paper.

3 Lightly toast the fennel seeds in a small dry frying pan, then crush to a powder using a pestle and mortar. Stir the cacao powder with the honey and boiling water to create a paste. Mix in the fennel powder and vanilla seeds.

4 In another, larger bowl, whisk the eggs until fluffy. Add the olive oil and carry on whisking for a good few minutes until the mixture is thick and creamy. Whisk in the cacao paste, then add the ground almonds and bicarbonate of soda and mix well with a spatula.

5 Tip the mixture into the cake tin. Sprinkle the salt on top. Bake for 25–35 minutes until cooked – the centre of the cake should still be slightly wet. To test, put a knife into the centre: it should come out with some traces of the cacao mixture on it. Leave to cool in the tin.

6 Serve the cake with the ice cream, sprinkled with extra cacao powder.

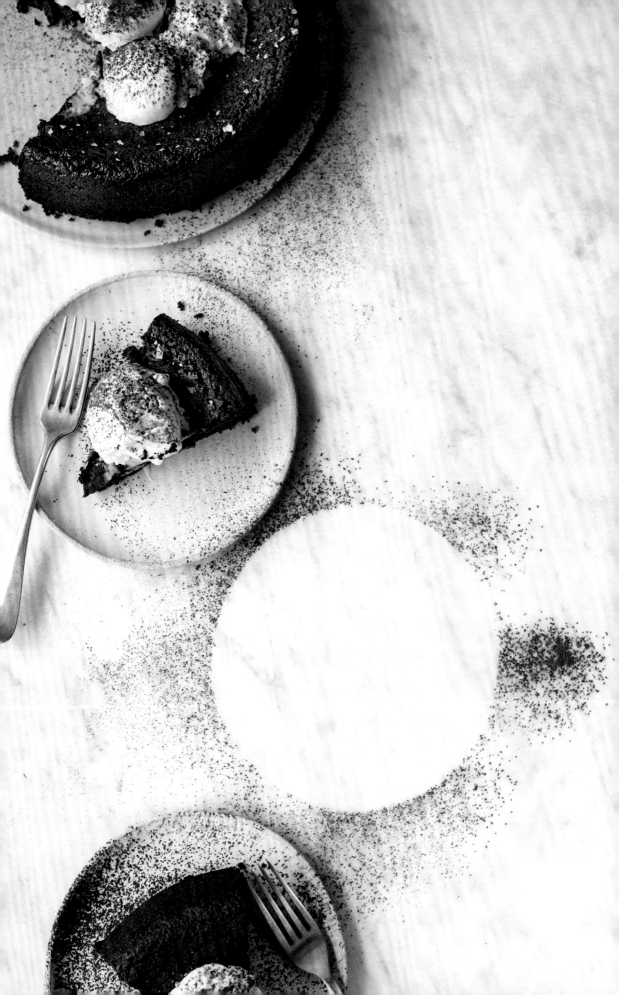

Rhubarb

Rhubarb may technically be a vegetable – a member of the Polygonaceae family, which also contains sorrel – but I am glad to say that the recipes that follow are unashamedly sweet. This is because rhubarb, which is triumphantly tart, needs sweetness to make it palatable and delicious.

There are two crops of rhubarb every year in the UK. The first, in January and February, is 'forced' rhubarb. This is grown under the darkness of upturned pots, which makes for a more tender crop. The second, or 'maincrop' rhubarb, grown outdoors between March and June, is more robust and has a more intense flavour.

Rhubarb is colourful and is easy to grow in even the smallest of gardens. It needs very little attention and will be one of the first vegetables to come through in the early spring. Although rhubarb plants are happiest in a sunny spot, I have managed to grow some in my north-facing garden – the relative lack of sunshine just means that the rhubarb tastes very sharp and needs an extra helping of honey to sweeten it.

If you do decide to grow your own, or if you buy rhubarb with its leaves on, make sure you chop the leaves off the thick stalks and discard them before cooking, as they contain poisonous oxalic acid.

Nutritional bonus
Rhubarb is a good source of **fibre** and of **calcium**. An adequate daily intake of this mineral is vital throughout life, to ensure good bone and teeth development and health.

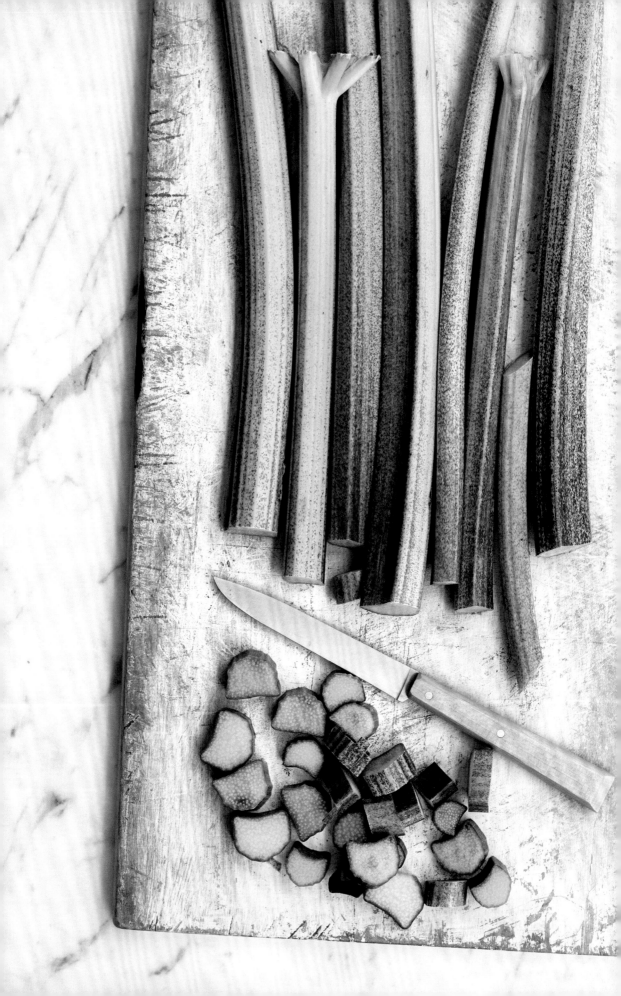

Rhubarb and peach crumble

Serves 4
555 calories per serving
In June and July both rhubarb and peaches are in season, so that's the best time of year to make this crumble. It is a delicious combination of sweetness and tartness, and the pink of the rhubarb alongside the deep gold of the peaches makes it a feast for the eyes too.

400g rhubarb, cut into 2.5cm pieces
100ml water
50g honey
1 cinnamon stick
4 peaches, sliced
Coconut yoghurt to serve

For the crumble
100g ground almonds
50g flaked almonds
1 tbsp coconut oil
2 tbsp gluten-free flour
2 tbsp honey
100g porridge oats

1   Preheat the oven to 200°C/Fan 180°C/Gas 6.
2   Put the rhubarb into a saucepan with the water, honey and cinnamon stick. Simmer on a low heat for 12–15 minutes until the rhubarb is tender but still holding together. Remove the cinnamon stick and tip the stewed rhubarb into a pie dish. Top with the peach slices.
3   To make the crumble, put the ground almonds, flaked almonds, coconut oil, flour, honey and oats in a large mixing bowl. Mix together well, making sure that all of the almonds, oats and flour are covered in the oil and honey – this will help to create a golden topping.
4   Scatter the crumble over the fruit. Bake for about 20 minutes until the crumble topping is golden. Serve immediately with a dollop of coconut yoghurt on each portion.

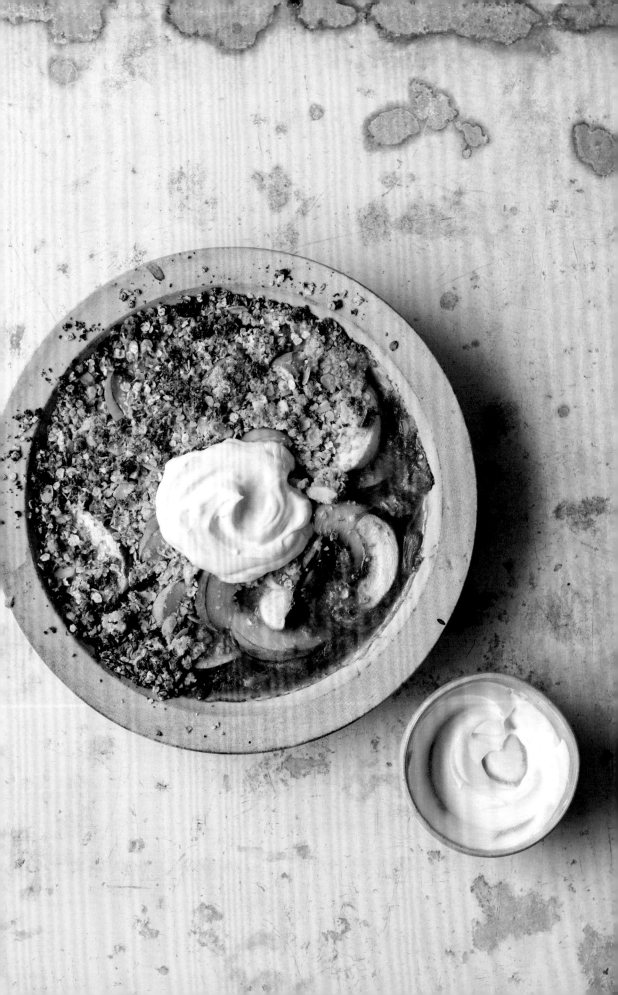

Quinoa porridge with rhubarb and berry compote

Serves 2
524 calories per serving
Stewing rhubarb with cardamom pods and golden syrup makes the most deliciously fragrant, sweet compote; the addition of raspberries brings an extra zing of tartness to it. Making porridge with quinoa means that as well as creaminess from the oats you gain an extra chewy bite.

100g quinoa
200ml rice milk
50g rolled oats
½ tsp ground cinnamon
A pinch of flaked sea salt
Coconut yoghurt to serve

For the compote
3 rhubarb sticks, chopped
1 tbsp golden syrup
5 cardamom pods
Zest and juice of 1 orange
100ml water
100g raspberries

1   First make the compote. Put the rhubarb into a saucepan with the golden syrup, cardamom pods, orange zest and juice, and water. Simmer for about 15 minutes until the rhubarb is soft. Stir in the raspberries and cook for a further 5 minutes until they have softened. Add a little more water if the pan gets too dry, but not too much – the compote should be thick, not runny. Remove the pan from the heat. Spoon out the cardamom pods and discard. Set the fruit compote aside.
2   To make the porridge, put the quinoa into another saucepan and cover with twice the amount of water. Bring to the boil, then simmer for 10 minutes. Stir in the rice milk and oats, and cook for a further 5 minutes. The quinoa will now be overcooked but will be the perfect texture for porridge. Add the cinnamon and salt and mix through.
3   Serve the porridge immediately, topped with the compote and some coconut yoghurt.

Rhubarb granita and banana ice cream sundae

Serves 2
599 calories per serving
Granita is a semi-frozen dessert that is typically made with fruit. This rhubarb version is refreshing and tart, perfect with sweet and creamy banana ice cream. Make sure to use the ripest bananas for the ice cream, as they will be the sweetest. Honeyed pecans are a lovely, crunchy topping.

3 very ripe bananas
500g rhubarb, roughly chopped
3 tbsp honey
100ml water
100g pecans, roughly chopped
A pinch of flaked sea salt

1   Peel the bananas, then put them into a freezer bag and leave in the freezer overnight.
2   To make the granita, place the rhubarb and 2 tablespoons of the honey in a saucepan with the water. Simmer for 15 minutes until the rhubarb is soft. Cool, then tip into a food processor and blitz until smooth. Pour the mixture into a shallow freezerproof container and place in the freezer.
3   After 30 minutes, use a fork to stir in any of the mixture that has frozen at the edges. Repeat this process four or five times, at 30-minute intervals, until the granita is semi-frozen all over with a granular texture and you are able to scrape off soft spoonfuls.
4   Toast the pecans in a dry frying pan until they are slightly browned. Remove from the heat and stir in the remaining honey and the salt. Tip the nuts on to greaseproof paper and leave to cool.
5   Remove the bananas from the freezer and put them into a food processor. Blitz until completely smooth and thick. This should take 3–5 minutes.
6   Fill each glass with a spoonful of pecans, then some banana ice cream, then granita. Repeat, finishing with a final sprinkle of granita.

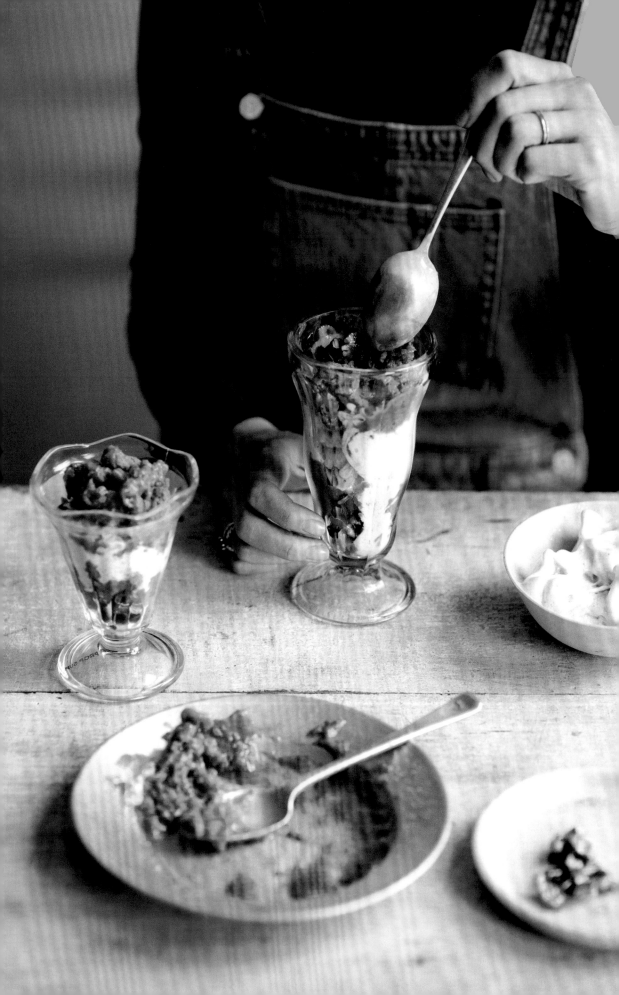

Rhubarb banana bread with compote

Serves 6

247 calories per serving

I love banana bread. In this recipe I've added a contrasting sharp taste of diced rhubarb. Served with coconut yoghurt and a home-made peach and rhubarb compote, the bread is great for afternoon tea when you have friends over. It will keep in an airtight container for up to three days.

2 bananas
50g honey
1 tbsp coconut oil
2 eggs, beaten
½ tsp ground cardamom
½ tsp ground cinnamon
140g gluten-free flour
½ tsp gluten-free bicarbonate of soda
1 rhubarb stick, finely diced
100g coconut yoghurt to serve

For the compote
2 peaches, diced
2 rhubarb sticks, diced
1 tbsp honey

1   Preheat the oven to 200°C/Fan 180°C/Gas 6. Line a 20 x 8cm loaf tin with greaseproof paper.

2   Peel the bananas and mash them in a bowl with a fork. Mix in the honey and then the coconut oil. Add the eggs and mix through. Add the cardamom, cinnamon, flour and bicarbonate of soda and gently fold in. Finally, fold in the diced rhubarb. Tip the mixture into the lined loaf tin. Bake for 20–25 minutes until golden on top and cooked through (test with a skewer, which should come out clean).

3   While the bread is baking, make the compote. Put the peaches, rhubarb and honey in a small saucepan with a splash of water and cook gently until the fruit has softened. Pour into a food processor and blitz until fairly smooth. Taste and add more honey if you would prefer a sweeter compote.

4   When the bread has finished baking, leave to cool in the tin for 5–10 minutes before turning out on to a wire rack to cool completely.

5   To serve, cut the banana bread into slices. Top each slice with a dollop of coconut yoghurt and a spoonful of compote.

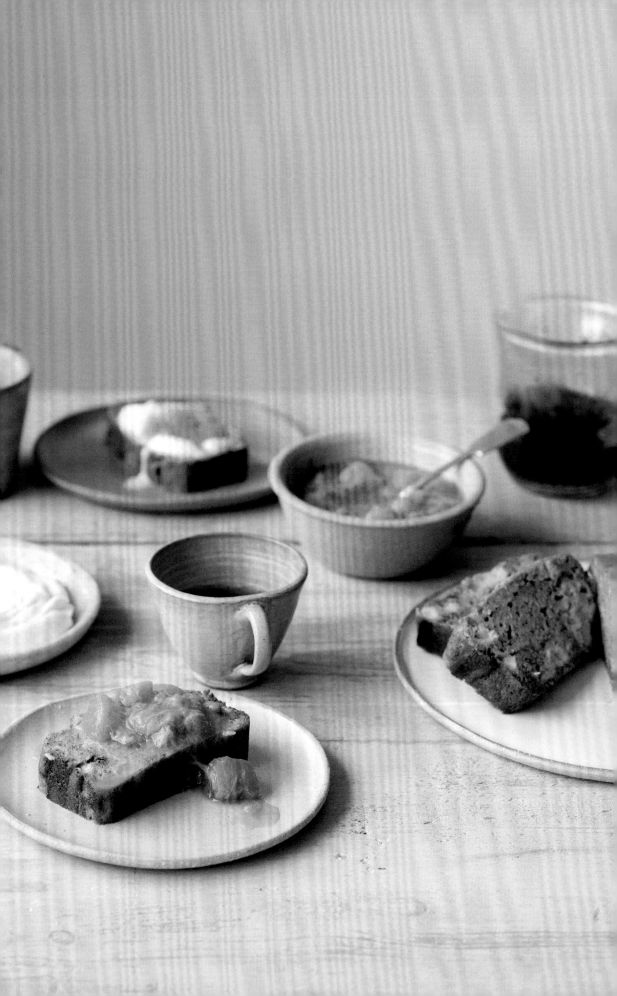

Radish

For me, the perfect radish is plump, crunchy and full of peppery flavour, a deep pink beauty that will bring a dash of colour to a salad. I am also rather partial to the more unusual approach of roasting radishes.

This small vegetable comes in a wide variety of shapes, sizes and rich colours (from red, bright pink or white to purple, yellow or multi-coloured). I especially like the mild 'French Breakfast' variety; it's long and thin with a white tip, and it makes an excellent garnish if you cut it into julienne.

When buying radishes, go for the smaller ones because larger radishes tend to lack flavour and they can often be more fibrous. If your radishes are looking a little tired and wrinkled, just pop them into a bowl of ice-cold water for a few minutes and their plumpness will soon be restored.

Nutritional bonus
Radishes are a source of **folate** and **vitamin C**. In addition, they are very low in calories, being 95 per cent water.

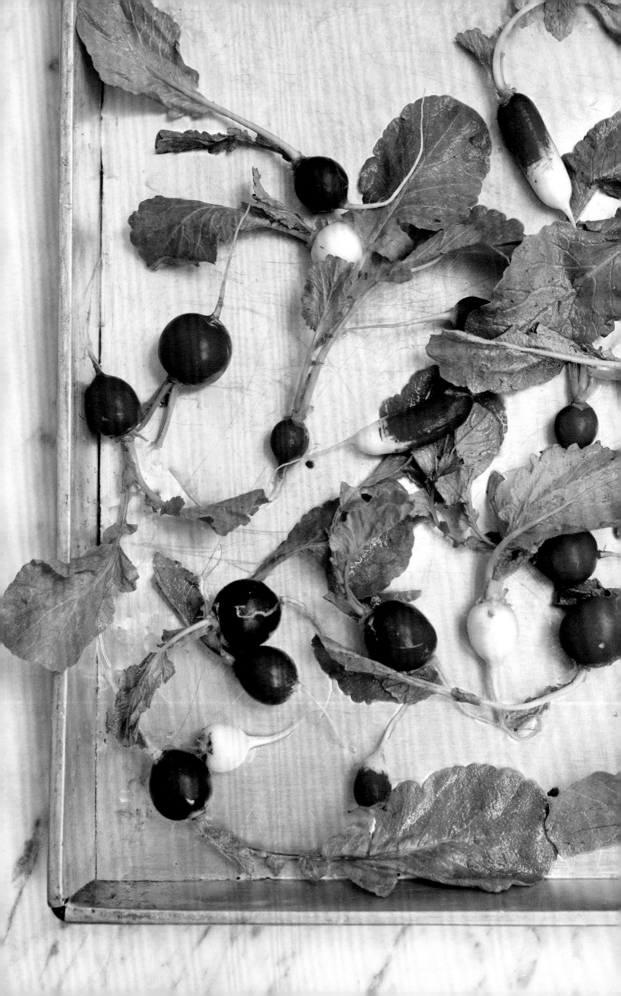

Radish and quinoa salad

Serves 2
474 calories per serving
The radishes in this quinoa salad not only add colour but also crunch and heat. The salad can be speedily thrown together for lunch or dinner, and it is even quicker if you keep cooked quinoa on standby in an airtight container in the fridge. (I would highly recommend doing this if you are often pressed for time.)

200g quinoa
200g radishes, sliced (keep fresh green leaves)
1 cucumber, diced
3 spring onions, finely sliced
1 large beef tomato, diced
1 tbsp tamari
1 tbsp chopped fresh mint
Juice of 1 lemon
30g pumpkin seeds
Flaked sea salt and cracked black pepper

1 Put the quinoa in a saucepan with a pinch of salt and cover with three times the amount of water. Bring to the boil, then simmer gently for 10–12 minutes until the quinoa is cooked and the tail has separated from the seed. Drain in a sieve and rinse under cold running water until cool.

2 Tip the quinoa into a large mixing bowl and add the radishes (along with any fresh green leaves), the cucumber, spring onions, tomato, tamari, mint and lemon juice. Season with salt and pepper, then mix together.

3 Toast the pumpkin seeds in a small dry frying pan over a medium heat until lightly golden. Scatter the seeds over the salad.

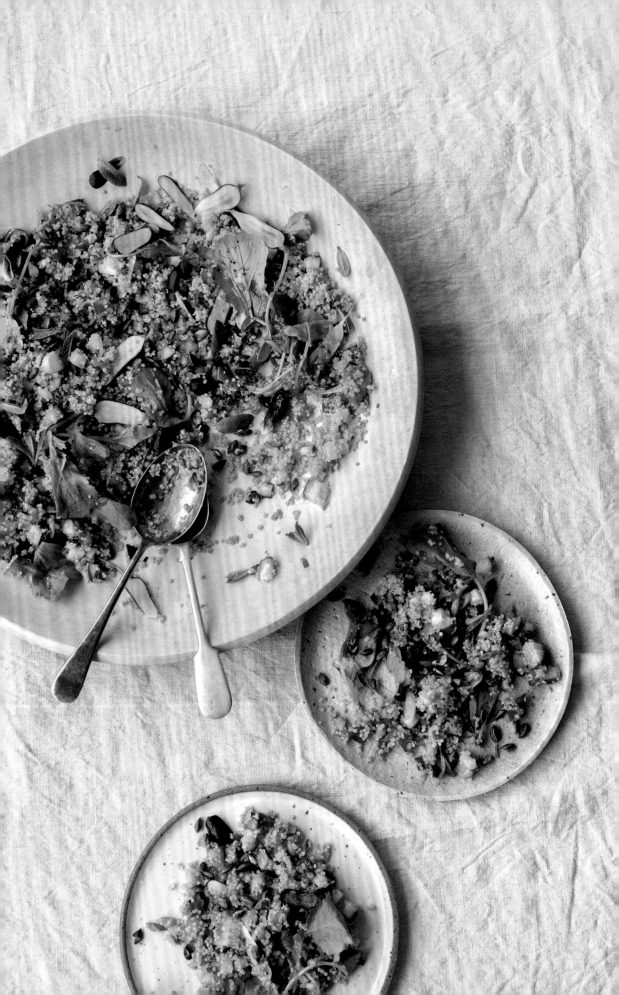

Warm salad with roasted radishes and courgettes

Serves 2
454 calories per serving

Roasting radishes is a game-changer: their skin becomes a delicate, crisp cocoon for the softened centre. Roasting the radishes along with white beans and baby courgettes makes a garlicky tray of deliciousness, the foundation for this tasty warm salad.

200g radishes
300g jarred white beans (haricot or cannellini),
   drained and rinsed
6 baby courgettes
4 garlic cloves (unpeeled)
5 fresh thyme sprigs
1 tbsp olive oil
5 fresh mint sprigs, leaves picked
A handful of fresh flat-leaf parsley
10 fresh chives

For the dressing
2 tbsp Dijon mustard
1 tbsp olive oil
Zest and juice of 1 lemon
Flaked sea salt and cracked black pepper

1 Preheat the oven to 200°C/Fan 180°C/Gas 6. Line a baking tray with greaseproof paper.
2 Place the radishes in a bowl of cold water and set aside while the oven heats up.
3 Drain the radishes and spread them on the tray with the white beans, baby courgettes, garlic cloves and thyme. Season with salt and pepper and drizzle over the olive oil. Roast for 30 minutes until the courgette are tender and the beans are slightly crisp.
4 Meanwhile, make the dressing by whisking all the ingredients together in a small bowl. Pick out the garlic cloves from the baking tray and squeeze the flesh into the dressing. Whisk again. Season to taste.
5 Chop the mint, parsley and chives together.
6 To serve, transfer the radish and bean mixture to a serving bowl, drizzle over the dressing and sprinkle with the herbs.

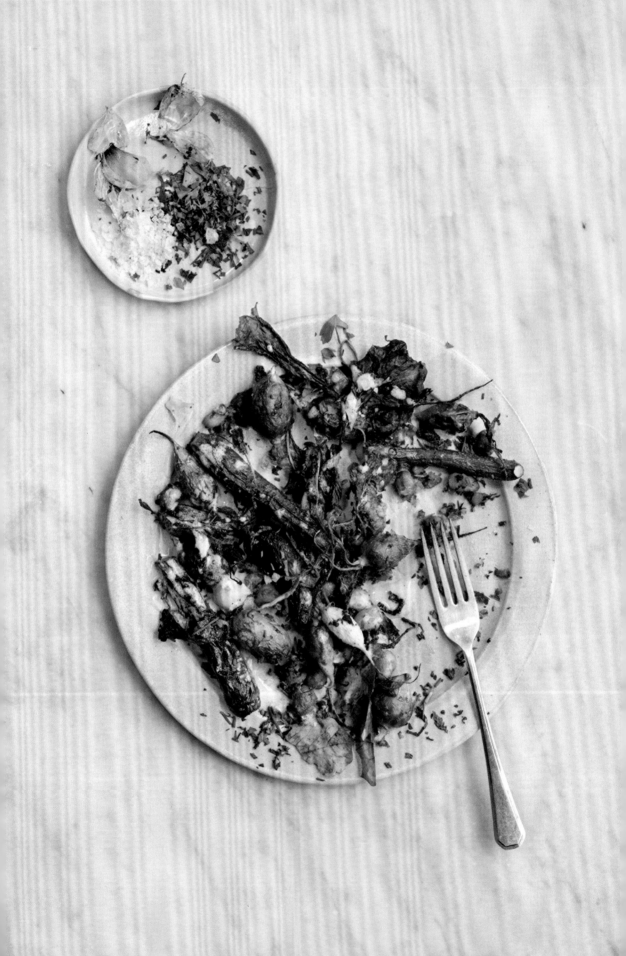

Radish, avocado and tofu 'voké' bowl

Serves 2
652 calories per serving

The Hawaiian salad called poké is typically served with rice but in my vegetable version ('voké') I've chosen to use quinoa as a lighter alternative. The creamy avocado and toasted seeds offer a great contrast of textures, and the bowl is finished in the most perfectly pink way with quick-pickled radishes and crisp ginger.

140g quinoa
A pinch of flaked sea salt
20g sunflower seeds
20g pumpkin seeds
1 tbsp tamari
1 tsp toasted sesame oil
1 avocado

For the pickled radishes
70g radishes, finely sliced
100ml water
1 tbsp honey
2 tbsp brown rice vinegar

For the shoyu sauce
2 tbsp grated fresh root ginger
100ml tamari
1 tbsp toasted sesame oil
A pinch of dried chilli flakes

For the tofu
200g firm tofu, cut into 2cm squares
1 green chilli, thinly sliced
100ml tamari
Zest and juice of 2 limes

For the stir-fried ginger
7.5cm piece of fresh root ginger
Rapeseed oil for frying

1   To make the pickled radishes, put the radishes into a saucepan with the water and honey and bring to a simmer. Remove from the heat. Stir in the brown rice vinegar and pour into a bowl. Leave to cool, then chill for about 30 minutes.

2   Meanwhile, whisk together the ingredients for the shoyu sauce in a small bowl. Set aside.

3   Place the tofu squares in a bowl with the green chilli, tamari, and lime zest and juice and toss together. Set aside.

4   Put the quinoa in a saucepan with the salt and cover with three times the amount of water. Bring to the boil, then leave to simmer gently for 10–12 minutes until the quinoa is cooked and the tail has separated from the seed. Drain in a sieve and rinse well under cold water, then leave to drain completely.

5   Toast the seeds in a dry frying pan until golden. Stir in the tamari and sesame oil. Remove from the heat and leave to cool, then tip into a bowl.

6   Peel and cut up the avocado.

7   For the stir-fried ginger, peel the ginger, then cut into long matchsticks. Heat a little oil in a small pan and flash-fry the ginger for a few minutes until it is slightly browned. Drain on kitchen paper.

8   Spoon the quinoa into serving bowls and add the tofu. Top with drained pickled radishes, avocado, stir-fried ginger and shoyu sauce. Finish with a sprinkling of tamari seeds.

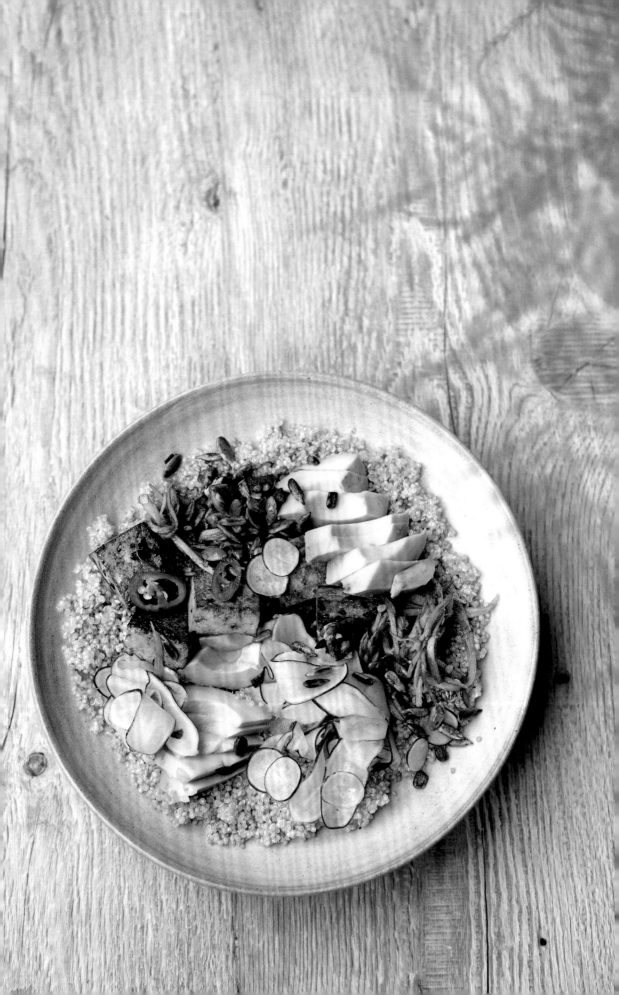

Pickled radishes

Makes a small jar (serves 2)
50 calories per serving

These are easy to make and will enhance almost anything with their sweet and tangy flavour. Keep the radishes in the fridge so you can use them at your leisure over the week.

200g radishes, quartered
100ml brown rice vinegar
2 tbsp honey
1 tsp flaked sea salt
1 tsp coriander seeds
1 tsp fennel seeds
1 red chilli, chopped
2 bay leaves
50ml water

1   Put all the ingredients into a small pan and bring to the boil. Once boiling, remove from the heat and pour into a Kilner jar. Leave to cool completely before putting on the lid.
2   Store in the fridge until you are ready to use the radishes. They will keep in the airtight jar in the fridge for about a week.

Crudités with dips

Serves 4
222 calories per serving

A crudité plate of fresh vegetables with bright dips is a joy to behold. I like to take my time preparing the vegetables, carefully picking the leaves off the radishes so that only the prettiest remain, and cleaning the baby carrots. If you keep all the vegetables in cold water before serving, they will be perfectly plump. Both of the dips are quick and easy and can be prepared up to a day in advance – just keep them covered and in the fridge until you're ready to serve them.

300g radishes
300g baby carrots, scrubbed
2 baby cauliflowers, cut into thin florets through the stem/stalk

For the spinach and butter bean dip
200g spinach
200g jarred butter beans, drained and rinsed
1 tbsp olive oil

For the red pepper and chickpea dip
1 tbsp olive oil, plus extra for frying
1 red pepper, seeded and roughly chopped
200g jarred chickpeas, drained and rinsed
1 tbsp smoked paprika
Flaked sea salt and cracked black pepper

1   Leave any bright, clean leaves on the radishes. Put the radishes into a bowl of cold water to soak. If there are green tops on the carrots, trim neatly to about 2.5cm in length.
2   To make the spinach and bean dip, put all the ingredients in a food processor or high-speed blender and blitz until smooth. Season with salt and pepper to taste.
3   For the red pepper and chickpea dip, heat a little oil in a small frying pan and fry the red pepper until slightly blackened. Tip into a food processor or high-speed blender and add the chickpeas, 1 tablespoon oil and the paprika. Blitz until smooth. Season.
4   Drain the radishes and arrange on a platter with the carrots and cauliflower. Serve with the dips.

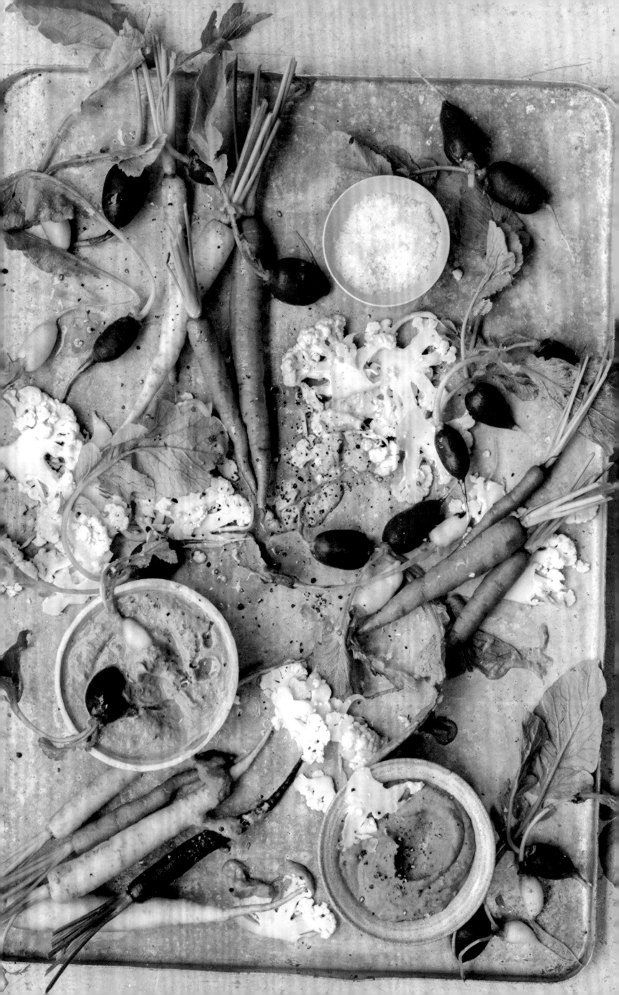

Cucumber

Like freshly cut grass, the smell of sliced cucumber is a nostalgic one for me. It reminds me of eating cucumber sandwiches, sipping Pimm's on long summer nights, and juicing hundreds of cucumbers for clients in the early days of founding Detox Kitchen.

Cucumbers are fairly easy to grow at home. Sow the seeds in good-quality compost in early June, ideally under a fleece, and make sure they are in full sun. Once the main stem has developed seven leaves, pinch out the growing tip. The mature cucumbers should be ready to harvest at the end of the summer.

The delicate taste of cucumber will not overpower other flavours; it will simply lend its crunchy texture, freshness and bright colour to a dish.

Nutritional bonus
Cucumbers are 95 per cent water, which means that you could get your daily water requirement through food by eating four cucumbers (you would, admittedly, have to be a very big fan of cucumber to do that).

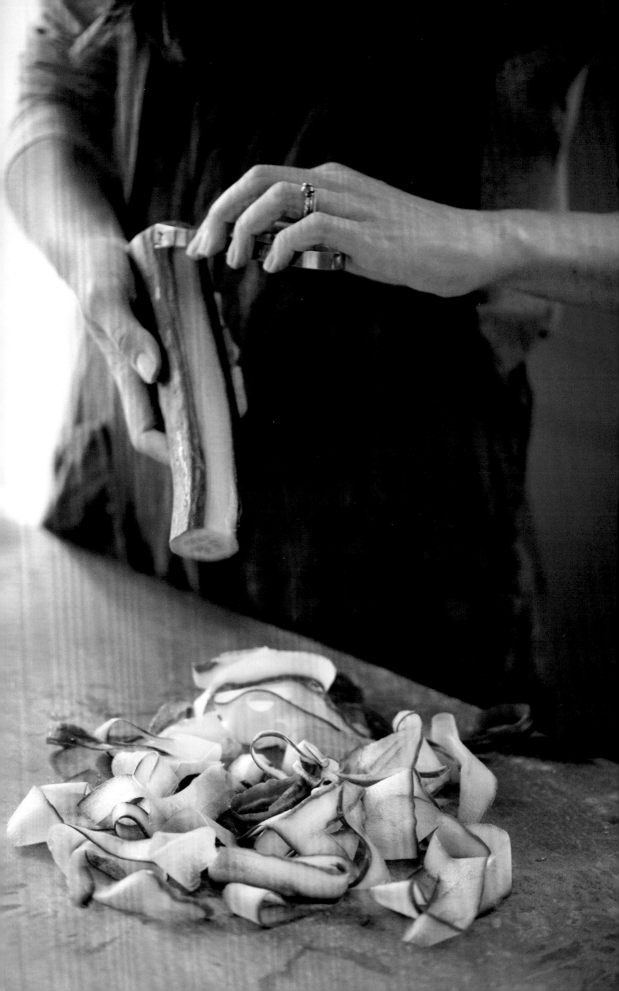

Cucumber and avocado gazpacho

Serves 2
184 calories per serving

I am partial to gazpacho in summer, particularly as the classic Spanish recipe for chilled tomato soup is a perfect pick-me-up after one too many Pimm's! My cucumber and avocado version is almost like a fresh, zingy smoothie and it can be served in a glass or in a small bowl as a starter.

2 cucumbers
1 avocado
A handful of spinach
1 spring onion, finely chopped
A small handful of fresh basil
Juice of 2 lemons
Flaked sea salt and cracked black pepper

1   Juice one of the cucumbers. Roughly chop the other cucumber. Place both the cucumber juice and the chopped cucumber in a food processor.
2   Halve the avocado and scoop out the flesh into the food processor. Add the spinach, spring onion, basil and lemon juice. Blitz to a thick soup consistency. Season to taste. Chill well before serving.

Mum's rice salad

Serves 2
604 calories per serving

My mum is the queen of rice salads. She always cooks the rice in the morning and cools it under running cold water, then sets it aside at room temperature until the evening. As well as giving the rice a deeper flavour, this approach means that throwing a salad together will always be quick and easy.

For this recipe you can use whatever vegetables or salad ingredients you happen to have – it's a great way to use up leftovers. The key is to chop the vegetables finely, starting with the cucumber and tomatoes. The secret ingredient is tamari, which is used to season the salad.

100g wild rice or brown rice
1 cucumber, seeded and finely diced
2 tomatoes, finely diced
100g radishes, thinly sliced
1 avocado, peeled and roughly chopped
½ yellow pepper, seeded and finely diced
1 spring onion, finely sliced
2 tbsp tamari
2 tbsp sunflower seeds
2 tbsp pumpkin seeds
1 tbsp cashew nuts
Flaked sea salt and cracked black pepper
Fresh coriander, roughly chopped, to garnish

1   Put the rice in a pan with a pinch of salt and cover with three times the amount of water. Bring to the boil, then simmer until the rice is tender – wild rice will take 30–35 minutes, brown rice 20–25 minutes. Drain and rinse under cold water. Leave at room temperature until you are ready to make the salad.
2   Put the cucumber, tomatoes, radishes, avocado, yellow pepper and spring onion in a large mixing bowl. Add the cooked rice, tamari and a good pinch of black pepper.
3   In a small dry frying pan, gently toast the seeds and cashew nuts until golden. Add these to the salad and mix through. Serve garnished with chopped coriander.

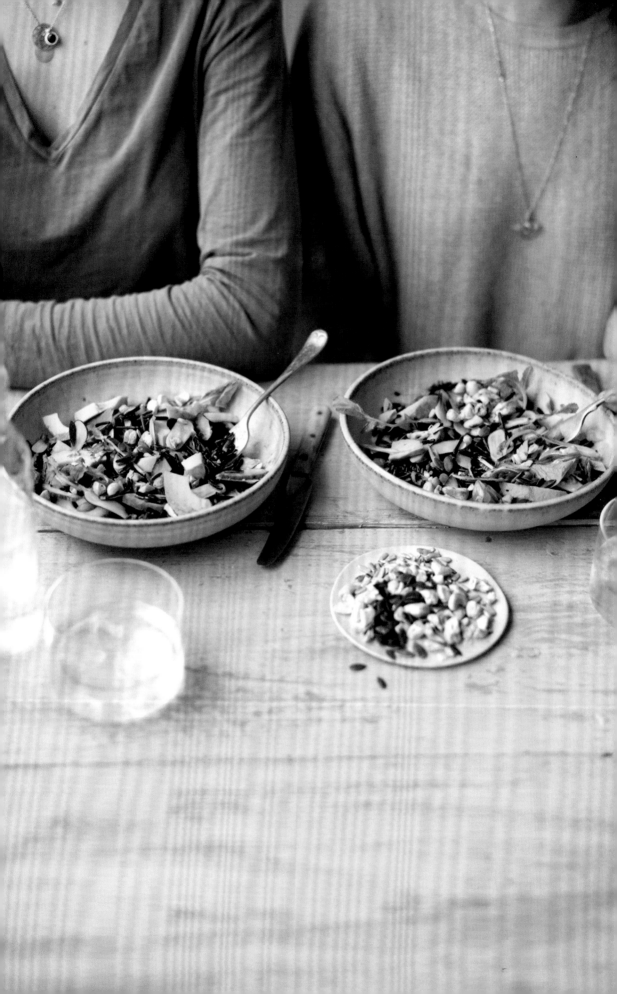

Cucumber and red pepper nori rolls

Serves 4
521 calories per serving

It takes skill to perfect most sushi, but not if it's the type that's only going to sit around for a few seconds before you devour it. The key is to pack the quinoa on to the nori sheet as compactly as possible so that it holds firm when you cut through the wrap.

400g quinoa
2 tbsp sunflower seeds
2 tbsp tamari
½ cucumber, cut into long matchsticks
½ red pepper, seeded and sliced
1 avocado, peeled and sliced
4 nori seaweed sheets (for nori wraps)
Flaked sea salt and cracked black pepper

For the satay sauce
1 tbsp smooth peanut butter
50ml coconut milk
1½ tsp tamari
¼ tsp toasted sesame oil

1   Put the quinoa in a pan with a pinch of salt and cover with three times the amount of water. Bring to the boil, then leave to simmer gently for at least 10–12 minutes – you want the quinoa to be slightly overcooked (you will know that it is overcooked when the tail or germ has separated from every seed). Drain in a sieve and set aside, which will allow for further cooking. When the quinoa is at room temperature, tip it into a bowl and put it into the fridge to cool completely.

2   Toast the sunflower seeds in a small dry frying pan until golden. Add the tamari and stir until all the seeds are covered. Remove from the heat and leave to cool.

3   To make the satay sauce, put the ingredients in a bowl and whisk together until smooth. (The sauce can be kept, covered, in the fridge for 3 days.)

4   When you are ready to make the rolls, set out all the prepared vegetables. Lay a bamboo sushi mat on a flat dry surface and place a nori sheet on top. Spoon 4 heaped tablespoons of quinoa on to the nori sheet and spread out flat to the edges – the layer of quinoa should be about 5mm thick.

5   In the centre place a row of cucumber, red pepper and avocado across the nori, which should take up about 5cm. Don't add too many vegetables or the nori sheet will be difficult to roll up. Top the vegetables with a few small dollops of satay sauce and sprinkle with some tamari seeds, salt and pepper. Fold the bottom of the nori sheet up towards the top, then pull the filling ingredients tightly together and continue to roll, using the mat to help, so that you form a neat cylinder.

6   Repeat to make three more rolls. Chill them for about 10 minutes, which will help the rolls to firm up and make them easier to cut.

7   When you are ready to serve, simply cut each roll across into four pieces.

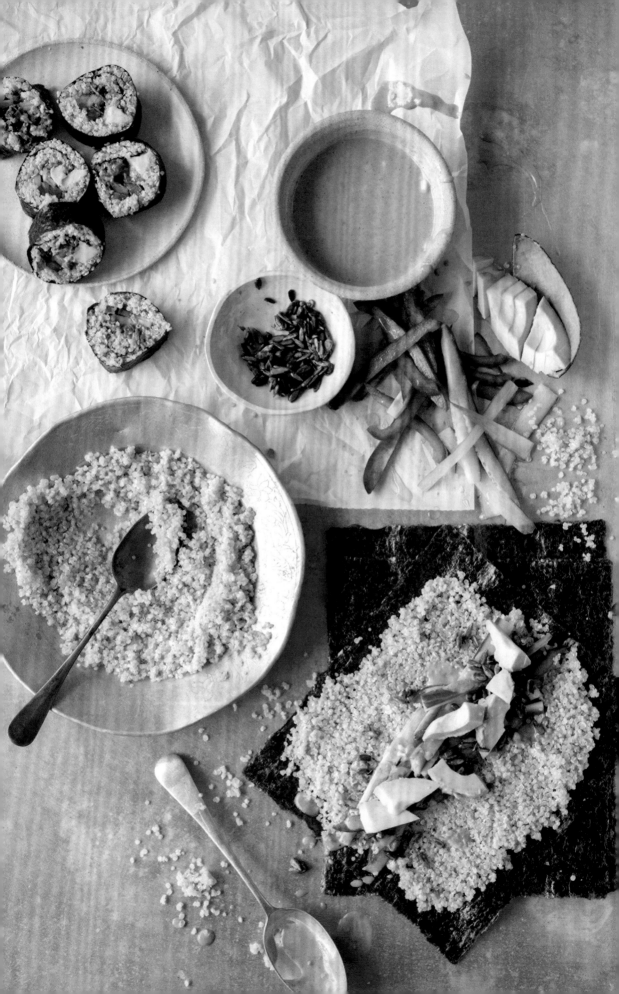

Cucumber, avocado and coconut smoothie

Serves 2
282 calories per serving
This smoothie has the perfect balance of fresh, bright flavours and smooth, creamy texture. The coconut yoghurt and avocado mean that it is brimming with good fats, and the cucumber gives a hydrating boost.

1 cucumber
1 avocado
2 tbsp coconut yoghurt
200ml coconut water
1 tsp maple syrup
Juice of 1 lime
3 ice cubes
Ground cinnamon (optional)

1   Juice the cucumber. Pour the juice into a blender.
2   Halve the avocado and scoop out the flesh into the blender. Add the yoghurt, coconut water, maple syrup, lime juice and ice cubes. Blitz until completely smooth.
3   Pour into two glasses and sprinkle with cinnamon, if desired.

Cucumber, fennel, spinach and courgette juice

Serves 2
81 calories per serving
I have to include a green juice in this book, as it is such a quick and easy way to get some extra nutrients into your diet. This is a favourite of mine, with parsley and mint, plus lime for an extra kick.

1 cucumber
½ fennel bulb
1 courgette
A handful of spinach
1 tbsp fresh flat-leaf parsley leaves
6 fresh mint leaves
Juice of 1 lime
3 ice cubes

1   Juice the cucumber, fennel and courgette.
2   Pour the juice into a blender and add the spinach, parsley, mint, lime juice and ice cubes. Blitz until completely smooth.

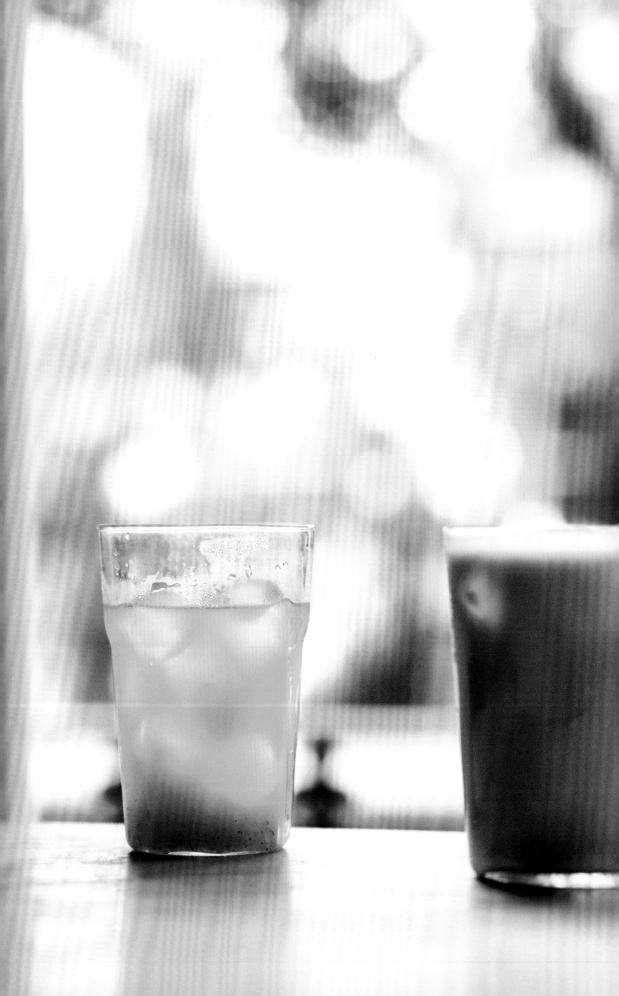

Spinach

Thanks to Popeye and his famous fondness for spinach, this vegetable saw a surge in popularity in the UK during the 1980s and we haven't really looked back. Perhaps this is because spinach is easy to grow, as well as being highly nutritious. It is available all year round, but the tastiest and most tender spinach is found in the spring.

One of my favourite cooking terms is *florentine*, simply because it means that any dish described as such will include spinach – as in 'eggs florentine'.

Although spinach is such a widely used ingredient, I seem to turn to the same cooking method time and time again, the 'add it to the dish and turn off the heat' approach. A lot of the flavour, colour and nutritional benefits of spinach are lost during prolonged cooking, whereas adding it at the last minute will ensure that the goodness and vibrancy are preserved. I also use a lot of raw spinach in salads, to give added texture and a nutritional boost.

I tend to use baby spinach – the leaves are smaller and more tender when they are young, so they work well eaten raw in a salad. When I buy a bag of spinach I often have some left over. I've found that if you don't want to use it up straight away it is fine to freeze it. You can then add the spinach to a soup or stew straight from the freezer.

Nutritional bonus

Legend has it that when scientists first analysed spinach for **iron** content, they put the decimal in the wrong place. Thus everyone thought that it was much richer in iron than it actually is. Whether or not the story is true, the iron content in spinach is still higher than that in many other vegetables. Spinach is also a great source of **potassium**, **magnesium**, **folate**, **calcium**, **carotene** (which is converted in the body to **vitamin A**) and **vitamin C**.

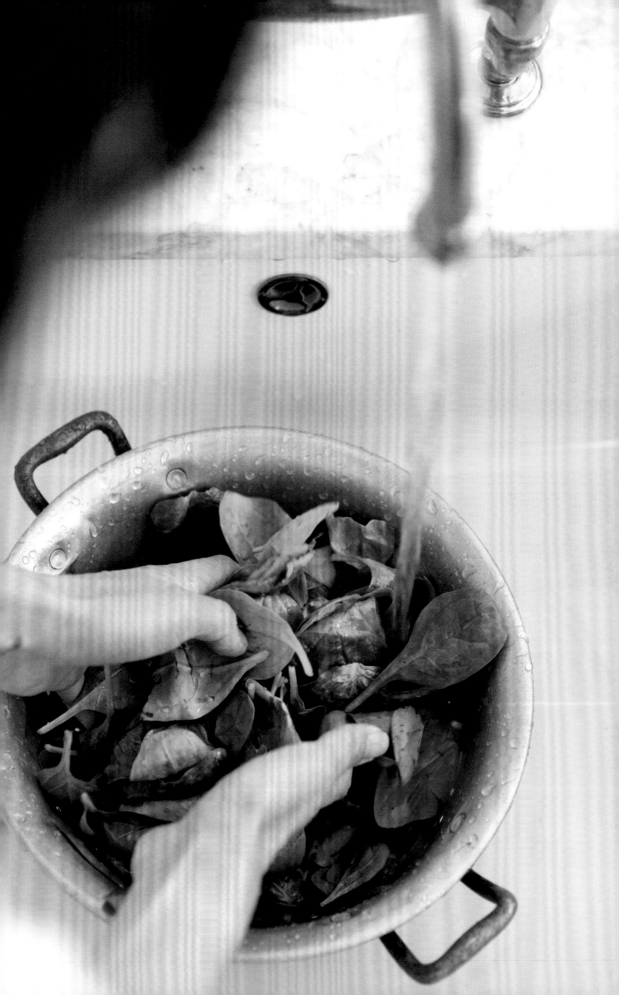

Flatbreads topped with spinach and egg

Serves 4
379 calories per serving
This is my take on a Florentine pizza. Instead of the traditional pizza base, I use flatbreads made from chickpea (gram) flour, which is coarser than normal flour and has a distinct nutty flavour that tastes, unsurprisingly, a lot like chickpeas. The bright green topping is made from spinach and butter beans, with a baked egg to finish.

A handful of caraway seeds
250g chickpea flour
125–175ml cold water
400g jarred butter beans, drained and rinsed
1 tbsp rapeseed oil, plus extra for frying
200g spinach
4 eggs
Toasted pumpkin seeds to sprinkle
Flaked sea salt and cracked black pepper

1   Toast the caraway seeds in a small dry frying pan until fragrant. Tip into a bowl and add the flour and a pinch each of salt and pepper. Gradually mix in enough water to create a thick batter. Chill for 2 hours.

2   Preheat the oven to 200°C/Fan 180°C/Gas 6.

3   To make the spinach mixture, place the butter beans, oil and a pinch each of salt and pepper in a food processor and blitz until smooth. Add the spinach and blitz again. Set aside.

4   Heat a little oil in a 20cm frying pan. Spoon in about a quarter of the batter, spreading it out with the back of the spoon to create a large pancake. Once golden on the base, flip over and cook the other side. As the flatbreads are cooked, transfer them to a baking tray.

5   When all the flatbreads are on the tray, smear the spinach mixture over them. Crack an egg on top of each. Bake for 2–3 minutes until the eggs are cooked. Season with salt and pepper. Sprinkle with pumpkin seeds and serve.

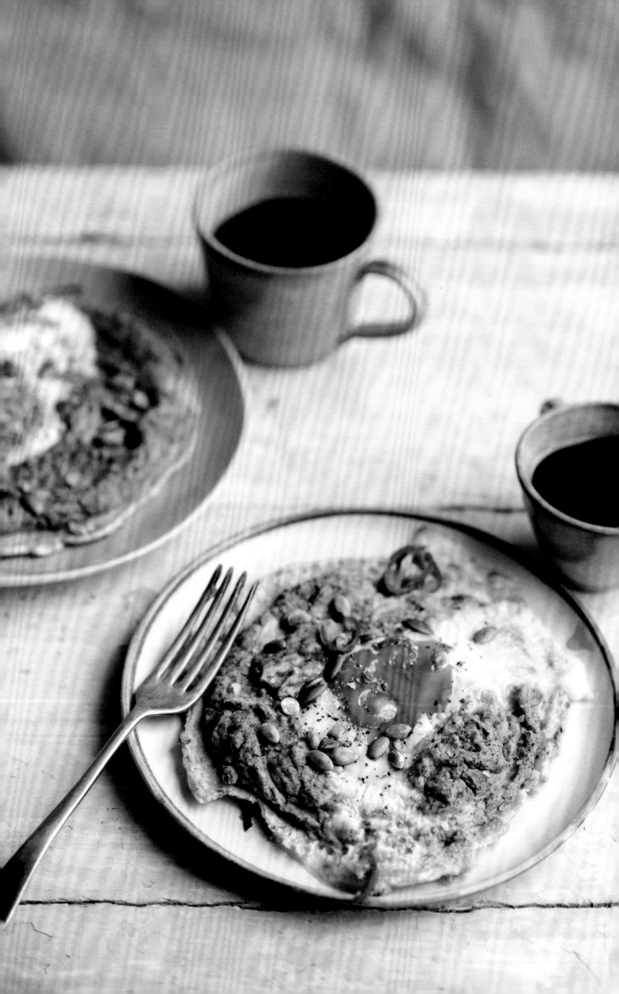

The ultimate chopped salad

Serves 2
430 calories per serving

This is a go-to salad when you're in a hurry but want to make something really nutritious and tasty. Chopped spinach, cucumber and tomatoes are mixed with sweetcorn, sliced mushrooms and toasted seeds. The salad is topped with a couple of soft-boiled eggs. This will feed two but I could easily eat the whole bowl myself.

2 eggs
250g spinach
1 cucumber, seeded and finely diced
2 vine tomatoes, cut into 1cm pieces
4 sun-dried tomatoes, diced
200g frozen sweetcorn, thawed
100g chestnut mushrooms, finely sliced
1 tbsp pumpkin seeds
1 tbsp sunflower seeds
1 tbsp roughly chopped cashew nuts

For the ranch dressing
150ml soya yoghurt
A handful of fresh chives, finely chopped
1 tsp dried parsley
1 tsp dried tarragon
¼ tsp garlic powder
¼ tsp onion powder
Flaked sea salt and cracked black pepper

1   Make the dressing by mixing together all the ingredients. Set aside.
2   Bring a pan of water to the boil. Add the eggs and cook for 6 minutes for soft-boiled (the white firm but the yolk still soft). Drain and cool under cold water. Set aside.
3   Shred the spinach finely and place in a bowl. Add the cucumber, tomatoes, sweetcorn and mushrooms.
4   Lightly toast the seeds and nuts in a small dry frying pan until golden. Add hot to the salad. Season with salt and pepper.
5   Divide the salad between two bowls. Peel the eggs and cut in half. Put one egg on each salad and drizzle over the ranch dressing.

Spinach kitchari

Serves 4
532 calories per serving

Kitchari, which means 'mixture', is an important dish in the Ayurvedic tradition of cooking. Here I've used the classic combination of brown rice and red lentils, but you can use any kind of lentil or rice you like.

My grandmother taught my dad to make this recipe and he has kindly passed it on to me. Whenever he's cooking kitchari, the smell of cardamom, cloves and lentils immediately transports me to a happy place. It's a warming dish that feeds the soul as much as the body.

300g red lentils
220g brown rice
Rapeseed oil for frying
1 red onion, diced
3 garlic cloves, finely chopped
2 tbsp grated fresh root ginger
6 cloves
4 cardamom pods
2 cinnamon sticks
3 bay leaves
½ tsp ground turmeric
500ml vegetable stock
200g baby spinach

1   Rinse the lentils and rice separately until the water runs clear. Set aside.
2   Heat a little oil in a large, heavy-based saucepan. Add the onion, garlic, ginger, cloves, cardamom, cinnamon sticks and bay leaves, and cook over a medium heat until the onion is slightly browned. Add the lentils and rice and stir them into the spices for 3 minutes so that all the grains are coated. Stir in the turmeric and vegetable stock. Bring to the boil, then turn the heat to low, put on the lid and simmer for about 40 minutes until the liquid is almost all absorbed and the rice and lentils are completely soft.
3   Pick out and discard the cloves, cinnamon sticks and cardamom pods. Stir in the spinach. Once the leaves have wilted, serve immediately.

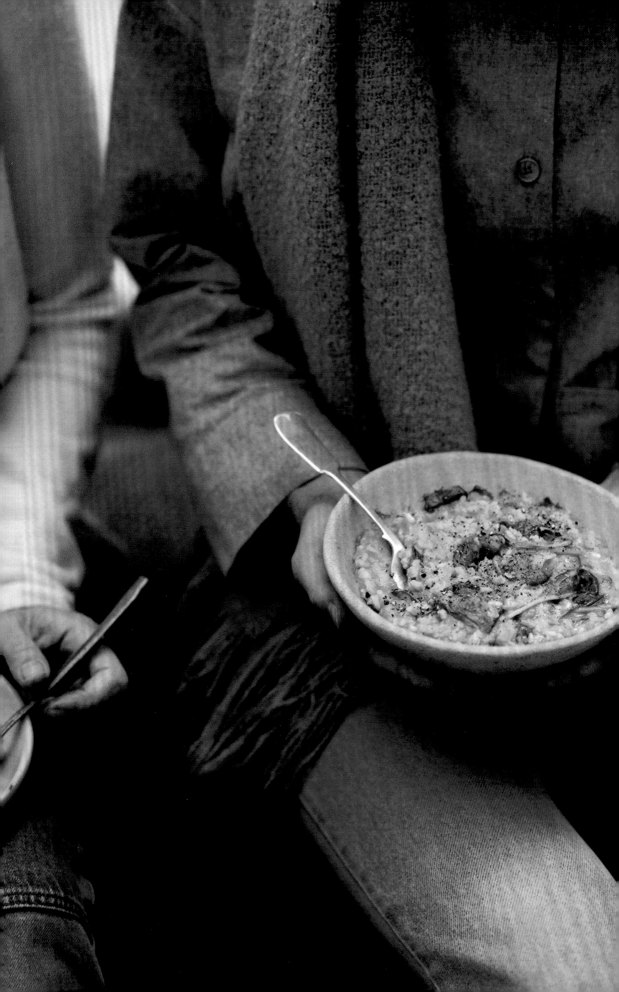

Kale

There are two types of kale, flat leaf and curly leaf. Curly leaf kale tends to be more readily available in greengrocers and supermarkets. When you are shopping, I'd advise you to choose kale with a small head, as the leaves will be more tender. This is particularly desirable if you're planning to eat the kale raw or just lightly sautéed.

Kale is hardy enough to add to stews, yet delicate enough in flavour to form the base of a salad. I find the best way to enjoy raw kale is to massage a bit of oil into the leaves, which softens them and makes them easier to digest.

Although it has had something of a resurgence in the UK in the past few years, kale has always been one of the most common green vegetables in Europe, where it has been cultivated for over 2,000 years. Its steady popularity over the centuries has been driven by the fact that it is easy to grow; it's abundant during the winter months, from December to April; and it is versatile to cook with (juiced, raw in a salad, sautéed, steamed, flash-fried or dried).

Nutritional bonus

Anything this green is bound to be good for you and it is no wonder that kale is often referred to as a 'superfood'. Its main attributes are a high level of **vitamin K**, which is important for bone health, plus good levels of **carotene**, which the body converts to **vitamin A**. Kale is also a great source of **vitamin C** and offers good supplies of **potassium, calcium** and **fibre**.

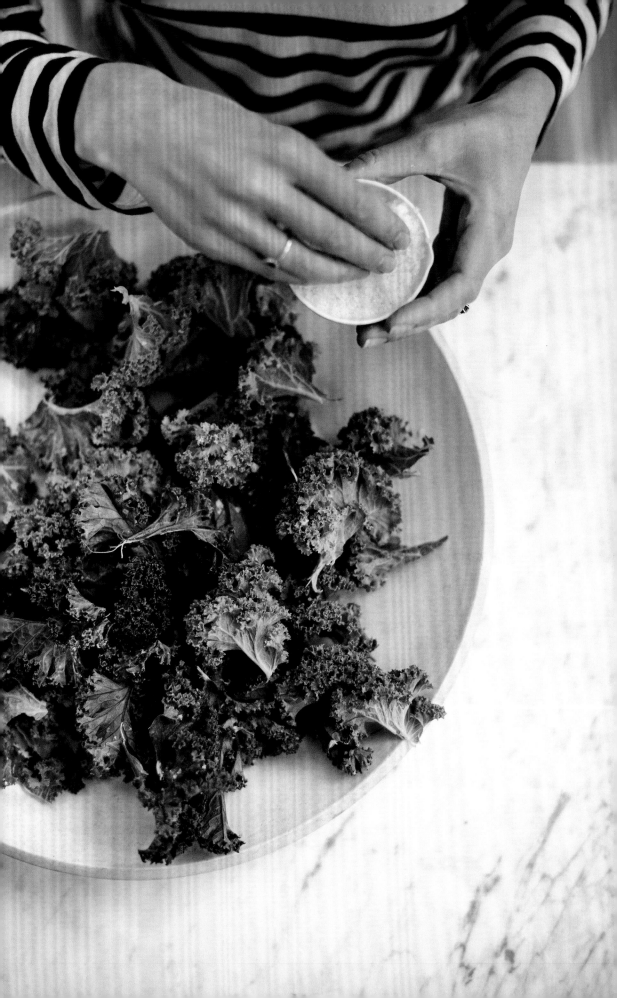

Kale pakoras

Serves 2

472 calories per serving

These pakoras are delicately spiced mouthfuls
of green goodness. The chickpea (gram) flour gives
them a nutty, rounded flavour and the chillies add
a little kick, which is soothed and balanced by the
coconut yoghurt and cucumber dip.

150g chickpea flour
1 tbsp ground cumin
1 tbsp ground coriander
1 tsp garam masala
2 green chillies, finely diced
200g kale
Rapeseed oil for frying
Dried chilli flakes for sprinkling

For the dip
3 tbsp coconut yoghurt
½ cucumber, peeled and finely diced
1 tbsp chopped fresh mint
1 tbsp chopped fresh coriander
Zest of 2 limes
Flaked sea salt

1   Combine the flour, spices, green chillies and
    a pinch of salt. Gradually mix in enough water
    to make a thick batter. Chill for 30 minutes.
2   To prepare the kale, pick the leaves off the
    tough stalks (discard the stalks), then roughly
    chop the leaves. Mix them into the batter.
3   To make the dip, mix all the ingredients
    together in a bowl. Season with a pinch
    of salt. Set aside.
4   Heat a little oil in a large frying pan. Add the
    batter to the pan in spoonfuls to create small
    pakoras (you'll need to cook them in batches).
    Cook until golden on both sides.
5   Serve with the coconut and mint dip plus
    a sprinkle of chilli flakes.

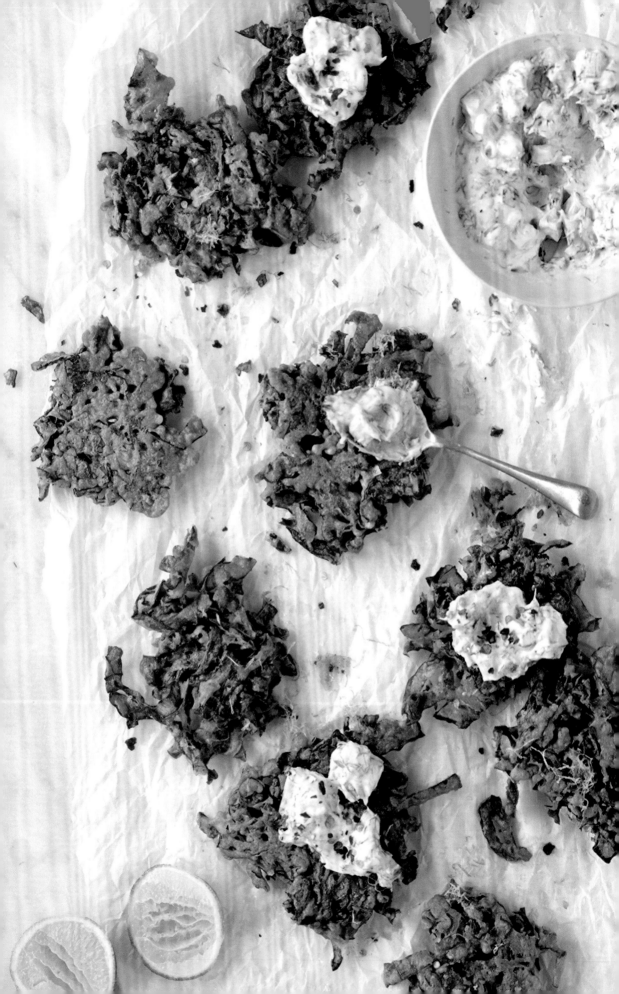

Kale, giant chickpea and celery stew

Serves 4
282 calories per serving

The humble chickpea will add body and texture to any recipe, especially if the chickpeas are of the giant variety. This kale and celery stew is the perfect dish for a quick weekday supper, or perhaps a Moroccan-inspired brunch at the weekend.

Olive oil for frying and drizzling
1 onion, diced
2 garlic cloves, finely chopped
250g jarred giant chickpeas, drained
3 celery sticks, cut into 1cm pieces
Zest and juice of 2 lemons
3 fresh thyme sprigs
2 bay leaves
1 preserved lemon, finely chopped
300ml vegetable stock
200g kale (tough stalks trimmed), roughly chopped
A small handful of fresh flat-leaf parsley, roughly chopped
Flaked sea salt and cracked black pepper

1   Heat 1 tablespoon olive oil in a saucepan over a medium heat and cook the onion and garlic until the onion is soft and translucent. Add the chickpeas, celery, lemon zest and juice, thyme sprigs, bay leaves, preserved lemon, vegetable stock, and some salt and pepper. Bring to the boil, then place the lid on the pan and simmer for about 10 minutes until the celery is tender.
2   Use a potato masher to gently mash all of the ingredients in the pan – you do not want to create a mush but you do want the chickpeas to start to fall apart.
3   Add the kale and cook until it has wilted. Serve sprinkled with chopped parsley and drizzled with a little olive oil.

Kale and chilli salad with cashews

Serves 2
440 calories per serving

This is an endlessly adaptable recipe, based on flash-frying kale with chilli and shallot. Here the creamy accompaniment is a cashew dressing, but you could also try making a simple dressing with sesame oil and lime instead. There is a wide variety of kale available, not just the green type. I like to mix it with other colours – purple, black or red kale – as it makes the dish more special.

1 tsp rapeseed oil
1 shallot, sliced
1 garlic clove, sliced
250g kale (tough stalks trimmed), chopped
1 red chilli, sliced

For the dressing
100g cashew nuts
200ml coconut milk
1 tbsp tamari

1   Preheat the oven to 200°C/Fan 180°C/Gas 6.
2   Spread the cashew nuts on a baking tray and toast in the oven for 10 minutes until golden. Tip them into a food processor and blitz, then add the coconut milk and tamari. Blitz again to your desired texture – I like to keep the dressing a little chunky.
3   Heat the oil in a large frying pan over a medium heat and cook the shallot and garlic until the garlic is golden. Add the kale and chilli and sauté for a few minutes until the kale has slightly softened.
4   Drizzle the dressing over the kale to serve.

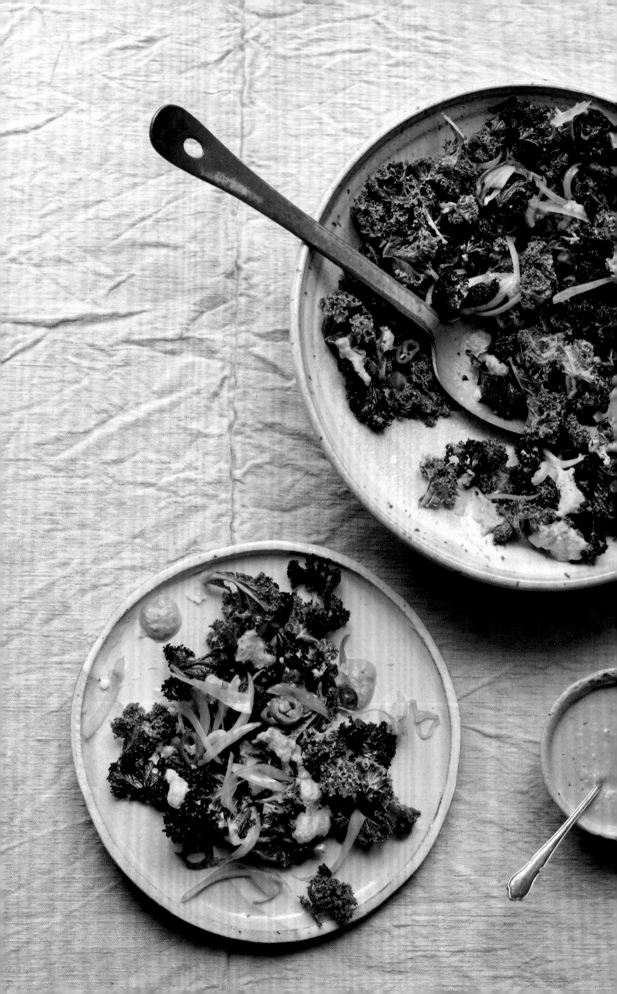

Kale and pea omelette with chilli sambal

Serves 1
725 calories per serving
Sautéing chopped kale gives it a good crisp texture that works well with peas and soft, fluffy eggs in this omelette. The chilli sambal on the side is very spicy and full of bold, bright flavours that will add a new dimension to your breakfast.

1 tsp rapeseed oil
150g kale (tough stalks trimmed), roughly
    chopped
100g podded fresh peas (or thawed frozen peas)
3 eggs
50ml rice milk
Fresh coriander, to garnish

For the chilli sambal
1 lemongrass stick
A thumb-sized piece fresh root ginger, roughly
    chopped
4 kaffir lime leaves
3 shallots, roughly chopped
2 red chillies, seeded and roughly chopped
1 tsp dried chilli flakes
1 tbsp rapeseed oil
1 tbsp tamari
50g honey
1 tsp smoked paprika
2 tbsp brown rice vinegar
Flaked sea salt and cracked black pepper

1   First make the sambal. Bash the lemongrass with a rolling pin, then roughly chop. Put the lemongrass in a food processor with the ginger, lime leaves, shallots, red chillies and chilli flakes and blitz to a paste.

2   Heat the oil in a small frying pan and sauté the paste over a low heat for about 10 minutes until fragrant, stirring constantly so the paste doesn't stick. Stir in the tamari, honey, smoked paprika and brown rice vinegar and cook for a few more minutes until the solids separate from the oil. Remove from the heat and allow to cool. (The sambal will keep in the fridge in an airtight container for 7 days.)

3   To make the omelette, heat the oil in a 25cm frying pan on a high heat and flash-fry the kale and peas for 1 minute to soften. Remove from the heat and transfer the kale and peas to a bowl (leave as much oil behind in the pan as possible). Crack the eggs into the bowl and add the rice milk and salt and pepper to taste. Whisk together.

4   Set the frying pan over a medium heat and add a few more drops of oil if necessary. When the oil is hot, tip in the kale and egg mixture and cook for 3–4 minutes until lightly golden on the base. Flip half of the omelette over to create a half-moon. Cook for a few more minutes until the omelette is cooked through.

5   Slide the omelette on to a serving dish and garnish with the coriander. Serve with the chilli sambal.

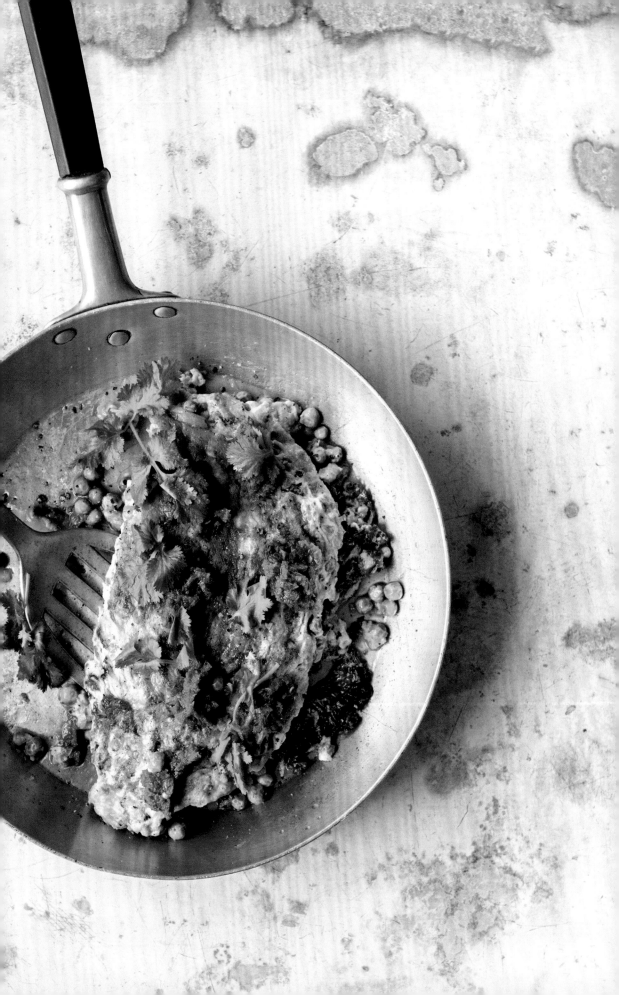

Watercress

'Peppery' is the word that springs to mind when describing watercress, yet all too often it gets overlooked in favour of its similarly peppery friend rocket. I often opt for the deep green leaves and stalks of watercress, however, as they add a really pungent flavour to my cooking and the stalks give salads extra lightness thanks to their crisp texture. Another reason to choose watercress over rocket is that it is a nutritional powerhouse.

Watercress should definitely feature on everyone's weekly shopping list, to be kept in the fridge and used over the next few days – in a salad (the watercress and roasted tomato salad on page 102 is flavourful and punchy), packed into a sandwich, in a risotto (see page 102) or blitzed into a smooth emerald-green soup.

Watercress is typically grown in shallow gravel beds fed by springs that provide a constant flow of water. To grow your own watercress at home, you just need to ensure that the plants are constantly submerged in water.

A simple method is to use a fairly thin plastic container (a washed takeaway tray would be fine). Punch holes in the bottom of the tray, then fill it with compost. Sit it in a slightly larger tray full of water. When the soil is saturated, sow the seeds, then keep the container covered with a clear plastic bag until the seeds have germinated. Continue to change the water in the base tray regularly so that the soil is kept constantly wet, and rinse it out every week to ensure the water doesn't get stagnant. If you want to do this outdoors, it is best to sow the seeds around April, when it is warm enough for them to germinate happily.

Once you have seedlings, you can remove the plastic bag and water the plants from above – and start harvesting the micro leaves.

Nutritional bonus

Throughout history, watercress has been associated with cleansing the blood. Although there is little evidence to support this, it is true that **iron** and **folate** are important nutrients for the production of healthy red blood cells, and **vitamin C** helps the body to absorb iron and folate from food. Watercress contains all these nutrients in abundance. It also contains **vitamin E** and **calcium**.

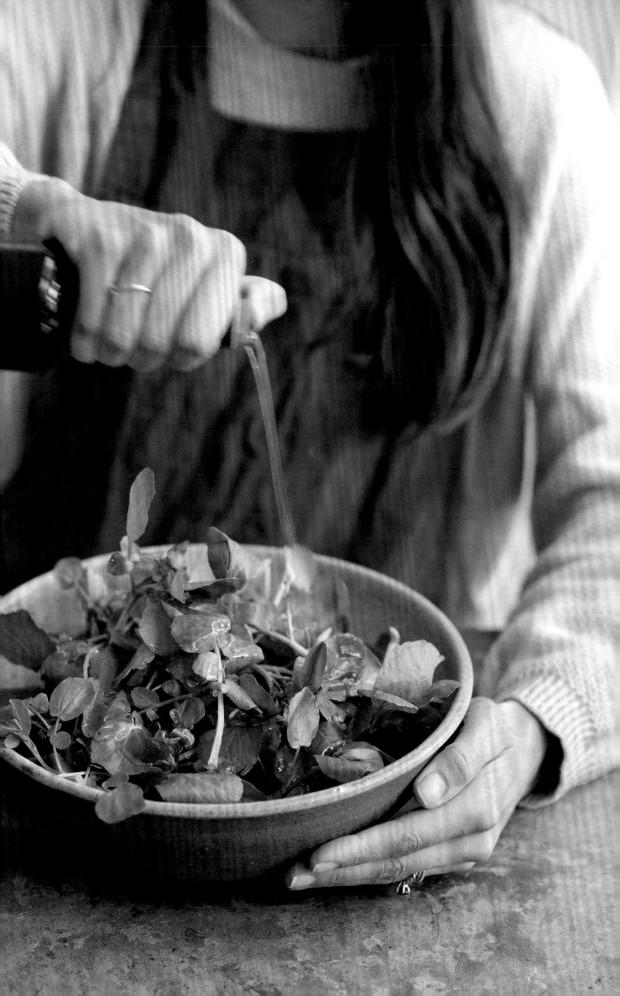

Watercress quiche

Serves 4
506 calories per serving

Quiche is a great make-ahead dish for feeding crowds, when it can be served with a quick salad. It's also an excellent addition to a picnic, being easy to transport and substantial – a welcome alternative to a soggy sandwich. I love adding watercress to a quiche filling as not only does it make it a pretty green, it's a really good way to add a burst of peppery flavour.

150g watercress
1 tsp olive oil, plus extra for frying
Zest and juice of 1 lemon
2 onions, diced
2 garlic cloves, finely chopped
100g podded fresh peas (or thawed frozen peas)
100g spinach
4 eggs
50ml oat milk
50g walnuts, chopped
50g nutritional yeast (yeast flakes)
Flaked sea salt and cracked black pepper

For the pastry
Rapeseed oil for greasting the tin
200g gluten-free flour, plus extra for dusting
2 tbsp coconut oil
4 tbsp ice-cold water

1   Preheat the oven to 200°C/Fan 180°C/Gas 6. Grease a 25cm loose-bottomed tart tin.
2   To make the pastry, put the flour and coconut oil in a bowl and, using your hands, mix them together to a breadcrumb consistency. Add a pinch of salt and the iced water and bring the dough together into a ball (the texture is similar to a bread dough). Wrap in cling film and chill for 20–30 minutes.
3   Roll out the dough on a lightly floured surface to about 3cm thick. Use to line the tart tin, making sure there are no gaps. As this pastry is not very stretchy, you might have to patch it together. Line with baking paper and fill with baking beans, then blind bake for 10 minutes. Remove from the oven and take out the baking paper and beans. Leave the pastry case to cool to room temperature.
4   To make the filling, put half of the watercress in a food processor with the oil and lemon zest and juice. Blitz to a green paste. Heat a little oil in a frying pan and sauté the onions and garlic until the onions are softened. Add the peas and spinach and cook for just a few minutes until the spinach is wilted. Remove from the heat. Add the remaining watercress together with the blitzed watercress and mix well. Season with salt and pepper to taste.
5   Whisk the eggs in a bowl with the oat milk and a pinch each of salt and pepper.
6   Spread the watercress mixture in the pastry case, then pour over the egg mixture. Scatter the chopped walnuts and nutritional yeast over the top. Bake for 30 minutes until the filling has set and the top is golden.

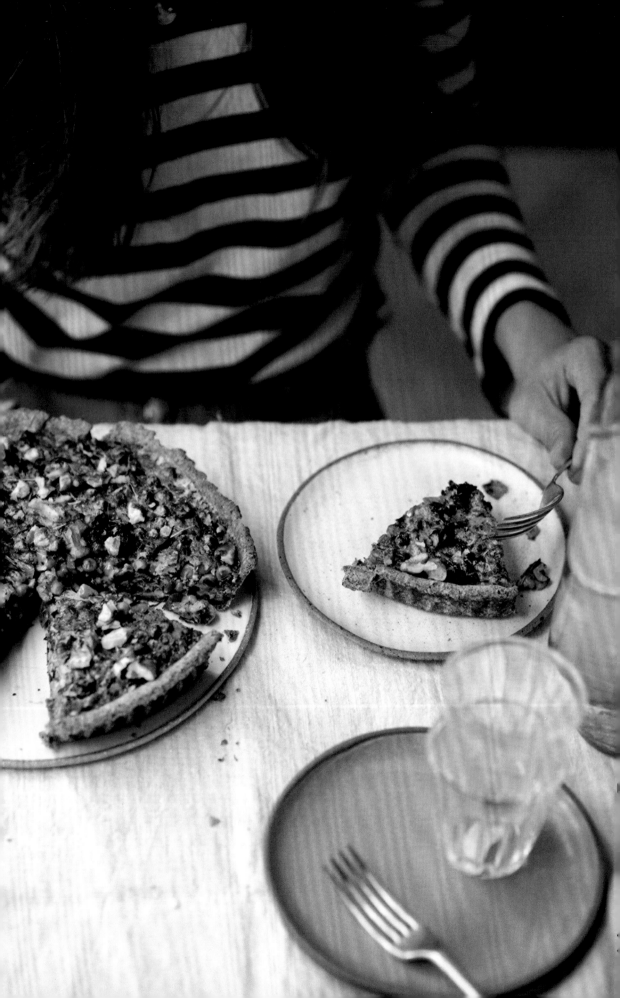

Watercress and roasted tomato salad

Serves 4
180 calories per serving
This salad can be served as an accompaniment for a main course but it's also great on its own as a light lunch. The peppery watercress and sweet roasted tomatoes make a delicious combination, which is enhanced by the heat of a garlicky mustard dressing. If you would like to add cheese, this goes particularly well with burrata.

300g tomatoes (a mixture of vine and heirloom)
4 garlic cloves
1 tbsp olive oil
Zest and juice of 2 lemons
3 fresh thyme sprigs
1 tbsp rapeseed oil
1 tbsp mustard (ready-made English or Dijon)
200g green beans
200g watercress
1 tbsp flaked almonds, toasted
Flaked sea salt and cracked black pepper

1. Preheat the oven to 200°C/Fan 180°C/Gas 6.
2. Cut all of the tomatoes in half and place them on a baking tray. Bash the garlic cloves to break them up, then add to the tray. Drizzle the olive oil over the tomatoes and sprinkle with the lemon zest and a pinch each of salt and pepper. Add the thyme sprigs. Roast for about 30 minutes until the tomatoes are soft and the garlic is golden.
3. To make the dressing, remove the roasted garlic cloves from the baking tray and put them into a food processor with the lemon juice, rapeseed oil, mustard and a pinch each of salt and pepper. Blitz together. Set aside.
4. Bring a pan of water to the boil and blanch the green beans for 1 minute until tender but still crunchy. Drain and rinse in cold water, then tip them into a bowl. Add the watercress and the dressing and toss together.
5. Arrange the watercress salad on a serving platter and add the roasted tomatoes. Sprinkle with the flaked almonds.

Watercress risotto with pumpkin seeds

Serves 2
486 calories per serving
The key to risotto is good stock and patience. The good stock is easy: my preferred version is made with onion, celery, fennel and bay leaves. In this recipe I've added brown rice vinegar, which gives a nice level of acidity. Patience can be a challenge, but it's needed once you start adding the stock to the rice. At the end a blitzed watercress paste is stirred in to transform this risotto into a deep green bowl of peppery goodness.

600ml vegetable stock
100ml brown rice vinegar
200g watercress
200g spinach
1 tbsp rapeseed oil
1 onion, diced
1 garlic clove, chopped
250g brown rice
50g sunflower seeds
50g pumpkin seeds
30g pine nuts
Flaked sea salt and cracked black pepper

1. Pour the vegetable stock into a saucepan and bring to a simmer over a low heat. Stir in the brown rice vinegar and remove from the heat.
2. Put the watercress and spinach in a food processor with a little of the vegetable stock mixture and blitz until smooth. Set aside.
3. Heat the oil in a heavy-based saucepan and cook the onion and garlic for 10 minutes until softened. Add the rice and sunflower seeds and stir to coat with the oil. Add half of the vegetable stock mixture and cook, stirring, until the rice has absorbed all the liquid. Add the remaining stock and continue simmering, stirring occasionally. Once the rice is almost cooked, stir in the blitzed watercress and spinach paste. Cook for a further 5 minutes. Season the risotto with a good pinch each of salt and pepper.
4. Toast the pumpkin seeds and pine nuts in a dry frying pan until golden. Serve the risotto sprinkled with the seeds and nuts.

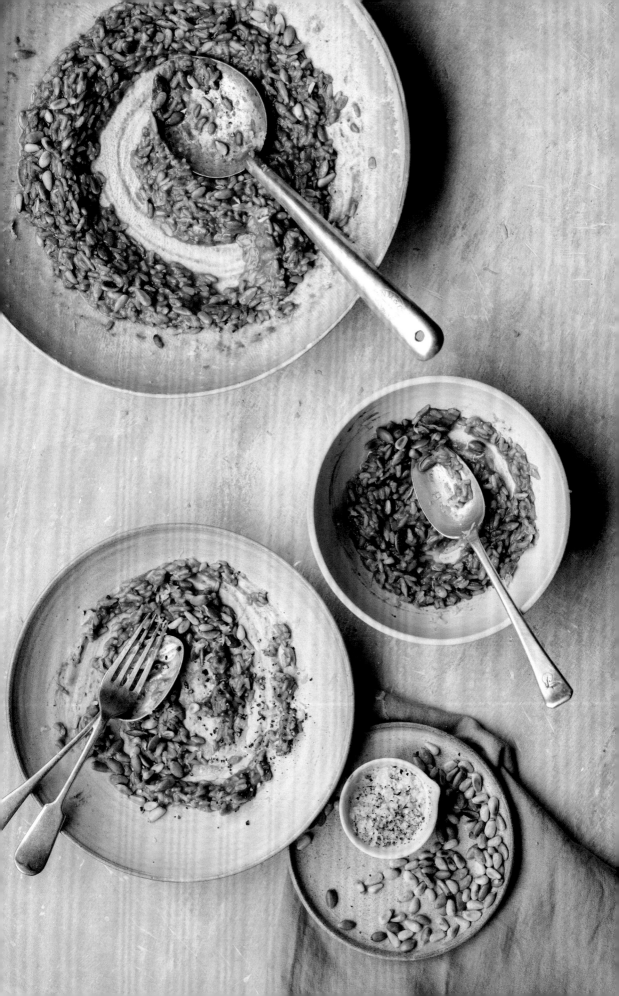

Pak choi

Pak choi (also called bok choy) is a variety of cabbage that is traditionally associated with Asian cooking. It is now available in many supermarkets, most often in the form of small or 'baby' pak choi. The white stems are crunchy with soft, dark green leaves at the top.

Pak choi is grown mostly in China – it is thought to be one of the longest-farmed vegetables in Asia – and thrives in colder weather. It is in season from October to March.

Because pak choi has a milder flavour than most of its relatives in the cabbage family, it lends itself to a wide variety of dishes. It is often stir-fried but you can also steam or blanch it, use it in a soup, or eat it raw. In the recipes here, I've paired it with bold flavours commonly found in Asian cooking, including soy, satay, chilli and ginger. Believe me, although it is mild, the pak choi really holds its own among them!

Nutritional bonus

Pak choi has traditionally been used in Chinese medicine to ease stomach pains, calm fevers and soothe coughs. It contains **vitamin K**, essential for the normal clotting of blood, as well as **calcium**.

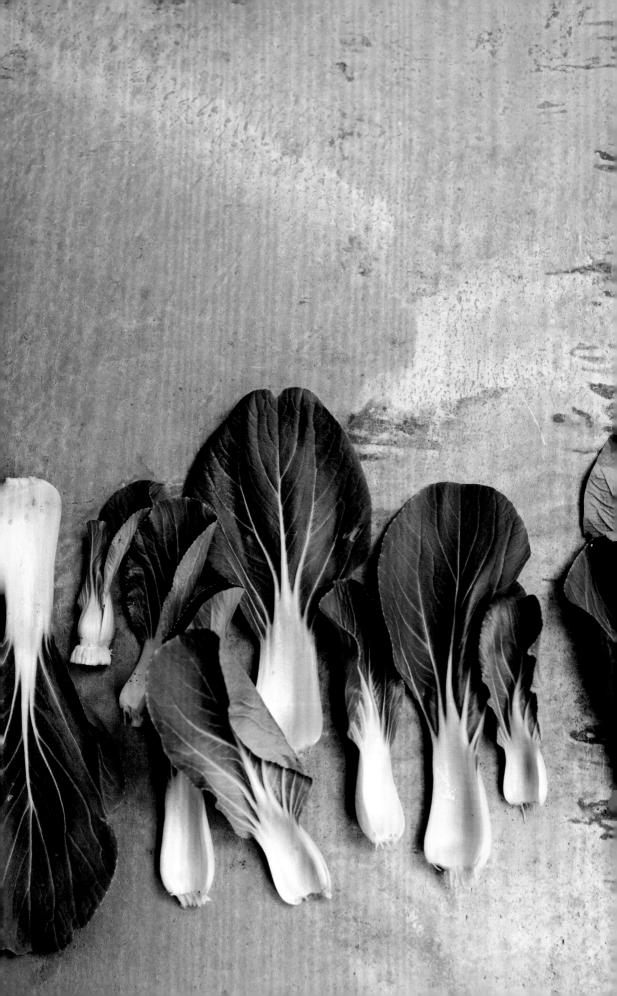

Korean-style pak choi and tofu

Serves 2

655 calories per serving

Korean food is a harmonious blending of sweet, spicy and sour flavours. This recipe, although very simple, demonstrates the core balance: pak choi acts as the perfect vehicle for sweet chilli and garlic flavours.

A thumb-sized piece fresh root ginger, grated

3 garlic cloves, sliced

1 tbsp honey

3 tbsp tamari

1 tbsp toasted sesame oil

1 tsp chilli powder

300g firm tofu, cut into sticks

1 tsp rapeseed oil

100ml water

4 small pak choi, cut into quarters through the stalk

Fresh coriander, to garnish

Brown rice and lime wedges to serve

1   Mix together the ginger, garlic, honey, tamari, sesame oil and chilli powder in a bowl. Add the tofu and turn to coat, then leave for a few minutes to allow the tofu to become infused with the spices.

2   Remove the tofu from the bowl (keep the marinade). Heat the rapeseed oil in a frying pan, add the tofu and cook until crisp and browned on all sides. Remove the tofu from the pan and set aside.

3   Add the reserved marinade and water to the pan and bring to the boil. Add the pak choi. Cook for a minute or so, tossing, until the pak choi is covered in the marinade and slightly wilted.

4   Place the tofu and pak choi on a serving platter and garnish with coriander. Serve with brown rice and lime wedges for squeezing over.

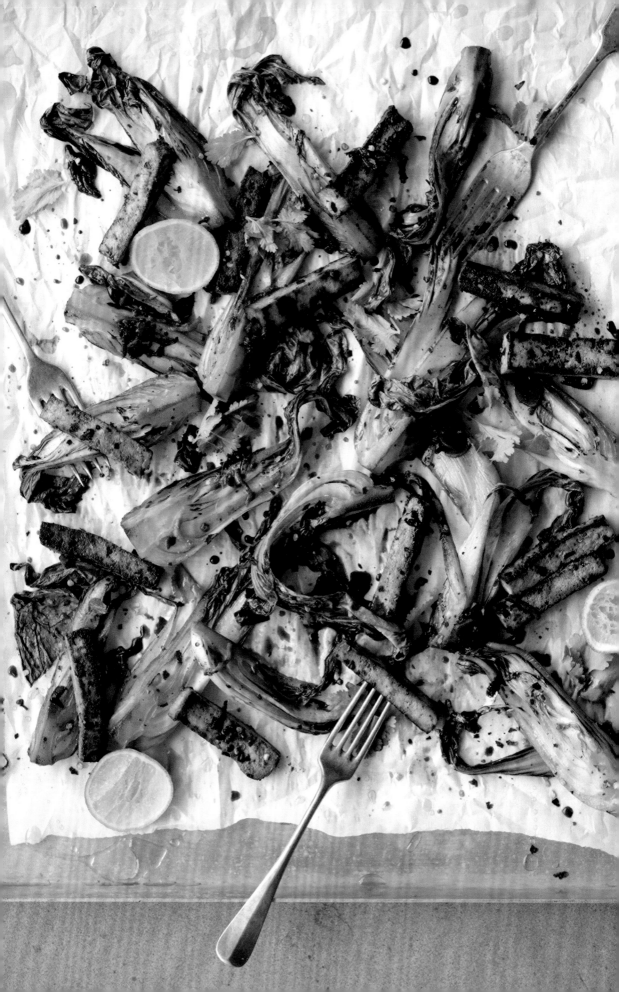

Pak choi and satay noodles

Serves 2
737 calories per serving

The pak choi and other greens in this dish have a delicate crunch, a lovely contrast with the smooth and spicy peanut sauce coating them. Even the noodles are green, as I've used courgette noodles in place of the traditional type.

3 courgettes
1 tsp toasted sesame oil
1 tbsp grated fresh root ginger
100g sugarsnap peas
2 spring onions, sliced
2 small pak choi, cut into quarters through
    the stalk
2 tsp black or white sesame seeds
1 red chilli, sliced
1 tbsp roughly chopped peanuts
Fresh coriander, chopped

For the sauce
4 tbsp smooth peanut butter
2 tbsp tamari
100ml coconut milk
1 tsp dried chilli flakes
Zest and juice of 2 limes

1   Put all the ingredients for the sauce in a bowl and whisk together until well mixed. Set aside.
2   Use a julienne peeler/cutter or spiraliser to make courgette noodles.
3   Heat the sesame oil in a wok and add the ginger, sugarsnap peas and spring onions. Stir-fry until slightly browned. Add the pak choi and stir-fry until the ends are slightly golden.
4   Add the sauce and courgette noodles to the wok and mix everything together so that all the noodles are covered in the sauce. Cook for a few minutes just to warm the noodles.
5   In a separate small, dry frying pan, toast the sesame seeds until golden and fragrant.
6   Serve the courgette noodles sprinkled with the toasted sesame seeds, fresh red chilli, chopped peanuts and coriander.

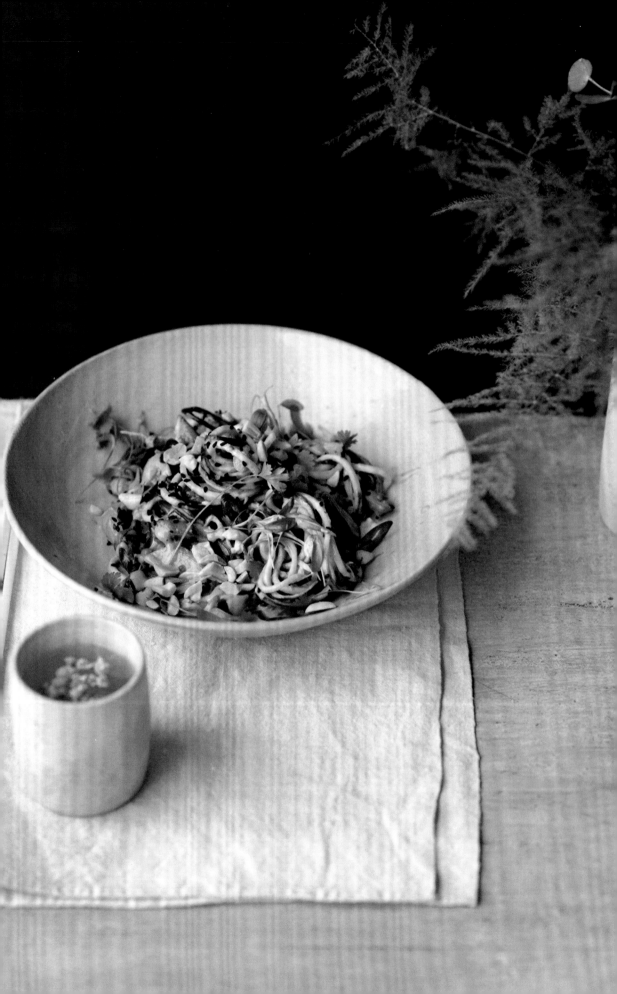

Asian-style broth with pak choi, ceps and quinoa

Serves 2

321 calories per serving

Making a broth is straightforward: the key is to have a good-quality vegetable stock and season well. I also like to season this Asian-style broth with tamari and lime juice to create a balance of piquancy and saltiness. The pak choi takes only minutes to cook in the broth but will nevertheless take on all its delicious flavours.

100g quinoa

2 tsp rapeseed oil

2 spring onions, sliced

A thumb-sized piece fresh root ginger, cut into fine matchsticks

1 garlic clove, finely chopped

1 carrot, cut into fine matchsticks

500ml vegetable stock

60g fresh ceps, sliced

2 small pak choi, cut into quarters through the stalk

2 tbsp tamari

Juice of 2 limes, plus lime wedges to serve

A small handful of fresh coriander, roughly chopped

Flaked sea salt

Micro coriander, to garnish

1   Put the quinoa in a pan with a pinch of salt and cover with three times the amount of water. Bring to the boil, then leave to simmer gently for 10–12 minutes until the quinoa is cooked and the tail has separated from the seed. Drain in a sieve and rinse under cold water. Set aside.

2   Heat 1 teaspoon of the oil in a saucepan over a medium heat, add the spring onions, ginger and garlic, and lightly sauté for 5 minutes. Add the carrot and cook for a further 3–5 minutes, stirring, until the carrot is lightly browned. Pour in the vegetable stock and simmer for about 15 minutes until the carrot is tender.

3   Meanwhile, in another frying pan, heat the remaining oil and sauté the sliced ceps over a medium heat for 4–6 minutes until softened. Add them to the pan containing the stock and vegetables along with the pak choi and cooked quinoa. Bring back to a simmer, then remove from the heat. Stir in the tamari, lime juice and chopped coriander.

4   Garnish with micro coriander and serve with wedges of lime for squeezing over.

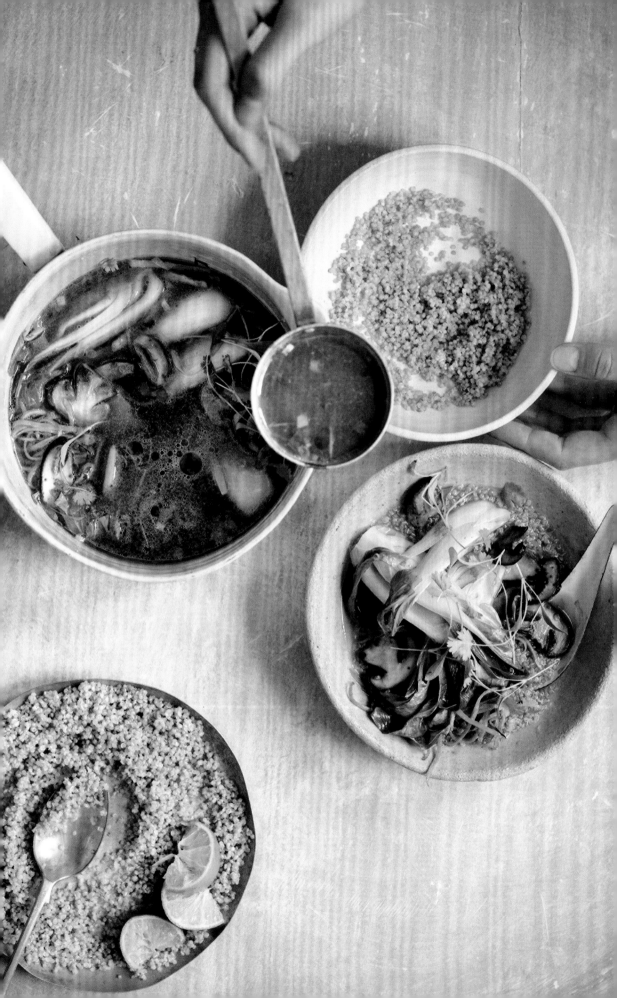

Cabbage

You may think you have a big extended family, but you've got nothing on the cabbage. Not only does the Brassica family include the familiar green, white and red varieties of cabbage, but it also encompasses broccoli, cauliflower, Brussels sprouts and pak choi.

Cabbage is a great addition to any barbecue – at my house you'll always find big wedges on the grill, as well as chopped cabbage in an accompanying salad (see my Thai-inspired slaw on page 116). White cabbage is the one most commonly used in a slaw because it can carry the heaviest, creamiest dressings, but I prefer red cabbage as it adds a pop of colour and has a crunchier texture.

When buying cabbage, you want to go for a head that is vibrantly coloured and heavy, with tightly packed leaves (loose leaves indicate an older vegetable). Cabbage is delicious all year round, but it comes into its own in February, especially Savoy or green cabbage.

Nutritional bonus

Cabbage is an amazing source of **fibre** and of **vitamins B6, C and K**, as well as a whole host of minerals including **potassium**. The deep purple pigmentation of red cabbage indicates the presence of a beneficial antioxidant called **anthocyanin**, which may help lower your risk of disease, including cancer, dementia and heart disease.

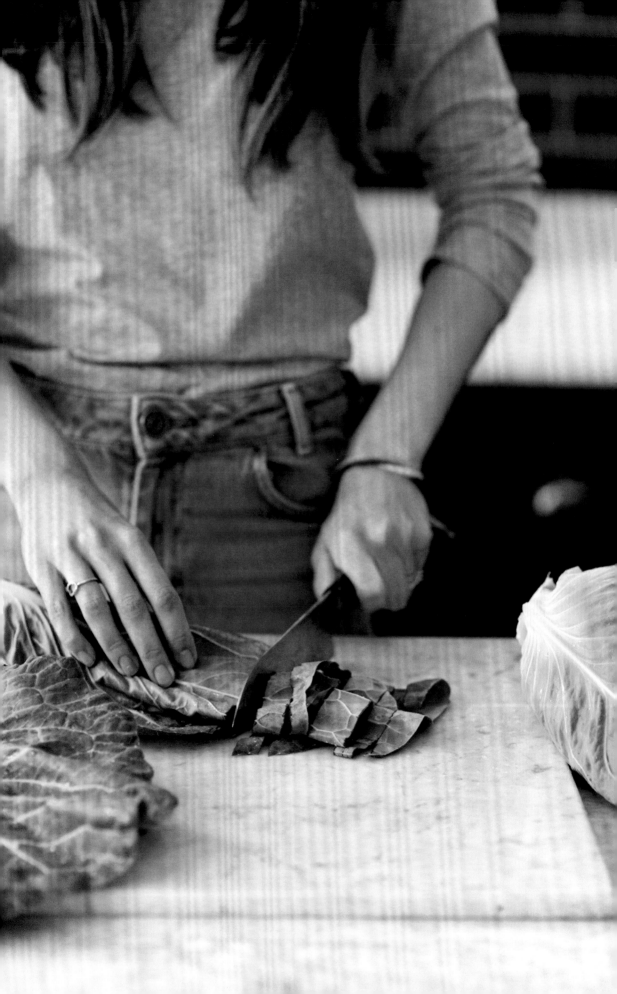

Green spring salad

Serves 2
550 calories per serving
To me, the best balance for an al fresco feast is one warm dish – usually a frittata or quiche – plus a grain salad and a green salad. This particular green salad features Savoy cabbage and it is filled with all the joys of spring, with purple sprouting broccoli sitting regally among the lighter green beans and peas. A classic English mustard and lemon dressing adds the perfect level of heat and fresh tartness.

150g purple sprouting broccoli
200g green beans
150g sugarsnap peas
1 avocado
100g podded fresh edamame beans (or thawed frozen beans)
½ Savoy cabbage, cored and finely shredded
1 tsp black sesame seeds

For the dressing
1 tbsp English mustard powder
Zest and juice of 1 lemon
2 tbsp rapeseed oil
1 tbsp brown rice vinegar

1   To make the dressing, whisk the mustard with the lemon zest and juice, then slowly whisk in the rapeseed oil followed by the rice vinegar. Set aside.
2   Bring a pan of water to the boil. Blanch the purple sprouting broccoli, green beans and sugarsnap peas for 1–2 minutes, just to take away the rawness but maintain the crunch. Drain and rinse under cold running water to cool quickly. Place the vegetables in a large mixing bowl.
3   Peel the avocado and chop the flesh roughly. Add to the bowl along with the edamame beans and cabbage. Pour the dressing over the vegetables and toss together thoroughly. Serve on a platter sprinkled with black sesame seeds.

Roasted cabbage and lentils

Serves 2
679 calories per serving
Sometimes white cabbages are huge, and this is a great way to use up any extra that you may have. The crunchy leaves of the cabbage and the small tender lentils are brought to life by a piquant caper and walnut dressing.

200g Puy lentils
500ml vegetable stock
1 bay leaf
½ small white cabbage (or ¼ large cabbage)
2 tbsp ras el hanout
1 tbsp olive oil, plus extra for dressing
1 garlic clove, finely chopped
1 tbsp capers
2 tbsp chopped walnuts
Juice of 2 lemons
A small bunch of fresh flat-leaf parsley, roughly chopped
Flaked sea salt and cracked black pepper
1 lemon, cut into thin slices

1   Place the lentils in a pan, cover with the stock and add the bay leaf. Bring to the boil, then simmer for 15–20 minutes until the lentils are cooked but still have a firmness to them. Drain (discard the bay leaf). Set aside.
2   Preheat the oven to 200°C/Fan 180°C/Gas 6.
3   Cut the cabbage into thin wedges, making sure to cut equally through the core so that each wedge still has some of this holding it together. Place the wedges on a baking tray. Sprinkle them with the ras el hanout, drizzle over the oil, and season with salt and pepper. Roast for 20 minutes.
4   Remove the baking tray from the oven and add the lentils, garlic, capers and walnuts. Roast for a further 15 minutes until the cabbage is lightly browned and the walnuts are crisp.
5   Remove from the oven. Add the lemon juice, parsley and an extra glug of olive oil. Toss everything together well. Serve each portion garnished with a few slices of lemon.

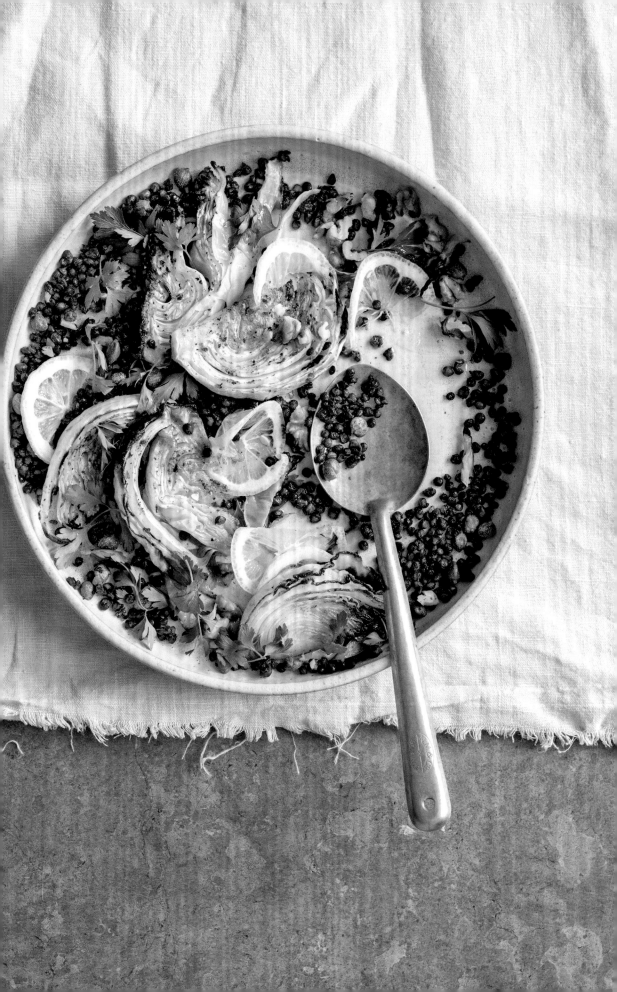

The best barbecue slaw

Serves 4
101 calories per serving
Purple-red cabbage, pink radishes, green kale,
spring onions and lettuce, bright orange mango...
this is what 'eating the rainbow' really looks like.
The true star of my best-ever slaw is the mango
dressing, which is sweet, salty and bold, and
brings the whole thing to life.

300g kale (tough stalks trimmed), shredded
½ Iceberg lettuce, shredded
½ small red cabbage, finely chopped
2 spring onions, sliced
200g radishes, sliced

For the dressing
1 mango
Juice of 2 limes, plus lime wedges to serve
2 tbsp tamari
2 tbsp brown rice vinegar
1 green chilli, sliced (optional)
Flaked sea salt and cracked black pepper

1   Combine the kale, lettuce and red cabbage
    in a bowl with the spring onions and radishes.
2   To make the dressing, peel the mango and cut
    all the flesh from the flat stone. Put the flesh in
    a food processor with the rest of the dressing
    ingredients and blitz until smooth. Season
    with salt and pepper to taste.
3   Drizzle the dressing over the vegetables and
    toss. Serve immediately, sprinkled with fresh
    chilli, if you like, and with lime wedges for
    squeezing over.

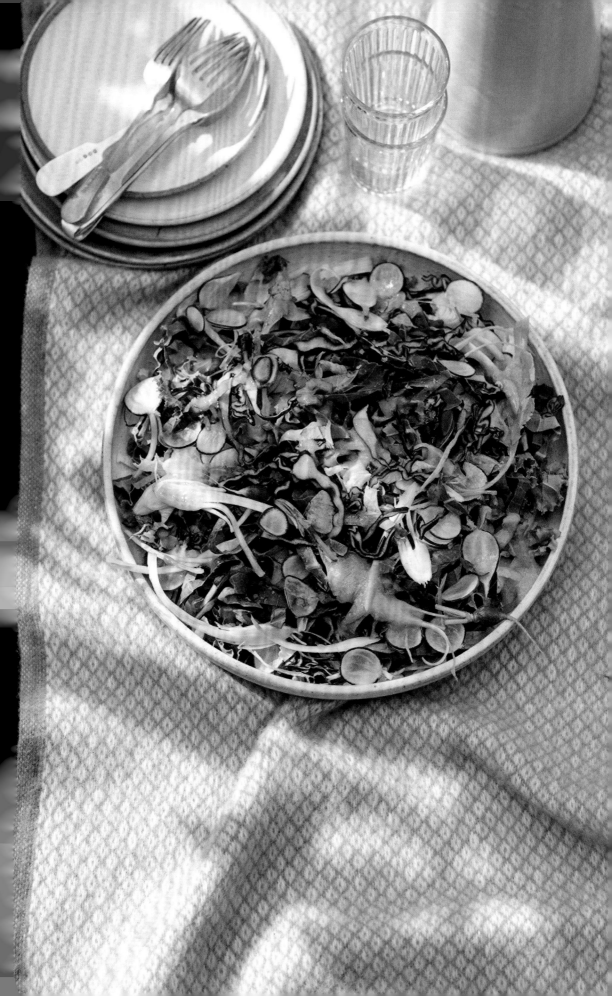

Brussels sprouts

The Belgians were early adopters of Brussels sprouts, and they've been cultivating them for hundreds of years, hence the name. I must say I love Brussels sprouts. I have been known to stir-fry a panful, season them just with salt and pepper, and then hide myself away to devour them in secrecy (the rationale here is questionable, as I'm sorry to say that my children are not fans).

I think my love for Brussels sprouts may have something to do with the fact that some people seem to hate them so much: I feel the need to stand up for the humble sprout. I adore the way that they grow along a stalk in neat rows, and it's wonderful to buy them this way at Christmas, which is when they are in season. They are plump little nuggets of savoury, crunchy deliciousness. I love them when they are roasted or sautéed or shredded to eat raw.

One very important tip: don't score the bottom of your Brussels sprouts if you're going to boil them, as this causes the sprouts to absorb too much water and then go mushy. Stop scoring and start loving.

Nutritional bonus

Brussels sprouts are part of the cruciferous family, which consists of nutritious vegetables that offer a unique composition of **antioxidants** that promote good health. Additionally, Brussels sprouts are low in calories, but full of **protein**, vitamins including **vitamin C** and **folate**, and minerals such as **potassium**.

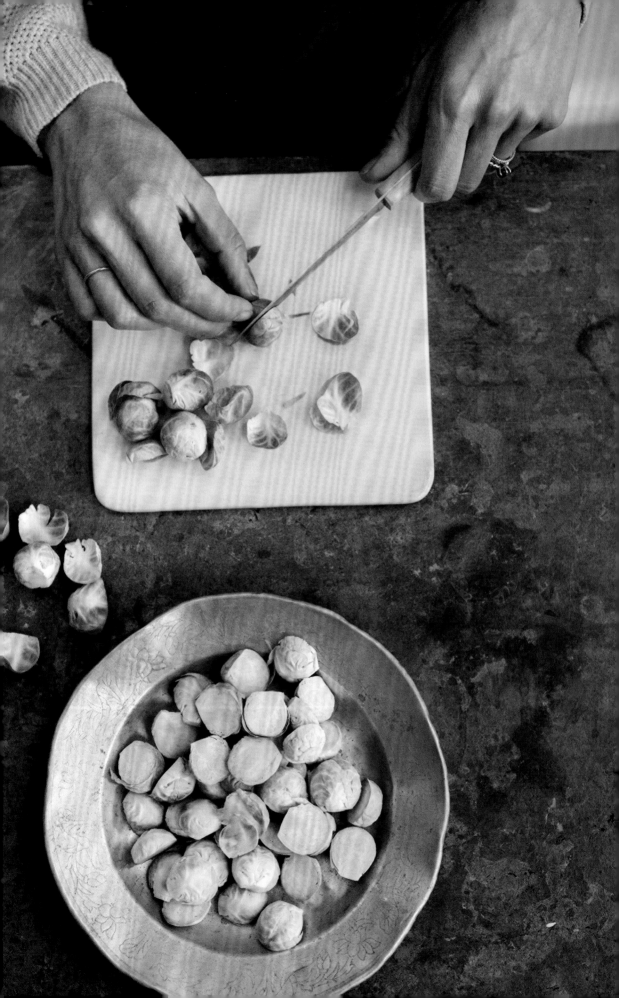

Sprouts and spelt rigatoni with tomato-cashew sauce

Serves 2
639 calories per serving

Brussels sprouts and pasta are an unexpectedly good match: a fork loaded with al dente pasta and a crisp little Brussels sprout promises a mouthful of comfort. Spelt rigatoni is a very good substitute for traditional pasta – it has a nice texture, not grainy. The cashews in the tomato sauce give it an indulgent creaminess.

100g cashew nuts
1 tbsp olive oil, plus extra for frying
200g cherry tomatoes
3 fresh basil sprigs
Zest of 1 lemon
200g Brussels sprouts, cut in half
180g spelt rigatoni
Flaked sea salt and cracked black pepper
Fresh basil leaves, to garnish

1   To make the sauce, soak the cashews in water for about 30 minutes. Drain and tip them into a food processor. Add the oil, tomatoes, basil, lemon zest, 1 teaspoon salt and a pinch of pepper, and blitz until quite smooth (obviously it won't be completely smooth as there will be pips from the tomatoes but that's fine). Pour into a saucepan and set aside.
2   Heat a little oil in a small frying pan and cook the Brussels sprouts until they are tender and lightly browned all over.
3   Cook the pasta according to the instructions on the packet (add a good pinch of salt to the water). Drain, keeping back some of the cooking water.
4   Gently heat through the cashew and tomato sauce. When the sauce is hot, add the sprouts, pasta and reserved cooking water and stir through. Serve garnished with basil leaves.

Brussels sprouts, peanut and pumpkin seed salad

Serves 2
642 calories per serving

This warm salad is the perfect way to spruce up Brussels sprouts. Long gone are the days of the over-boiled, slimy mini-cabbages – here it's all about lightly browned, crunchy little gems. The toasted peanuts and pumpkin seeds work magic, bringing out the savoury nuttiness of the sprouts.

40g dried cranberries
Zest and juice of 1 lemon
150g quinoa
2 spring onions, finely sliced lengthways
Rapeseed oil for frying
250g Brussels sprouts, cut in half
1 tbsp pumpkin seeds
2 tbsp roughly chopped peanuts
Flaked sea salt and cracked black pepper
Fresh coriander, roughly chopped, to garnish

1   Put the cranberries in a small bowl and add the lemon juice and a pinch of salt. Leave to soak.
2   Put the quinoa in a pan with a pinch of salt and cover with three times the amount of water. Bring to the boil, then leave to simmer gently for 10–12 minutes until the quinoa is cooked and the tail has separated from the seed. Drain in a sieve and tip into a mixing bowl. Add the soaked cranberries, the spring onions, lemon zest and a pinch of pepper. Mix well.
3   Heat a little oil in a frying pan and sauté the Brussels sprouts until lightly browned. Add the pumpkin seeds, peanuts and a pinch each of salt and pepper. Cook, stirring, for a minute longer to brown the seeds and peanuts.
4   To serve, place the quinoa on a large serving platter, top with the Brussels sprouts mixture and garnish with some chopped coriander.

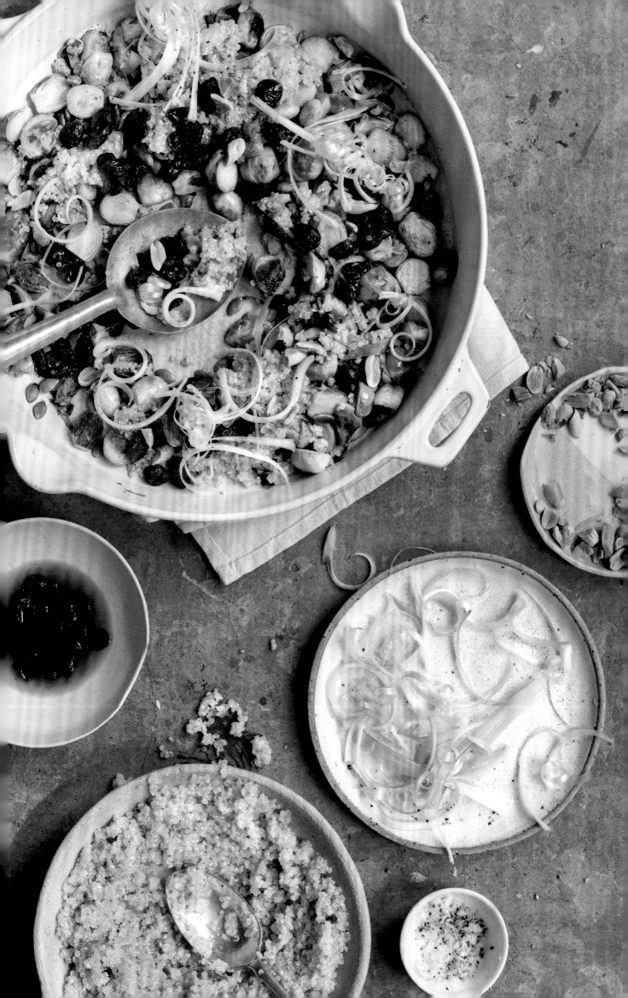

Brussels sprout and coconut dal

Serves 2
689 calories per serving
A Christmas-time winner, this dal is made with lentils, coconut milk and ginger, among other things. It's particularly good for Boxing Day, to sweep away those roast-dinner cobwebs.

1 tbsp rapeseed oil
300g Brussels sprouts, finely sliced
1 tbsp grated fresh root ginger
200g red lentils
150g cherry tomatoes
1 tsp sweet paprika
1 tsp ground cumin
400ml vegetable stock
200ml coconut milk
100g cashew nuts
A small handful of fresh coriander,
   roughly chopped
1 lemon, cut into wedges

1 Heat a little of the oil in a saucepan, add half of the sprouts and stir-fry for a few minutes. Add the ginger, lentils, tomatoes, paprika and cumin, and stir everything together. Pour in the vegetable stock. Bring to the boil, then simmer for 15 minutes until the lentils have completely broken down. Stir in the coconut milk and simmer the dal for 5 more minutes.
2 In a separate frying pan, heat a little oil and add the rest of the Brussels sprouts. Sauté for a few minutes until slightly browned. Add the cashew nuts and cook for a further few minutes, stirring, until they are browned.
3 Spoon the dal into bowls and top with the sautéed sprouts and cashew nuts and some chopped coriander. Serve with lemon wedges for squeezing over.

Spiced stir-fried Brussels sprouts with tofu

Serves 2
769 calories per serving
If you are wondering what to pair with Brussels sprouts, simply think about how you would cook cabbage – and suddenly culinary inspiration will strike. This is a really simple dish inspired by a classic cabbage stir-fry, which will win over anyone who usually dislikes sprouts or tofu.

1 tbsp rapeseed oil, plus extra for frying
1 tbsp toasted sesame oil
1 tbsp brown rice vinegar
1 tsp ground ginger
1 tsp ground coriander
1 tbsp five-spice powder
2 tbsp honey
2 tbsp tamari
Juice of 1 lime
200g tofu, cut into sticks
150g brown rice
300g Brussels sprouts, finely shredded
4 spring onions, finely sliced
2 garlic cloves, sliced
1 tbsp grated fresh root ginger
1 avocado, peeled and sliced
Fresh coriander, roughly chopped

1 Mix together the oils, vinegar, ground spices, honey, tamari and lime juice. Add the tofu and toss to coat, then leave to marinate.
2 Meanwhile, put the rice in a saucepan with a pinch of salt and cover with three times the amount of water. Bring to the boil, then simmer for 20–25 minutes until the rice is tender and fluffy. Drain.
3 Heat a little oil in a non-stick frying pan, add the spring onions, garlic and fresh ginger, and sauté over a medium heat for a few minutes. Drain the tofu (keep the marinade), then add to the pan along with the Brussels sprouts and cook until the tofu is slightly browned on all sides. Add the reserved marinade and cook for a few minutes until bubbling.
4 Serve the sprouts and tofu with the rice, sliced avocado and chopped coriander.

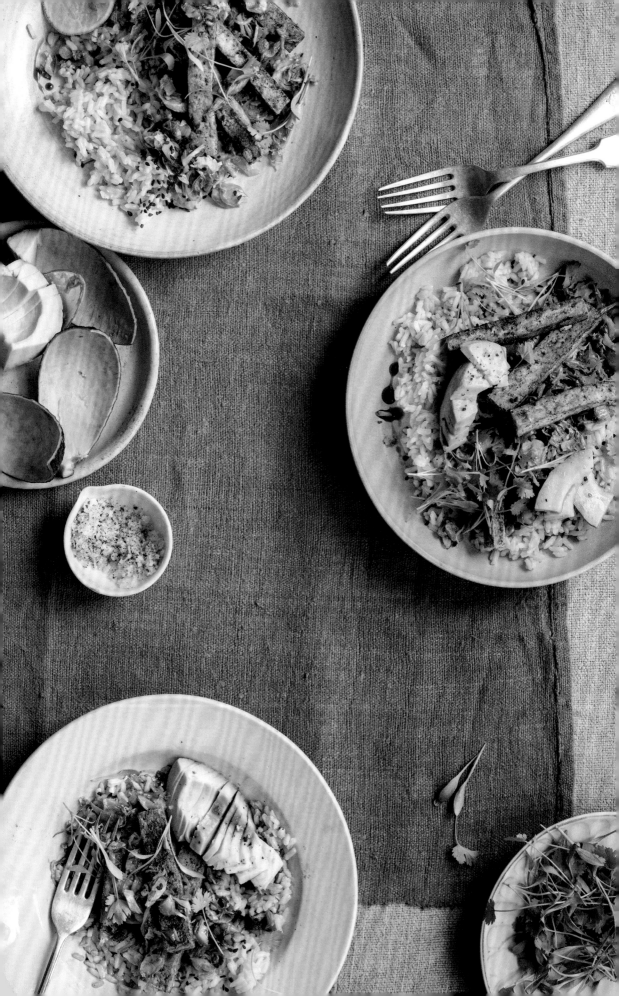

Broccoli

I often find that the best ingredients need very little enhancement, and that is certainly true of broccoli. The roasted broccoli recipe on page 128 is a fantastic example of this, where the earthy, savoury flavour of the broccoli is brought to life simply by adding fresh chillies and lime.

We often think of broccoli as an ingredient to be boiled and popped on the side of the plate. But it can be a star. It lends itself to bold Asian and Middle Eastern flavourings, and it can be eaten raw, quickly blanched or steamed, roasted, griddled or stewed.

It's always worth remembering that vegetables from the same botanical family will tend to cook well together. With broccoli we're talking brassicas such as cabbage and cauliflower. Broccoli and cauliflower are a particularly good pairing, as demonstrated by my lentil stew on page 132.

It pains me to say this, but my son is not a fan of broccoli. However, I have managed to sneak it into his diet with my trusty recipe for broccoli bread on page 126. A favourite with my kids, it tastes nutty and wholesome but is made predominantly of blitzed broccoli. Smothered in an easy artichoke spread, it is a perfect snack.

Nutritional bonus

Broccoli is a nutrient-dense vegetable. Like most greens, it is a rich source of both soluble and insoluble **fibre**, as well as **antioxidants**, and it contains **calcium** – something that, as a vegetarian, I always look for in plant foods. Broccoli also provides a good source of **vitamins C and E**.

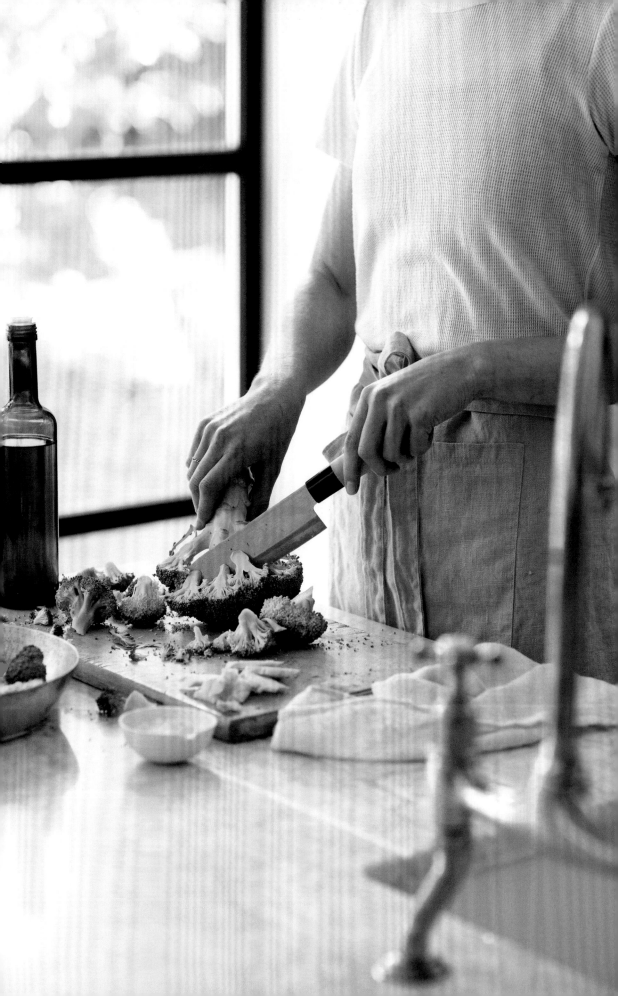

Broccoli bread with artichoke spread and radishes

Serves 6

202 calories per serving

Broccoli bread is not technically a bread, as it doesn't contain gluten, wheat or yeast, but it does rise, it is light and fluffy, and it is truly delicious smothered with a spread or dipped into a soup. Imagine it as more of a focaccia than a standard loaf because you make it in a baking tray. The accompanying artichoke spread is a favourite of mine – I always make extra to keep in the fridge for the week ahead.

500g broccoli

4 eggs

100g ground almonds

5 radishes, thinly sliced

Zest of 1 lemon

For the artichoke spread

200g jarred artichoke hearts packed in oil, drained

1 garlic clove, roughly chopped

1 tsp rapeseed oil

A small handful of fresh chives, roughly chopped

Flaked sea salt and cracked black pepper

1   Preheat the oven to 200°C/Fan 180°C/Gas 6. Line a 24 x 18cm baking tray with greaseproof paper and set aside.

2   Cut the broccoli into small pieces and place in a food processor. Blitz until the broccoli is the consistency of cous cous (you might need to do this in batches). Transfer to a bowl and add the eggs, ground almonds and a pinch each of salt and pepper. Mix together.

3   Tip the mixture into the prepared baking tray. Spread and flatten it with your hands to a layer about 1cm thick. Bake for 20–25 minutes until lightly golden and cooked through. Remove from the oven and allow to cool before cutting into six pieces. (The broccoli bread is at its best served on the day it is made, but will keep in an airtight container in the fridge for up to 3 days and can be toasted.)

4   To make the spread, line another baking tray with greaseproof paper. Place the artichoke hearts and garlic on the tray, drizzle over the oil and season with salt and pepper. Roast (at the same temperature as the bread) for about 20 minutes until golden. Remove from the oven and allow to cool.

5   Transfer the artichokes and garlic to the (clean) food processor and blitz to a coarse consistency – you want to keep some texture in the spread rather than it being very smooth. Tip the mixture into a bowl and finish by mixing through the chives.

6   Slather the artichoke spread over the broccoli bread. Top with the radishes and sprinkle with the lemon zest, salt and pepper.

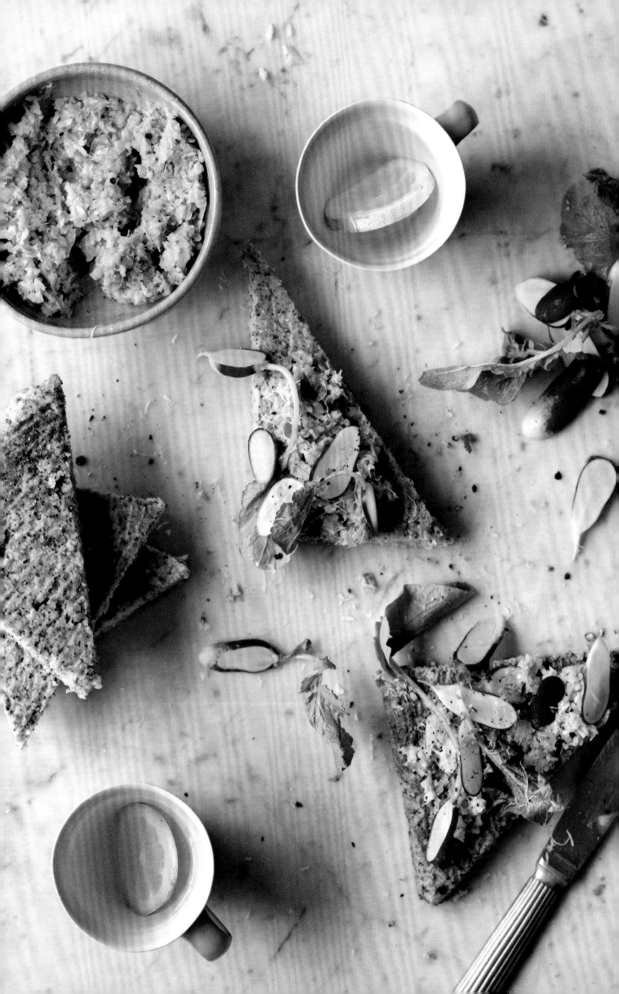

Roasted broccoli with chilli

Serves 2
239 calories per serving

Roasting is one of the best ways to cook broccoli, as it maintains its crunch while developing a more savoury flavour and the tips become crisp and golden. Paired with red chillies, garlic, lime juice and tamari, this is a great recipe. It can be served as a side dish, as part of a platter of salads or even as a starter. I also like to mix through Puy lentils or brown rice for a more substantial meal.

3 garlic cloves (unpeeled)
2 red chillies, finely chopped
1 tbsp olive oil, plus extra for drizzling
Juice of 2 limes
2 tbsp tamari
500g broccoli
A small handful of fresh coriander, roughly
  chopped
Flaked sea salt and cracked black pepper

1 Preheat the oven to 200°C/Fan 180°C/Gas 6. Line a baking tray with greaseproof paper.
2 Place the garlic cloves on the tray and roast for about 20 minutes until completely soft. Set aside to cool (leave the oven on), then squeeze the garlic flesh from its skin into a bowl. Add the chillies, olive oil, lime juice, tamari and a pinch of pepper. Mix well.
3 Cut the broccoli into florets, keeping as much of the stem/stalk as possible – you want to create florets with pretty long, pointed stems. Spread the broccoli on the baking tray you used for the garlic, drizzle with olive oil, and season with salt and pepper. Roast for about 10 minutes until the broccoli is tender but still has a bite to it.
4 Place the broccoli in a bowl and gently mix through the garlic and chilli dressing along with the coriander.

Broccoli and coconut soup

Serves 2
434 calories per serving
This is an ever-evolving soup recipe – you can have it chunky or smooth, spicy or tangy, rich or light, depending on the quantity of the ingredients you use. This is a smooth version, with pieces of crunchy rye bread and cashew nuts on top.

500g broccoli
Rapeseed oil for frying
2 spring onions, sliced
1 tbsp grated fresh root ginger
2 lemongrass sticks
300ml vegetable stock
200ml coconut milk
2 handfuls of spinach
A good pinch of celery salt
1 tbsp tamari
1 slice rye bread, broken into small pieces
50g cashew nuts
1 tsp dried chilli flakes
Zest of 1 lime
Cracked black pepper

1   Cut the broccoli florets off the stalk and set aside. Roughly dice the stalk.
2   Heat 1 tablespoon oil in a large saucepan, add the spring onions and ginger, and sauté for a few minutes. Bash the lemongrass sticks with a rolling pin to release the flavour, then add to the pan with the diced broccoli stalk and vegetable stock. Bring to the boil. Reduce the heat and simmer for about 15 minutes until the broccoli pieces are tender.
3   Add the broccoli florets along with the coconut milk, spinach, celery salt, a pinch of black pepper and the tamari. Simmer for a further 5 minutes until the florets are tender. Remove and discard the lemongrass. Using a hand blender, blitz everything together until smooth.
4   Heat a little oil in a small frying pan and fry the rye bread with the cashew nuts until golden.
5   Ladle the soup into bowls and top with the rye bread, cashew nuts, chilli flakes and lime zest.

Super green salad with tahini and ginger

Serves 2
547 calories per serving
Tahini is a sesame paste typically used in Middle Eastern cooking. The flavour can be overpowering but here it is balanced by the saltiness of tamari, the acidity of lime and vinegar, and the heat of fresh root ginger in a creamy dressing. Blanched broccoli salad is the perfect vehicle to deliver it!

1 tbsp sesame seeds
500g broccoli, cut into florets
200g sugarsnap peas, cut in half
100g podded fresh edamame beans (or thawed frozen beans)
1 small Hispi (sweetheart) cabbage, finely sliced
2 fresh mint sprigs, leaves picked and roughly chopped
A small handful of fresh coriander, roughly chopped

For the dressing
2 tbsp tahini
1 tbsp rapeseed oil
2 tbsp water
2 tbsp tamari
2 tbsp brown rice vinegar
Juice of 1 lime
1 tbsp grated fresh root ginger

1   To make the tahini dressing, put all of the ingredients in a small food processor and blitz until smooth. Set the dressing aside.
2   Toast the sesame seeds in a dry frying pan until golden. Tip into a bowl and set aside.
3   Bring a pan of water to the boil. Drop in the broccoli florets and cook for about 3 minutes until they are tender but still have a crunch. Drain the broccoli and rinse under cold water to stop the cooking. Put the broccoli in a large mixing bowl and add the sugarsnap peas, edamame and cabbage. Add the dressing and toss to coat all the vegetables.
4   Tip on to a serving platter and sprinkle with the toasted sesame seeds, mint and coriander.

Broccoli carpaccio with hoisin sauce

Serves 2
510 calories per serving
Raw broccoli slathered in hoisin sauce is a unique combination of flavours. I often find that shop-bought hoisin sauce tastes far too sweet and is not sharp enough, so I make my own. It is fresh, rich, tangy and bold, a tribute to the flavours of Chinese food. You can keep the sauce in the fridge for up to a week, and it works as well in a stir-fry as it does in a salad. This is perfect as a side dish or a salad on its own.

500g broccoli, finely sliced
1 red chilli, sliced
2 spring onions, sliced
Black and white sesame seeds
Flaked sea salt and cracked black pepper

For the hoisin sauce
100g pitted dates
2 tbsp almond butter
100ml tamari
2 tbsp brown rice vinegar
Juice of 1 lemon
1 tbsp toasted sesame oil
1 tbsp grated fresh root ginger
½ tsp hot paprika
1 tsp five-spice powder

1   To make the hoisin sauce, put the dates in a bowl and cover with boiling water. Leave to soak and soften for 20 minutes, then drain, keeping about 100ml of the soaking water. Tip the dates into a food processor with the reserved soaking water and blitz until smooth. Add the rest of the sauce ingredients and blitz until smooth again.
2   Spread out the sliced broccoli on a salad platter and sprinkle with the red chilli, spring onions and sesame seeds. Serve with the hoisin sauce to be stirred through.

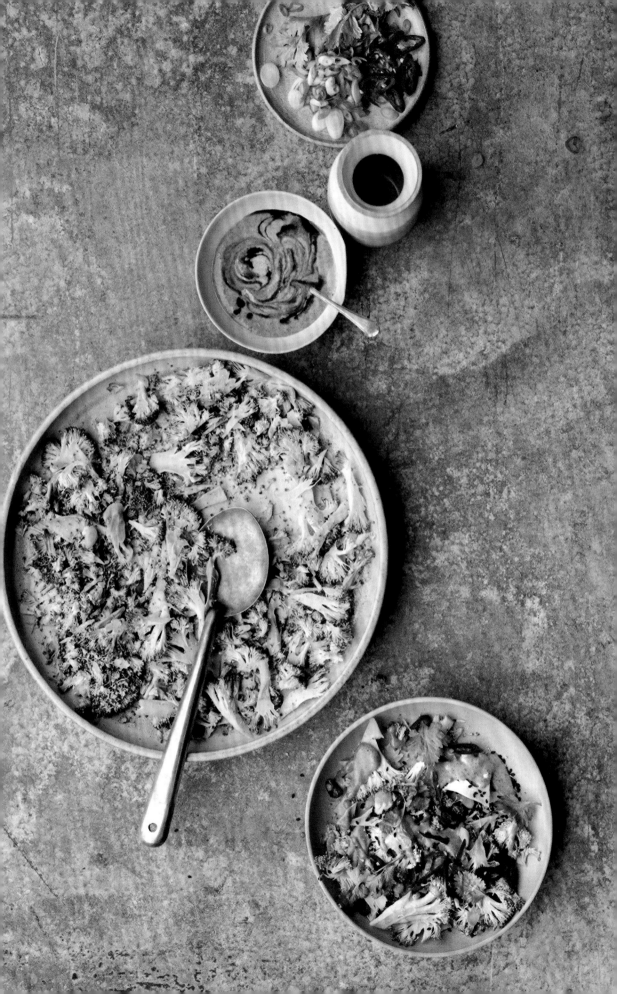

Broccoli and red lentil stew with preserved lemons

Serves 4
508 calories per serving

This is a Sunday night stew, full of goodness to set you up for the week ahead. It takes no effort whatsoever; you just need half an hour or so to let it simmer and then you will be rewarded with a hot bowl of steaming deliciousness. The broccoli and cauliflower are added about 5 minutes before the stew is ready to serve, which is just enough time for them to soften and take on the flavours of the stew while maintaining a good bite.

300g red lentils
200g wild rice
600ml vegetable stock
1 tsp garam masala
½ tsp dried mixed herbs
3 cloves
3 cardamom pods
½ cauliflower, cut into florets
250g broccoli, cut into florets
100g frozen peas, thawed
A small handful of fresh coriander, roughly chopped
1 large preserved lemon, finely sliced
Flaked sea salt and cracked black pepper

For the 'steak' seasoning
25g flaked sea salt
25g celery salt
50g garlic powder
50g onion powder
50g smoked paprika
25g cracked black pepper
25g dried chilli flakes

1   First make the steak seasoning by combining all of the ingredients in a mixing bowl. (The quantities here make much more seasoning mix than you need for this recipe, but it has many other uses, such as for the cauliflower steak recipe on page 142 and the spiced root vegetable rosti recipe on page 210. Stored in an airtight container, the steak seasoning will keep well for 3 months.)

2   Put a heavy-based saucepan on a medium heat and add the lentils, rice, vegetable stock, garam masala, 1 teaspoon steak seasoning, the mixed herbs, cloves and cardamom pods. Season with a pinch each of salt and pepper. Cover and simmer for about 30 minutes until the rice and lentils are cooked.

3   Add the cauliflower and broccoli and cook for a further 5–10 minutes until the vegetables are tender. Remove from the heat.

4   Stir through the peas, coriander and half of the preserved lemon, then leave to sit, covered, for a few minutes so that the peas heat through. Serve the stew in big bowls with the rest of the preserved lemon scattered over.

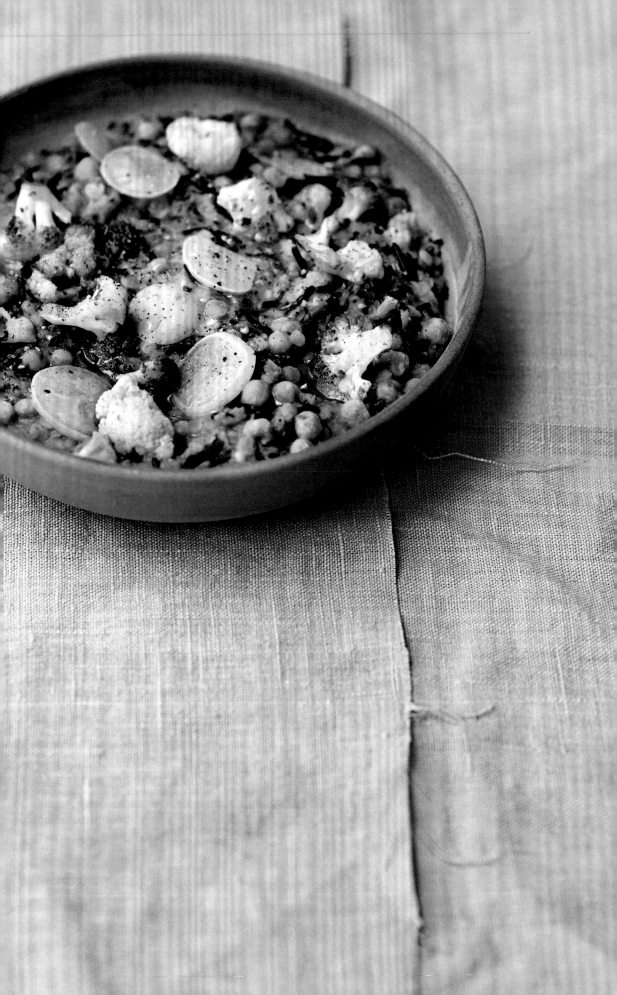

Cauliflower

Cauliflower comes into season in December and lasts until March. The humble white variety is surprisingly easy to grow at home – I grew my first cauliflower last year. Having sown the seed in late spring, I planted it out in late summer and we ate it in February. A good tip when you are buying cauliflower in the shops is to check the colour of the base, as this will give you an indication of how recently it's been picked – the whiter it is, the fresher.

Cauliflower is a versatile vegetable and it's an absolute staple in my weekly shop. It makes the easiest crudités, as you can simply tug off individual florets and they are ready to serve with a tasty dip. Or, if you roughly chop the florets, they can be thrown into a salad to give it instant crunch and substance.

You can use cauliflower to make a raw 'cous cous' (see page 140) or steamed 'rice' (see page 146) – both of these are excellent side dishes that will soak up the juices of stews and curries in a most delicious way. Roasted in thick wedges, cauliflower 'steaks' can be topped with a warm green lentil salad (see page 142). The unusual cauliflower pizza base on page 144, meanwhile, is an excellent alternative to the usual dough base.

There is a particularly beautiful variety of cauliflower called 'Romanesco' that I would recommend you try to track down. Its pointed lime-green florets have an almost architectural quality because of the way they are packed together in a complex fractal pattern. You'll find that 'Romanesco' has a slightly sweeter flavour than regular cauliflower, but it can be treated in exactly the same way when you cook with it.

Nutritional bonus

Cauliflower is a powerhouse of vitamins and minerals. It contains a phytochemical called **sulforaphane**, which has recently been a subject of intense research by scientists, as it is believed that it may help lower the risk of cancer. Sulforaphane is also thought to help protect the stomach lining against *Helicobacter pylori*, a bacteria that is linked to bloating. Cauliflower also contains dietary **fibre**, which supports a healthy digestive system.

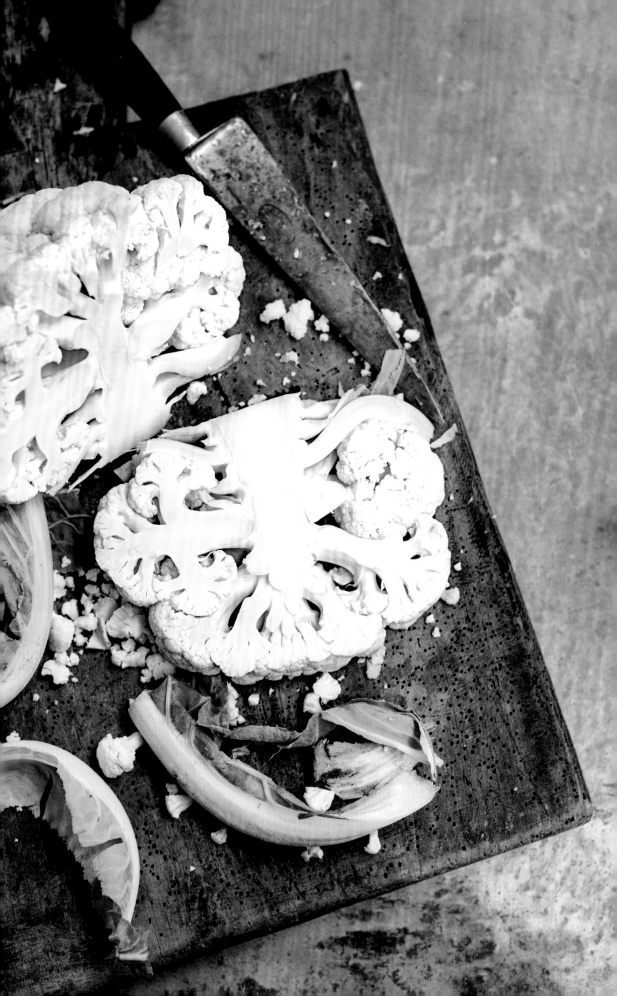

Cauliflower tortillas

Serves 4

496 calories per serving

These tortillas are great if you are feeding some hungry people. With five different toppings to mix and match, they are a fun dish to share. You can prepare the pickled onions, black beans and ranch dressing well in advance, so all you need to do at the last minute is fry the battered cauliflower and make the avocado salsa. Warm the tortillas through and you are good to go!

2 eggs

150g gluten-free flour

1 cauliflower, cut into small florets

12 small corn tortillas

Fresh coriander, chopped, to garnish

Lime wedges to serve

For the pickled onions

½ red onion, finely sliced

Juice of 1 lemon

1 tsp honey

For the ranch dressing

150ml soya yoghurt

A handful of fresh chives, finely chopped

1 tsp dried parsley

1 tsp dried tarragon

¼ tsp garlic powder

¼ tsp onion powder

For the black beans

Rapeseed oil for frying

1 spring onion, chopped

1 garlic clove, finely chopped

1 red pepper, seeded and diced

400g tinned black beans, drained and rinsed

For the avocado salsa

1 avocado, peeled and diced

1 spring onion, sliced

1 large tomato, diced

A small handful of fresh coriander, finely chopped

1 gherkin, finely chopped

Flaked sea salt and cracked black pepper

1   Prepare the pickled onions by placing the onion in a bowl with the lemon juice, honey and ½ teaspoon salt and leaving to soak.

2   In another bowl, mix together the ingredients for the ranch dressing. Set aside for about 20 minutes.

3   For the black beans, heat a little oil in a frying pan and fry the spring onion and garlic until the garlic is golden. Add the red pepper and black beans and cook on a low heat, stirring frequently, until the beans begin to break down. Remove from the heat and set aside.

4   Combine all the ingredients for the avocado salsa in a bowl and set aside.

5   Whisk the eggs and flour together to make a thick batter. Season with salt and pepper to taste. Add the cauliflower florets to the batter, turning them to make sure each is completely coated. Place a good glug of oil in a frying pan set over a medium heat. When the oil is very hot, add the battered cauliflower and fry until golden all over (do this in batches). Drain on kitchen paper.

6   Cook the tortillas in a dry frying pan to slightly brown on both sides and soften.

7   To assemble, smear the black bean mixture over the tortillas. Add the cauliflower and the avocado salsa and drizzle over the ranch dressing. Top with pickled onions and coriander. Serve with lime wedges for squeezing over.

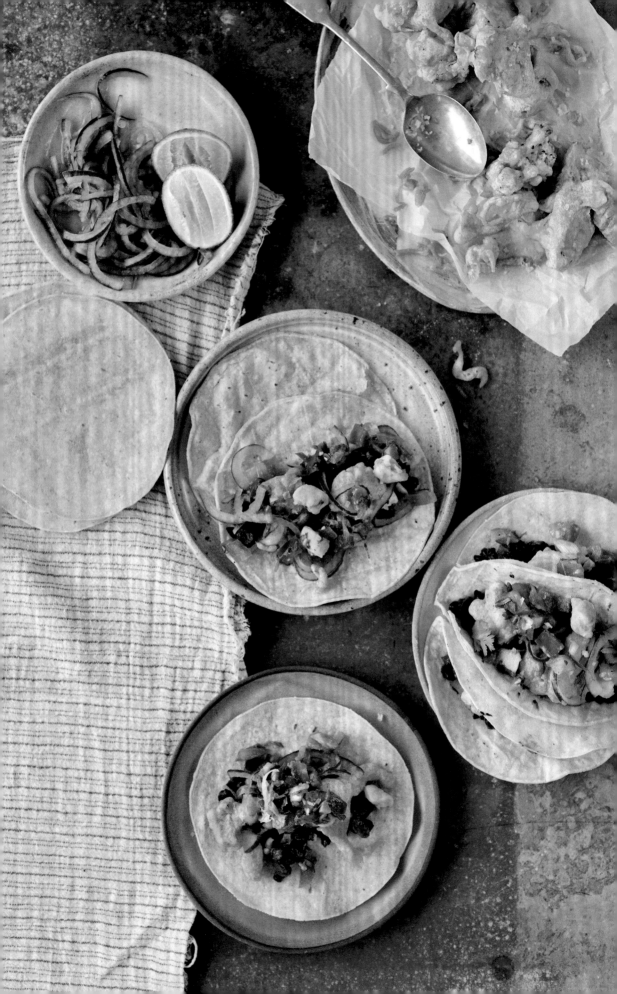

Cauliflower frittata

Serves 4
218 calories per serving
A frittata is the Italian answer to the Spanish
tortilla. Cauliflower works well in a frittata as it
cooks quickly but still maintains its shape. I like
to sprinkle over some pumpkin seeds at the end
for extra crunch.

6 eggs
100ml water
Rapeseed oil for frying
1 large onion, finely sliced
1 cauliflower, cut into thin florets (cut through
   the stem/core so the pieces are small
   and fine)
1 tsp ground cumin
1 tsp smoked paprika
50g pumpkin seeds
Flaked sea salt and cracked black pepper

1   Preheat the oven to 200°C/Fan 180°C/Gas 6.
2   Beat the eggs with the water and some salt
    and pepper in a large bowl. Set aside.
3   Heat a little oil in a 25cm ovenproof frying pan
    and fry the onion gently until softened. Add the
    cauliflower along with the cumin and paprika
    and cook, stirring, for 1–2 minutes until the
    cauliflower is well coated in the spices. Add
    a splash of water and cook until the water
    has evaporated.
4   Add a little more oil to the pan and turn the
    heat to high. Pour in the egg mixture and cook
    for a minute, then sprinkle over the pumpkin
    seeds. Transfer the pan to the oven and cook
    for 10–12 minutes until the frittata is golden
    and set. Serve hot.

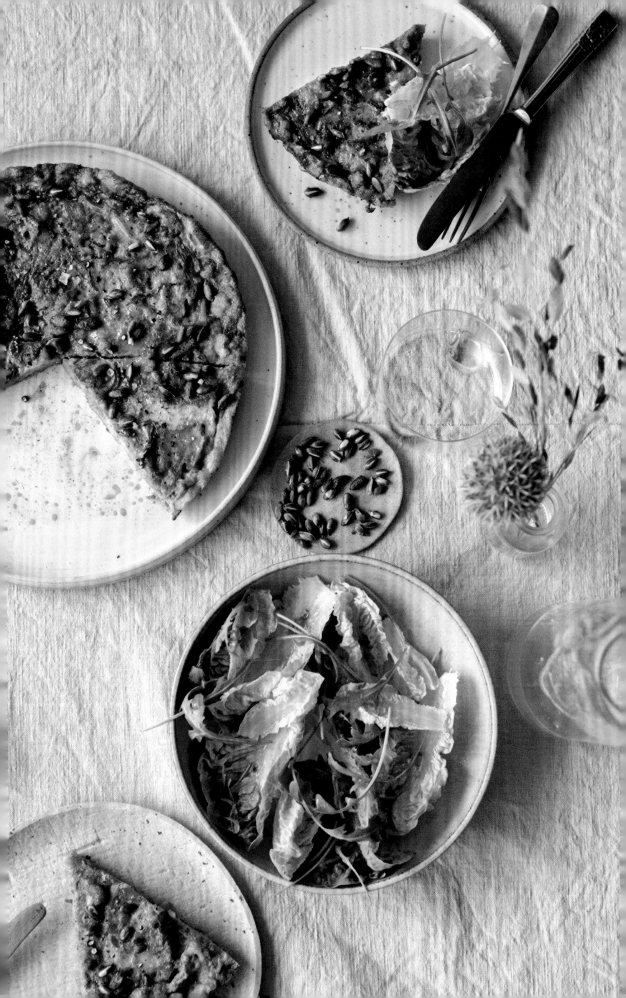

Cauli cous cous and cranberries

Serves 2
395 calories per serving

Cauliflower 'cous cous' with cranberries is great as either a main or side dish. The cous cous absorbs all the flavours of the other ingredients, so every mouthful tastes rich and vibrant. I generally find dried cranberries to be a little too sweet, but after soaking in lemon juice they achieve a balance of sweet and sour that gives a nice punch to a dish.

100g dried cranberries
½ red onion, diced
1 tsp hot paprika
Juice of 3 lemons
1 cauliflower
3 fresh mint sprigs, leaves picked and roughly
    chopped
A small handful of fresh flat-leaf parsley,
    roughly chopped
½ cucumber, peeled, seeded and diced
100g cherry tomatoes, cut in half
1 tbsp olive oil
50g walnuts, chopped
Flaked sea salt and cracked black pepper

1   Put the cranberries and onion into a bowl and season with the paprika and a pinch each of salt and pepper. Cover with the lemon juice. Leave to marinate for about 30 minutes so the cranberries and onion become infused with the lemon and paprika flavours.

2   Cut the cauliflower into florets and dice the stem/core. Put all the cauliflower in a food processor and blitz until it resembles cous cous. (You might need to do this in batches.)

3   Tip the cauliflower into a large mixing bowl and add the soaked cranberry mixture along with its juice. Add the herbs, cucumber, tomatoes, oil and some salt and pepper and mix well. Serve on a platter sprinkled with the walnuts.

Cauliflower fritters with sweet and sour sauce

Serves 4
305 calories per serving

This is my mum's recipe, an adaptation of a Ken Hom sweet and sour pork dish that she cooks on special occasions. Cauliflower is a great meat substitute as it holds its texture well and it has a satisfyingly savoury flavour. Mum has spent nearly 30 years perfecting her version of the sauce and it is a great pleasure to share it with you now.

2 carrots, diced
300ml vegetable stock
1 tbsp honey
1 tbsp tamari
1 tbsp tomato paste
2 tbsp white wine vinegar
4 spring onions, sliced
½ red pepper, seeded and diced
½ green pepper, seeded and diced
1 tbsp cornflour
2 tbsp cold water
4 fresh lychees, peeled (or pineapple chunks, if you prefer)

For the fritters
2 eggs
150g gluten-free flour
1 cauliflower, cut into small florets
Rapeseed oil for frying
Flaked sea salt and cracked black pepper

1   Bring a pan of water to the boil. Blanch the carrots for 4 minutes until just tender but still with a crunch. Drain and set aside.

2   Pour the vegetable stock into a saucepan and bring to the boil. Add the honey, tamari, tomato paste, white wine vinegar and some salt and pepper. Add the blanched carrots along with the spring onions and red and green peppers. Mix well, then leave to simmer.

3   Put the cornflour in a cup and mix with the cold water to make a paste. Whisk this paste into the simmering mixture and continue to cook for a few minutes, stirring, until the sauce has thickened. Stir in the lychees and remove from the heat.

4   Whisk the eggs and flour together in a bowl to make a thick batter. Season with salt and pepper. Add the cauliflower florets to the batter, turning them to make sure each piece is completely coated. Heat a good glug of oil in a frying pan set over a medium heat. When the oil is very hot, add the cauliflower and fry until golden all over (do this in two batches). Drain on kitchen paper.

5   Add the fritters to the sauce and bring quickly to the boil, then serve immediately.

Cauliflower steak with warm green lentil salad

Serves 2
703 calories per serving
In this dish a warm lentil and caper salad sits on a base of roasted cauliflower slices. The classic mustard dressing adds a delicious heat that brings all the earthy, rich flavours together.

1 cauliflower
2 tsp rapeseed oil
1 tsp 'steak' seasoning (see page 132)
Flaked sea salt and cracked black pepper

For the salad
150g green lentils or Puy lentils
100g cherry tomatoes, cut in half
70g lentil sprouts
½ red onion, finely sliced
1 tbsp capers
50g sultanas

For the dressing
1 tsp ready-made English mustard
Zest and juice of 1 lemon
1 tbsp rapeseed oil

To garnish
1 tbsp flaked almonds, toasted
A handful of fresh coriander, roughly chopped

1   Preheat the oven to 200°C/Fan 180°C/Gas 6. Line a baking tray with greaseproof paper.
2   Slice the cauliflower vertically into four 2.5cm 'steaks', cutting straight down through the stem/core. Lay the steaks flat on the lined baking tray. Drizzle over the rapeseed oil, then sprinkle with the steak seasoning and a little salt and pepper. Roast for 20–25 minutes until lightly golden – the edges of the cauliflower steaks should be a slightly darker golden colour than the centres.
3   Meanwhile, make the lentil salad. Put the lentils into a medium saucepan and cover with at least three times the amount of water. Bring to the boil, then simmer until the lentils are tender – this can vary greatly but should take 15–25 minutes.
4   While the lentils are cooking prepare the rest of the salad. Put the tomatoes, lentil sprouts, onion, capers and sultanas in a mixing bowl. Make the dressing by whisking together the mustard, lemon zest and juice, oil, and a pinch each of salt and pepper.
5   Once the lentils are cooked, drain them and add to the other salad ingredients. Mix through the dressing.
6   To assemble the dish, put the cauliflower steaks on plates and top with the salad. Garnish with flaked almonds and coriander.

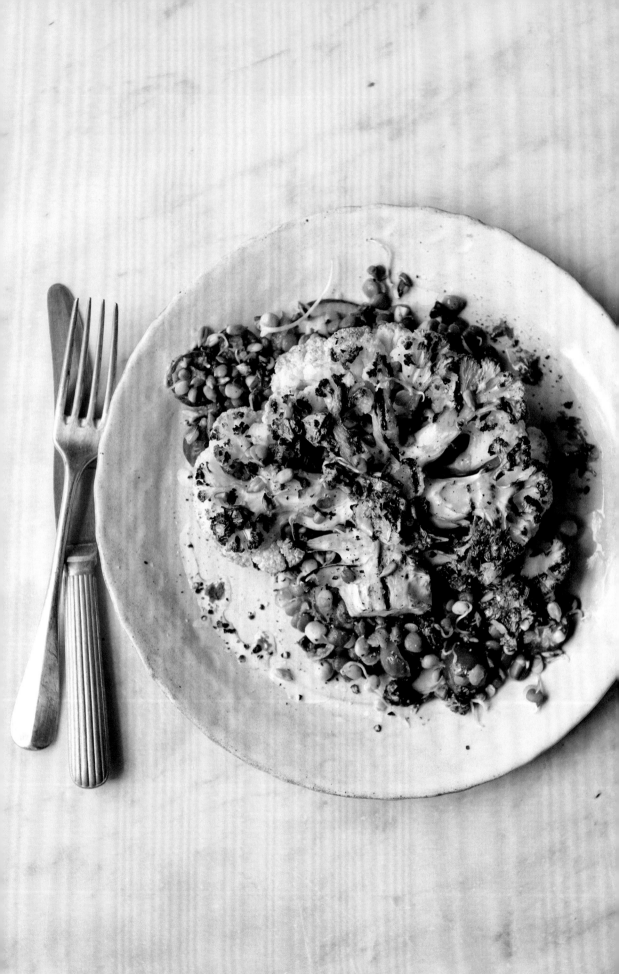

Cauliflower pizza with lemon-infused tomatoes

Serves 2
631 calories per serving

A perfect cauliflower pizza has a crispy base and the key to that is making sure it is pressed out as thinly as possible. The tomatoes for this pizza topping are infused with lemon zest, creating a sweet round flavour with a touch of zing.

2 large plum tomatoes, cut lengthways into thin wedges
½ red onion, cut into wedges
Zest of 1 lemon
1 tsp olive oil, plus extra for frying and drizzling
Fresh basil leaves, to garnish

For the tomato sauce
2 garlic cloves, finely chopped
150g cherry tomatoes
1 tsp dried oregano

For the cauliflower base
1 cauliflower, cut into florets
100g ground almonds
75g gluten-free flour
1 egg
1 tsp dried mixed herbs
1 tsp dried basil
½ tsp celery salt
Flaked sea salt and cracked black pepper

1   Put the tomatoes, red onion, lemon zest, oil and 1 teaspoon salt in a bowl and mix well. Set aside.

2   To make the tomato sauce, heat a little oil in a small pan over a medium heat and fry the garlic until golden. Add the tomatoes, oregano and a pinch each of salt and pepper. Cook for 10 minutes, stirring occasionally, until the tomatoes are softened. Allow to cool, then transfer to a small food processor and blitz to a paste.

3   To make the pizza base, put the cauliflower florets in a (clean) food processor and blitz to the consistency of rice. Tip into a bowl and add the remaining base ingredients. Mix well. The mixture should hold together.

4   Preheat the oven to 200°C/Fan 180°C/Gas 6. Line a baking tray with greaseproof paper.

5   Tip the cauliflower mixture on to the lined baking tray and flatten with your fingers to create two round pizza bases about 1cm thick. If you have time, place the tray in the fridge to chill for 20–30 minutes – chilling will help the bases hold together better and be crisper.

6   Spread the tomato sauce over the bases, then top with the lemon zest-infused tomatoes and onion. Sprinkle with a pinch of salt and drizzle over a little oil. Bake for 25–30 minutes until the tomatoes are soft and the base is crisp. Garnish with fresh basil leaves and serve.

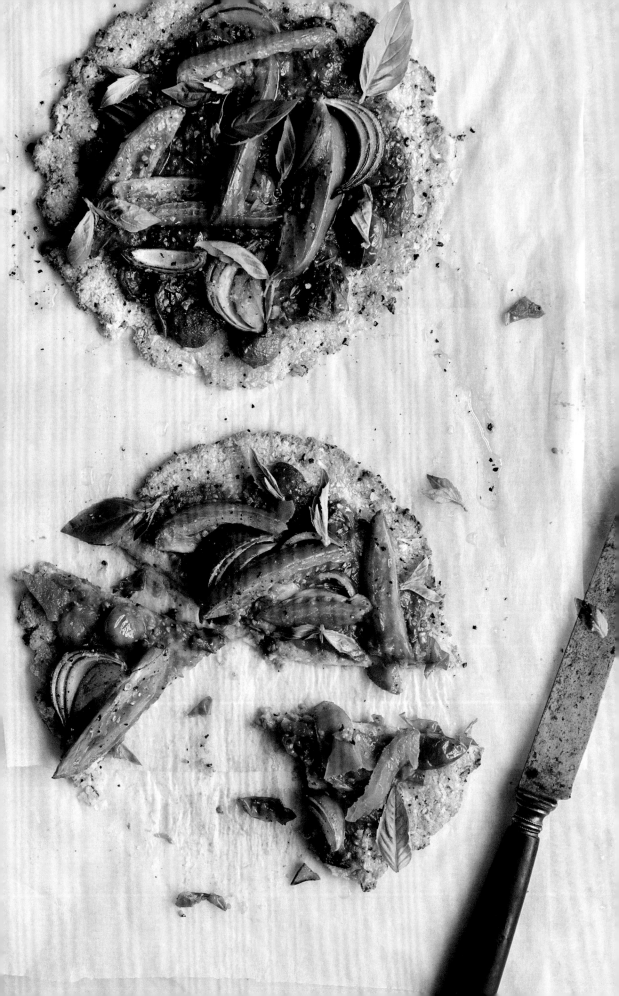

Tomato and aubergine curry with cauliflower rice

Serves 4
157 calories per serving

Cauliflower rice is wonderfully easy to make. It is also filling and its lovely light texture efficiently soaks up the juices of whatever it's served with. Here it partners a tomato and aubergine curry, proving its worth as a brilliant alternative to rice or cous cous.

1 tbsp rapeseed oil
1 onion, finely sliced
1 garlic clove, finely chopped
A thumb-sized piece fresh root ginger
   (unpeeled), grated
6 vine tomatoes, quartered
400g tinned chopped tomatoes
2 tbsp curry powder
1 small fennel bulb, cored and finely sliced
½ small aubergine, cut into chunks
100ml water
1 small cauliflower
1 tsp ground cumin
Zest and juice of 1 lemon
Flaked sea salt and cracked black pepper
A small handful of fresh coriander, roughly torn,
   to garnish

For the pickled onions
½ red onion, thinly sliced
Juice of 1 lemon

1. Preheat the oven to 200°C/Fan 180°C/Gas 6. Line a baking tray with a sheet of foil.
2. Heat a little of the oil in a saucepan over a medium heat and add the onion, garlic and ginger. Sauté for 5–10 minutes until the onion is soft and translucent. Add the fresh and tinned tomatoes and the curry powder. Stir well, then simmer for 20 minutes; add a little water if the mixture becomes too thick.
3. Add the fennel and aubergine along with the measured water. Mix together, then place the lid on the pan and simmer for 15–20 minutes until all the vegetables are tender. Season to taste.
4. While the curry is simmering, prepare the cauliflower rice. Break or cut the cauliflower into florets. Put them into a food processor and blitz to the consistency of cous cous. Tip on to the foil-lined baking tray. Add a drizzle of oil and sprinkle with the ground cumin, lemon zest and juice, and a pinch each of salt and pepper. Fold up the foil to create a package – the cauliflower will steam in this. Place in the oven and cook for 15–20 minutes.
5. Meanwhile, make the pickled onions. Put the onion in a bowl with the lemon juice and leave to soak for about 20 minutes – the onions will go bright pink.
6. Serve the curry on top of the cauliflower rice with the pickled onions and a sprinkling of chopped coriander.

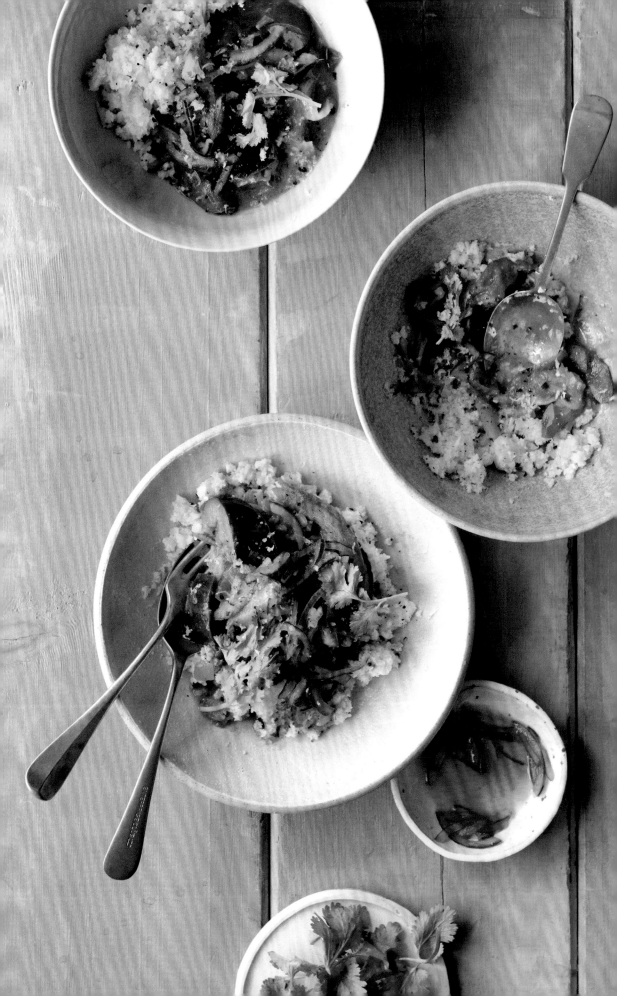

Okra

Also known as 'ladies' fingers', okra is a green flowering plant that belongs to the same family as hibiscus and cotton. With its nutty flavour and firm texture, it is one of those vegetables that you will quickly become enchanted by – as long as you cook it right the first time. But watch out! Just one splash of water can transform this lovely vegetable into a slimy mess that is far from appealing.

Okra is originally from Africa but it is now widely used throughout the world, notably in the Caribbean and India – which is not really surprising, as the mild taste lends itself brilliantly to bold flavours and spices.

When shopping, I always go for the smallest okra, as they tend to have the best texture and flavour. The greenest and firmest ones will usually be freshest.

Nutritional bonus
Recent studies suggest that including okra in your diet can have a positive effect on the early management of diabetes because of the high level of **fibre** and **antioxidants** that okra contains. It is also a great source of **calcium**, **magnesium** and **folate**.

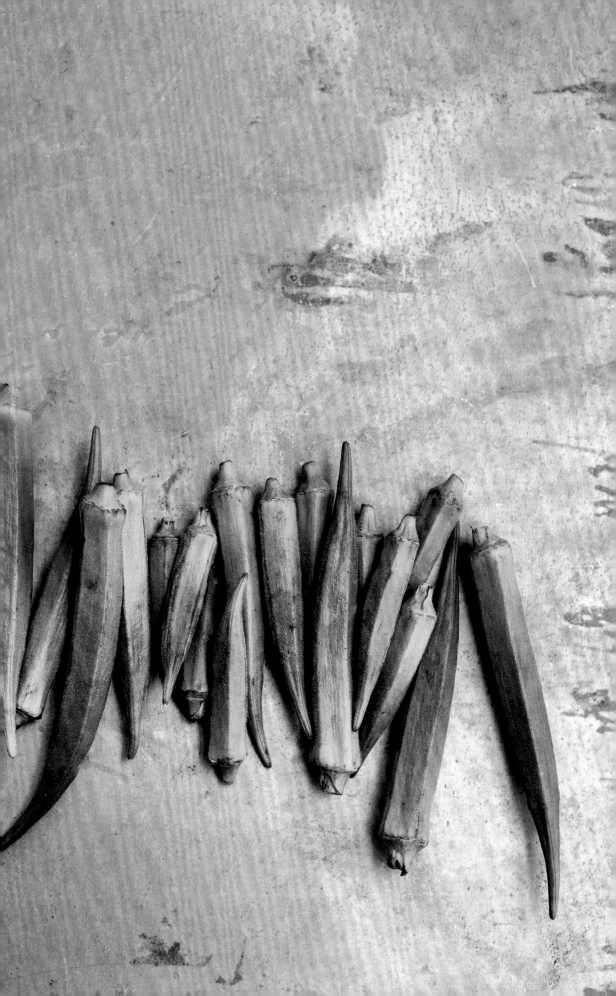

Okra and dal

Serves 2

667 calories per serving

Okra is the perfect companion to a dal – you often find them together in the classic Indian repertoire. Here fried okra with tempered spices makes a delicious topping for a smooth, creamy dal. The dish is great on its own but if you want to make it more filling, serve it with brown rice or quinoa.

Rapeseed oil for frying
1 onion, diced
2 tbsp grated fresh root ginger
1 tsp ground cumin
1 tsp garam masala
200g Puy lentils
500ml vegetable stock
100g red lentils
½ tsp mustard seeds
½ tsp fennel seeds
200g okra, cut into 1cm pieces
A small handful of fresh coriander, roughly
    chopped, to garnish
1 lemon, cut into quarters, to serve

1   To make the dal, heat 1 teaspoon oil in a small saucepan over a medium heat and sauté the onion and ginger until the onion is translucent. Add the cumin, garam masala, Puy lentils and stock and stir to mix. Bring to the boil, then leave to simmer for 15–20 minutes until the lentils are softened.

2   Stir in the red lentils and cook for a further 10 minutes until both types of lentil are soft and falling apart. Remove from the heat and keep warm.

3   Heat a drop of oil in a small non-stick frying pan and add the mustard seeds, fennel seeds and okra. Cook, stirring often to prevent the spices from catching, for 5–10 minutes until the okra is lightly browned.

4   Tip the cooked dal into a bowl, top with the okra and garnish with the fresh coriander. Serve with lemon wedges for squeezing over.

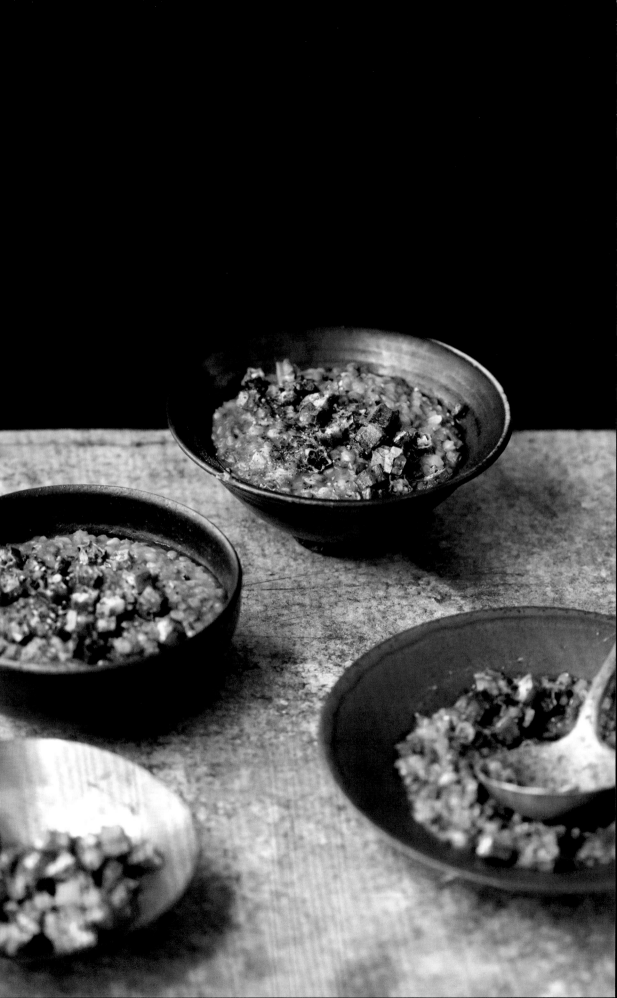

Spiced okra curry

Serves 2
316 calories per serving

This simple recipe for an okra and tomato curry flavoured with garam masala can be whipped up in less than 30 minutes. It is a great weekday supper or can be part of an Indian-style feast at the weekend. I often serve the curry with kale pakoras (see page 92) and the tomato and onion salad on page 262. Use plump, sweet tomatoes in the curry because they will give you a rich sauce to complement the earthy okra.

1 tbsp rapeseed oil
1 onion, diced
2 garlic cloves, finely chopped
1 tbsp grated fresh root ginger
200g okra, cut into 1cm pieces
200g vine tomatoes, diced
1 green chilli, sliced
1 fennel bulb, cored and thinly sliced
1 tbsp garam masala
A small handful of fresh dill, roughly chopped
Zest of 1 lemon
Brown rice to serve

1   Heat the oil in a saucepan over a medium heat, add the onion, garlic and ginger, and cook until the onion is translucent. Add the okra and cook, stirring occasionally, for 5–7 minutes until it is slightly browned (it's important that the okra be browned at this stage to ensure that it does not go mushy when you add the tomatoes).
2   Add the tomatoes, green chilli and fennel and stir well. Simmer on a low heat, stirring often, for about 15 minutes until the tomatoes have broken down and are soft.
3   Stir in the garam masala, dill and lemon zest. Cook for a few more minutes, then remove from the heat. Leave to stand for 5 minutes before serving with brown rice.

Okra and egg-fried rice

Serves 2
437 calories per serving

I love egg-fried rice for dinner. Sautéed okra, which has a wonderful texture, goes brilliantly with the fluffy rice mixture. For subtle saltiness, I tend to season the rice with tamari rather than salt.

150g brown rice
1 tsp rapeseed oil
1 onion, diced
2 garlic cloves, finely chopped
200g okra, cut into 1cm pieces
3 eggs
1 tbsp tamari
Juice of 1 lemon
A pinch of dried chilli flakes
A handful of fresh coriander, roughly chopped
2 spring onions, finely sliced
Flaked sea salt and cracked black pepper

1   Put the rice in a pan with a pinch of salt and cover with three times the amount of water. Bring to the boil, then leave to simmer gently for 20–25 minutes until the rice is tender and fluffy. Drain well.
2   Heat the oil in a non-stick frying pan over a medium heat and sauté the onion and garlic until softened. Add the okra and stir-fry for 5 minutes until they are slightly crisp. Add the cooked rice and fry, leaving the rice to catch slightly on the pan before stirring each time, to create some crispier bits.
3   After a few minutes, crack the eggs straight into the pan and stir to mix them into the rice and okra. Keep stirring until the eggs are cooked. Add the tamari, lemon juice, chilli and a pinch of pepper.
4   Serve immediately topped with the coriander and spring onions.

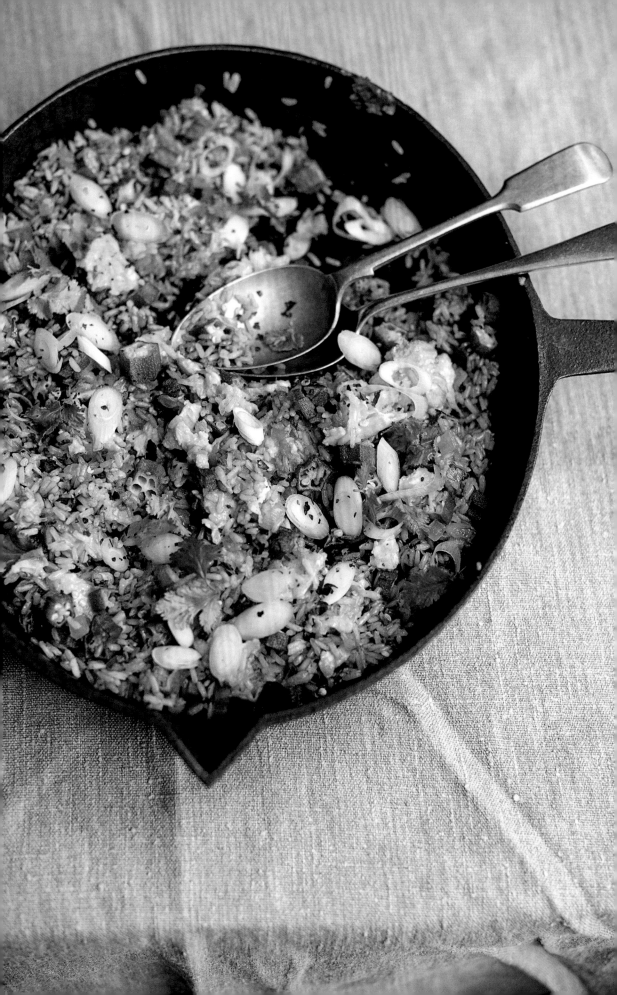

Butternut squash

First things first. Yes, a butternut squash is not technically a vegetable because it contains seeds. But let's be honest, it would seem odd to refer to it as anything else – and so it has a place here.

Butternut squash grows on a large vine. The big bulbous squashes hang down like impressive grapes and it's quite a spectacular sight. While its close relatives cucumber and courgette are at their best in the summer, butternut squash is in peak season during the colder months.

The owners of my local grocer's always make an effort to overload the outside shelves with piles of squash when they are in season, all different in size, shape and colour. It marks the start of autumn – and tends to inspire me to buy some wood for my log burner and pop a big pan of hot chocolate on the stove.

When selecting your butternut squash, take a tip from my good friend Alice, who advises to go for a heavy one, as this indicates it will have the richest and sweetest flavour when you come to cook it.

Butternut squash tastes great with Asian-style flavours – spices, chillies and coconut – and it is also commonly used in classic European risottos, stews and soups. Within an American-inspired flavour palette, it's delicious paired with cinnamon and nutmeg.

Nutritional bonus

Butternut squash is a great source of **carotene**, which the body turns into **vitamin A**, and of **complex carbohydrates** and **fibre**, two nutrients that work in harmony: carbohydrates (here in the form of glucose) are a key source of energy, while fibre works to control the rate at which your body absorbs the glucose.

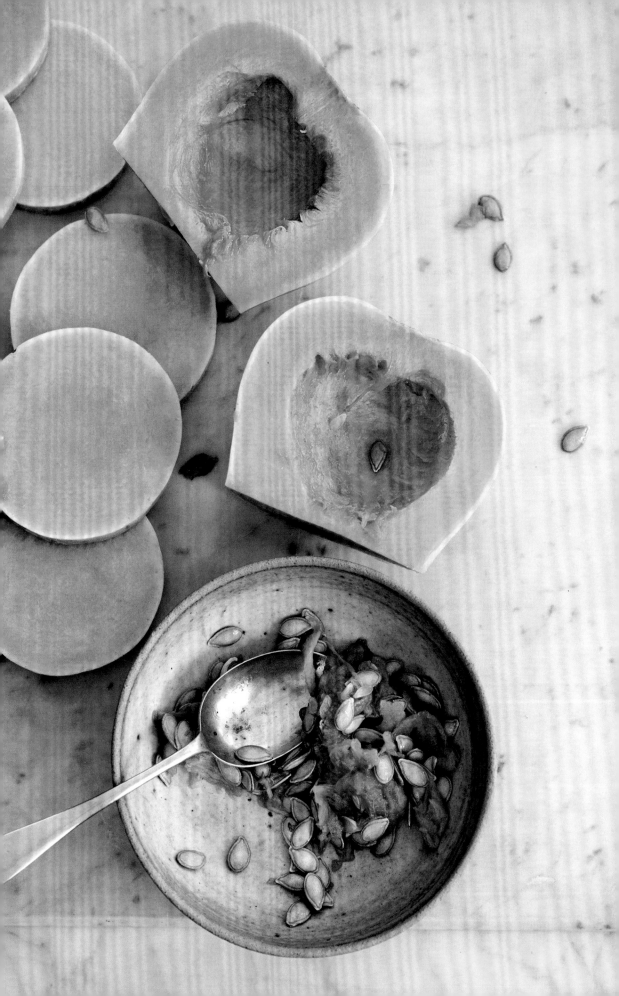

Butternut squash and rosemary soup

Serves 2

303 calories per serving

Butternut squash with rosemary is a classic flavour combination: the woody, floral nature of rosemary brings out the earthy sweetness of the squash. This beautifully coloured, silky-smooth soup has pumpkin seeds and some extra toasted rosemary scattered on top for crunchiness.

1 butternut squash
Rapeseed oil for drizzling and frying
8 fresh rosemary sprigs
½ red onion, diced
2 celery sticks, diced
1 carrot, diced
1 red pepper, seeded and roughly chopped
400ml vegetable stock
A handful of pumpkin seeds
Flaked sea salt and cracked black pepper

1   Preheat the oven to 200°C/Fan 180°C/Gas 6.
2   Peel the butternut squash, then cut it in half lengthways and remove the seeds and fibres. Roughly dice the flesh and spread it out on a baking tray. Drizzle with oil and sprinkle with salt and pepper. Lay five rosemary sprigs on top. Roast for 25–35 minutes until the squash is completely soft.
3   Meanwhile, put the onion, celery, carrot and red pepper in a saucepan with a little oil. Cook over a low heat for about 10 minutes until the onion has softened. Add the stock and a pinch of salt. Bring to the boil, then simmer until the carrots are very tender.
4   Remove the butternut squash from the oven and discard the rosemary. Add the squash to the saucepan. Using a hand blender, blitz all of the ingredients together until completely smooth. Season with salt and pepper to taste.
5   Pick the leaves from the remaining rosemary. Heat a little oil in a small frying pan and gently cook the pumpkin seeds with the rosemary leaves until the seeds are golden.
6   To serve, ladle the soup into bowls and garnish with the pumpkin seeds and rosemary.

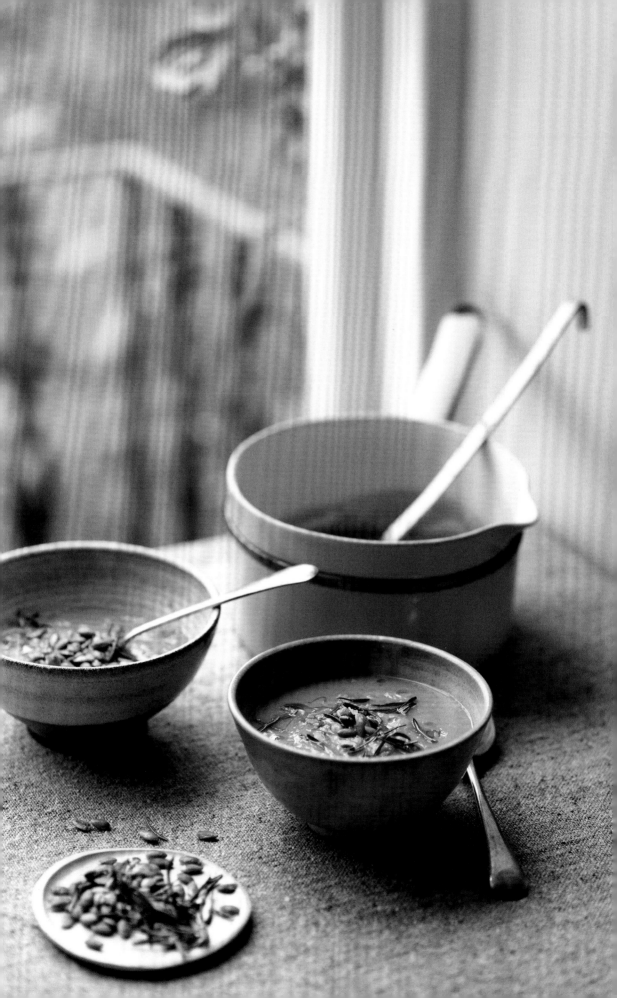

Roasted butternut squash with tahini and tamari seeds

Serves 2

634 calories per serving

Roasted squash with tahini dressing is a signature Detox Kitchen dish during the autumn and early winter months, when squash is at its best. Pickled onions add sharpness, while the tamari seeds offer saltiness and crunch. Be sure to use a large serving platter and add each topping with care, as you are creating art on a plate.

1 small butternut squash
Rapeseed oil for drizzling and frying

For the pickled onions
1 red onion, sliced
Juice of 1 lemon

For the tamari seeds
30g sunflower seeds
30g pumpkin seeds
5g sesame seeds
1 tbsp tamari
1 tsp toasted sesame oil

For the tahini dressing
1 tbsp tahini
1 tbsp rapeseed oil
1 tsp honey
40ml water
Juice of 1 lime
Flaked sea salt and cracked black pepper

1 Preheat the oven to 200°C/Fan 180°C/Gas 6.
2 Cut the butternut squash in half lengthways. Remove the seeds and fibres. Cut the halves across into half-moons 1cm thick. Place them on a roasting tray, drizzle with oil and season with salt and pepper. Roast for 20–25 minutes until tender. Remove from the oven and allow to cool. (Leave the oven on.)
3 Meanwhile, make the pickled onions. Heat a little oil in a small frying pan and fry the onion over a low heat for 5 minutes to soften (it should not be browned). Tip the onion into a bowl and squeeze over the lemon juice. Set aside for at least 10 minutes – the onion will go bright pink.
4 Line a baking tray with greaseproof paper. Mix all the seeds with the tamari and sesame oil. Scatter over the tray and bake for 10 minutes until crisp.
5 To make the dressing, put all the ingredients into a small food processor and blitz to make a smooth paste.
6 Arrange the butternut squash on a serving dish. Scatter over the pickled onions. Drizzle over the tahini dressing and sprinkle with the tamari seeds.

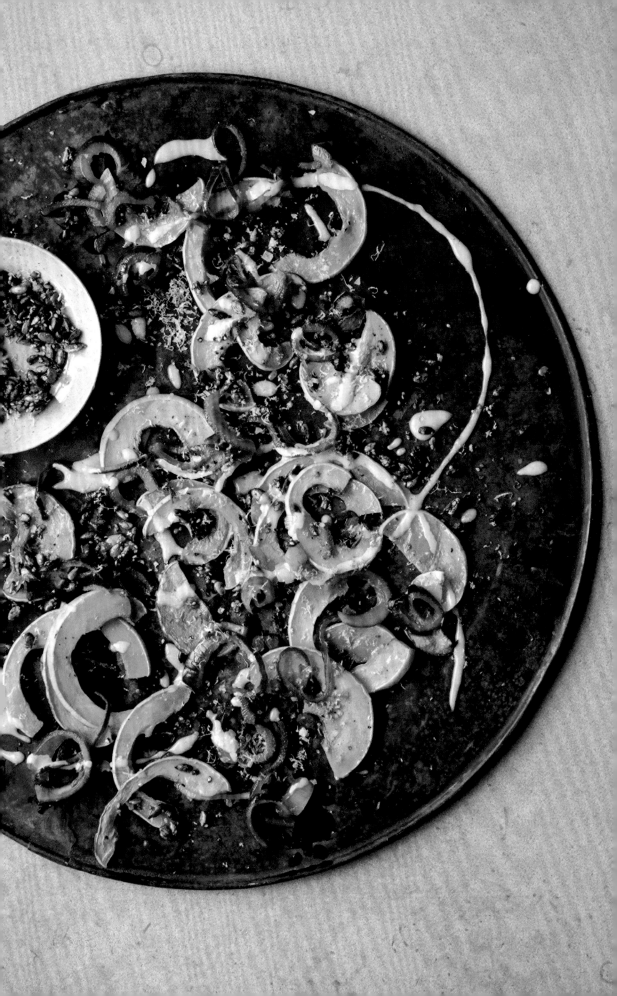

Butternut squash tacos

Serves 2

576 calories per serving

This is a take on corn tacos – the straight part of butternut squash is cut into thin discs to act as 'tortillas'. The rest of the squash is used in the filling, along with onion, garlic, chilli and spring greens. Topped with a rich cashew nut cream, you will be surprised by how filling yet more-ish these vegetable tacos are.

1 butternut squash
1 tbsp rapeseed oil
1 onion, diced
1 garlic clove, finely chopped
100g spring greens, thinly sliced
1 green chilli, sliced
Fresh coriander, to garnish

For the cashew cream
100g cashew nuts
½ tsp ground cumin
Juice of 2 limes

For the spiced seeds
70g pumpkin seeds
30g sunflower seeds
½ tsp smoked paprika
A pinch of chilli powder
2 tbsp tamari
Zest of 1 lime
Flaked sea salt and cracked black pepper

1 First make the cashew cream. Put the cashew nuts into a bowl and add just enough water to cover them. Leave to soak for 30 minutes, then tip the nuts and water into a food processor. Add the ground cumin, lime juice, and a pinch each of salt and pepper. Blitz to a smooth paste. Set aside.

2 Toast the pumpkin seeds and sunflower seeds in a small dry frying pan until golden. Remove from the heat and stir in the smoked paprika, chilli powder, tamari and lime zest. Tip into a bowl and set aside.

3 Peel the butternut squash, then cut across in half. Set the rounded half aside. Finely slice the remaining straight part of the squash into eight rounds – try to make them as thin as possible, aiming for about 1mm. Set a ridged griddle/grill pan on a high heat. Once the pan is hot, griddle the squash slices for a few minutes on each side until slightly softened with black charred marks.

4 To make the filling, dice all the rest of the butternut squash (discard seeds and fibres from the rounded part). Heat the oil in a frying pan over a medium heat, add the onion and garlic, and cook until lightly browned. Add the diced butternut squash and cook gently for about 10 minutes until it has softened, adding a little water if necessary to prevent it from sticking. Add the spring greens, green chilli and salt and pepper to taste. When the spring greens have wilted, remove from the heat.

5 To serve, top the butternut squash 'tortillas' with the filling, sprinkle with the seeds and top with a few dollops of cashew cream.

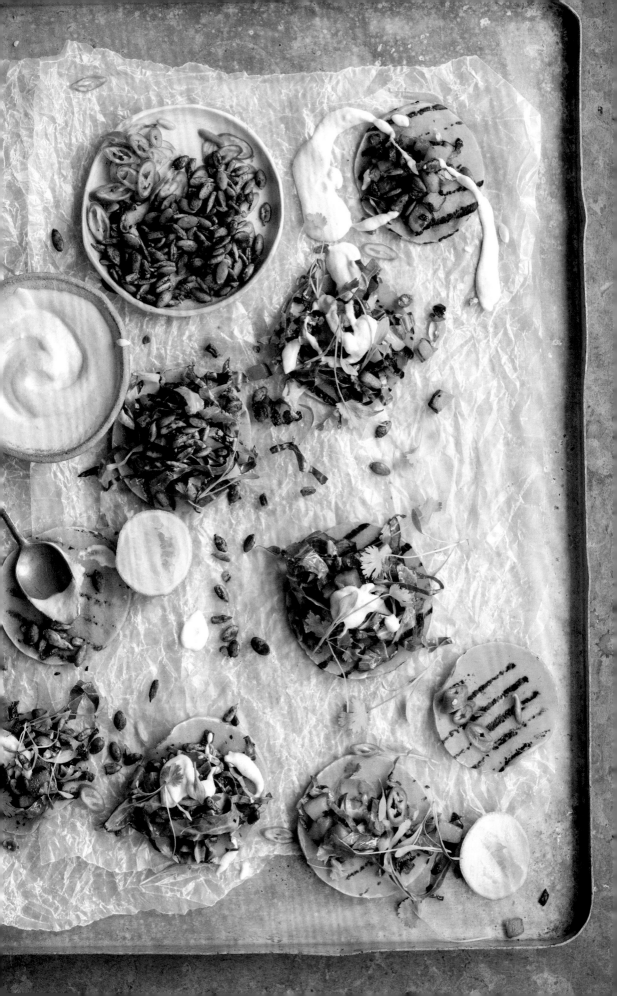

Za'atar-roasted butternut squash with lime yoghurt

Serves 2

414 calories per serving

Popular in Middle Eastern cooking, za'atar is a herb with long green leaves that has a similar taste to thyme. It is also the name of a herb and spice blend. You can buy this at the shop but it is very easy to make your own. The herbs in the za'atar blend bring out the sweetness of roasted butternut squash here, and the sumac element complements this with its sharpness. The creamy sumptuousness of a lime yoghurt dressing brings all the flavours together.

1 butternut squash

1 tbsp olive oil

Zest of 1 lemon

A small handful of fresh flat-leaf parsley, roughly chopped, to garnish

For the za'atar

4 tsp sesame seeds

4 tbsp finely chopped fresh oregano

4 tsp dried marjoram

4 tsp ground sumac

1 tsp flaked sea salt

4 tsp ground cumin

For the dressing

4 tbsp coconut yoghurt

Zest and juice of 2 limes

1 spring onion, finely chopped

Flaked sea salt and cracked black pepper

1   Preheat the oven to 200°C/Fan 180°C/Gas 6.

2   To make the za'atar, set a small dry frying pan over a medium heat and toast the sesame seeds until just golden. Tip them into a food processor or spice grinder. Add the remaining za'atar ingredients and blitz to a powder. (The quantities here make about 50g za'atar, which is more than you need for this recipe, but the spice mix has many other uses, for example in the recipes for roasted pumpkin on page 170 and stuffed marrow on page 286. The za'atar can be stored in an airtight jar in the fridge for 2 weeks.)

3   Cut the butternut squash in half lengthways and remove the seeds and fibres. Cut each half across into 1cm slices and place them on a baking tray. Drizzle with the oil and sprinkle over 2 tablespoons of the za'atar along with the lemon zest and a pinch each of salt and pepper. Roast for 25–35 minutes until tender.

4   To make the dressing, put the coconut yoghurt in a bowl and mix through the lime zest and juice, the spring onion, and a pinch each of salt and pepper.

5   Remove the butternut squash from the oven and place on a serving platter. Drizzle over the yoghurt dressing and sprinkle with parsley.

Creamy butternut squash curry

Serves 4
406 calories per serving
This rich, creamy curry can easily be made the
night before and stored in the fridge – I always
think a curry tastes better the next day anyway.
For side dishes, try the fried okra on page 150, the
cauliflower rice on page 146 and the tomato and
onion salad on page 262.

1 butternut squash
2 tsp rapeseed oil
2 onions, chopped
3 garlic cloves, chopped
2 tbsp grated fresh root ginger
3 cardamom pods
3 cloves
5 fresh curry leaves
100ml water
1 red pepper, seeded and sliced
1 yellow pepper, seeded and sliced
200g cherry tomatoes
200ml vegetable stock
200ml coconut milk
A small handful of fresh coriander,
   roughly chopped, to garnish

For the spice paste
1 tbsp fennel seeds
1 tbsp cumin seeds
1 tsp coriander seeds
½ tsp mustard seeds
2 tbsp rapeseed oil
100g cashew nuts
1 tsp ground ginger
½ tsp ground turmeric
½ tsp ground cinnamon

1 To make the spice paste, put the fennel seeds,
cumin seeds, coriander seeds and mustard
seeds in a dry frying pan and toast over a
medium heat for a few minutes until fragrant.
Tip into a small food processor (or use a spice
grinder or a pestle and mortar) and blitz to a
powder. Add the oil and cashew nuts and blitz
to a smooth paste. Transfer the paste to a bowl
and stir in the ground ginger, turmeric and
cinnamon. Set aside.

2 Peel the butternut squash, then cut in half
lengthways and remove the seeds and fibres.
Cut the squash into chunks. Heat half the oil
in a large saucepan, add the onions, garlic and
fresh ginger, and sauté until the onions are
translucent. Add the spice paste, cardamom
pods, cloves and curry leaves and cook for
a minute or so, stirring constantly, then add
the water and remaining oil. Cook on a high
heat until the excess liquid has evaporated.

3 Add the squash, peppers, cherry tomatoes and
vegetable stock. Bring to the boil, then simmer
for 20–25 minutes until the squash is tender.
Stir in the coconut milk and simmer gently for
a further 10 minutes. Remove the cardamom
pods and cloves before serving the curry
sprinkled with chopped coriander.

Butternut squash and sweet potato gnocchi with broccoli

Serves 4
292 calories per serving
The key to making good gnocchi is to dry out the potatoes by roasting them, and to chill the dough well so it's easy to roll. Gnocchi are filling and you need only a few per serving, which is why I have teamed them with a light but gloriously flavoured accompaniment of flash-fried broccoli and chilli.

1 small sweet potato (unpeeled)
1 small butternut squash
Rapeseed oil
4 tbsp gluten-free flour, plus extra for dusting
½ tsp grated nutmeg
A good handful of fresh sage leaves

For the broccoli
1 tsp rapeseed oil
500g broccoli, finely chopped
1 red chilli, seeded and finely sliced
Flaked sea salt and cracked black pepper

1   Preheat the oven to 200°C/Fan 180°C/Gas 6.
2   Prick the sweet potato with a fork and place on a small baking tray. Bake for 35–45 minutes until completely soft.
3   Peel the butternut squash, cut in half lengthways and remove the seeds and fibres. Chop into 2.5cm pieces and spread on another baking tray. Drizzle over a little oil. Place in the oven and roast for 30–40 minutes until completely soft.
4   Remove the sweet potato from the oven and allow to cool slightly before peeling. Discard the skin and place the sweet potato flesh in a bowl. Mash well until smooth.
5   Tip the roasted butternut squash into a food processor. Blitz until completely smooth. Add to the sweet potato along with 1 tablespoon of the flour, the nutmeg, 1 teaspoon oil, and a pinch each of salt and pepper. Mix through. Continue mixing in the flour, a tablespoon at a time, until the mixture comes together into a dough. Wrap the dough in cling film and leave to rest in the fridge for at least an hour.
6   Divide the dough into four balls. On a floured surface, roll and shape one of the balls into a long sausage, about 1cm thick. Cut across into 3cm pieces. Repeat with the remaining balls of dough. Lightly dust the pieces (gnocchi) with flour and place back in the fridge to chill.
7   Bring a pan of water to the boil. Add a good amount of salt. Drop in some of the gnocchi (it's best to cook in batches) and simmer until they rise to the surface of the water. Remove the gnocchi with a slotted spoon and place on a piece of kitchen paper. Pat them with the paper to remove as much moisture as possible.
8   Once all the gnocchi are cooked, heat a little oil in a frying pan over a high heat. Add the gnocchi and fry until they are golden all over – try not to touch them too much as they are very delicate. A few minutes before they have finished cooking, add the sage. Keep hot.
9   To cook the broccoli, heat the oil in another pan, add the broccoli, chilli and some salt and pepper, and cook, stirring, for a few minutes until tender but still crisp. Add to the gnocchi and mix together gently, then serve.

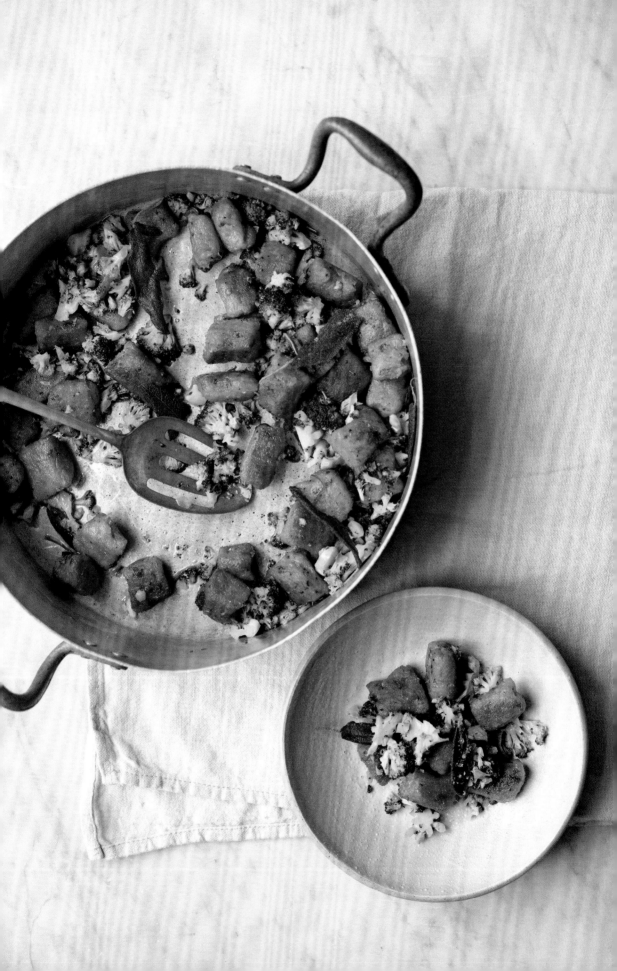

Pumpkin

Pumpkin is inextricably linked with Halloween, and to be honest the only time we eat it at home is during the six-week period from October to November when my local greengrocer stocks pumpkins to the high heavens in an abundant and beautiful display.

I must admit that I am not the biggest fan of pumpkin carving, however. I lack the patience to create anything truly impressive and always end up carving the same jagged-toothed, round-eyed ghoul. But what I do love is roasting slices of uncarved pumpkin to eat with black rice (see page 170). This is both simple and delicious, as well as showing the Halloween colours of orange and black.

In the US pumpkin is typically used more in sweet dishes than it is here in the UK – the ever-popular pumpkin pie, for example, is a traditional part of the feast at Thanksgiving. My version features cherries and maple syrup, with an almond-oat pastry

When buying a pumpkin, always go for one that is heavy and small to medium in size, because this will often be the freshest. I cannot resist sharing an amazing fact with you: the biggest pumpkins ever recorded weighed over a tonne. The record continues to be broken on a fairly regular basis, and the seeds from just one of these huge vegetables can sell for more than £1,500.

Nutritional bonus
Pumpkin is an excellent **complex carbohydrate**, with good levels of **fibre** and low levels of sugar and calories. When you eat pumpkin, this perfect balance of nutrients makes you feel fuller for longer. Pumpkin is also a rich source of **carotenoids** (the compounds that give it its bright orange colour), including **beta carotene**, which the body converts into **vitamin A**.

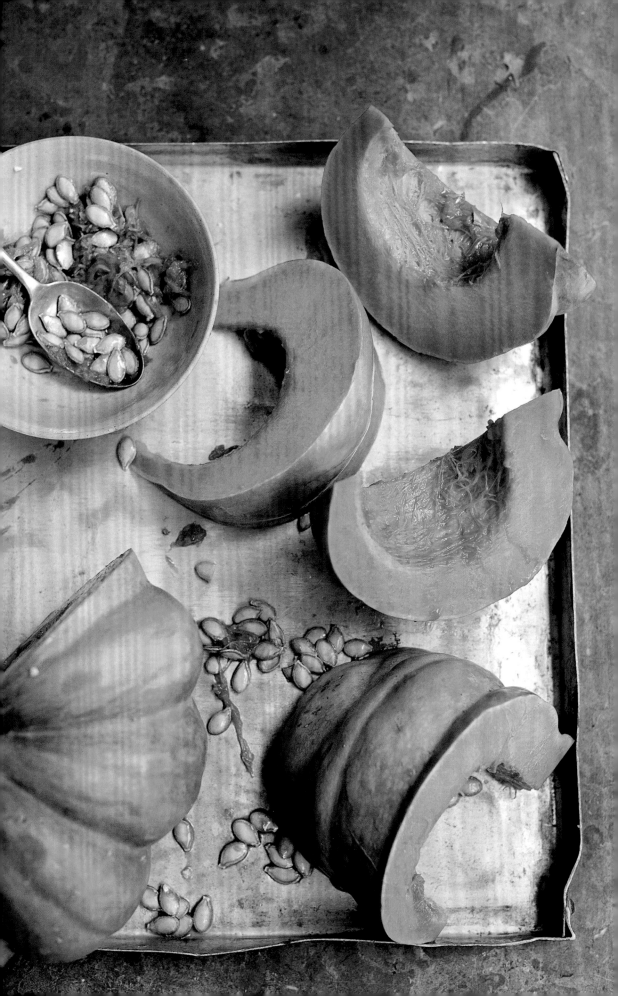

Pumpkin feijoada

Serves 4
288 calories per serving
The stew known as feijoada is one of Brazil's national culinary treasures and it is often made for large gatherings of family and friends. It is traditionally based on meat but this vegetarian version with pumpkin and black beans is just as good and hearty.

200g brown or wild rice
1 tbsp rapeseed oil
1 onion, diced
2 garlic cloves, finely chopped
2 tbsp grated fresh root ginger
1 tsp ground coriander
1 red pepper, seeded and sliced
1 yellow pepper, seeded and sliced
1 small pumpkin, peeled, seeded and cut into
    2.5cm pieces
300ml vegetable stock
400g tinned black beans, drained and rinsed
Zest and juice of 2 limes, plus lime wedges
    to serve
100g cherry tomatoes, cut in half
1 tsp smoked paprika
A small handful of fresh coriander
Flaked sea salt

1 Put the rice in a pan with a pinch of salt and cover with three times the amount of water. Bring to the boil, then simmer until tender – brown rice will take 20–25 minutes, wild rice 30–35 minutes. Drain and keep hot.

2 While the rice is cooking, heat the oil in a saucepan over a medium heat and sauté the onion, garlic and ginger until the onion is soft. Add the ground coriander, the red and yellow peppers and pumpkin and cook for a few more minutes, stirring. Pour in the stock. Bring to the boil, then leave to simmer for 10 minutes until the pumpkin is soft.

3 Add the black beans, the lime zest and juice, cherry tomatoes and smoked paprika and stir well. Simmer for a few more minutes until the beans are hot.

4 Meanwhile, pick the coriander leaves and set aside. Finely chop the stalks. Add them to the pan and mix into the feijoada.

5 Serve the feijoada with the rice, coriander leaves and lime wedges for squeezing over.

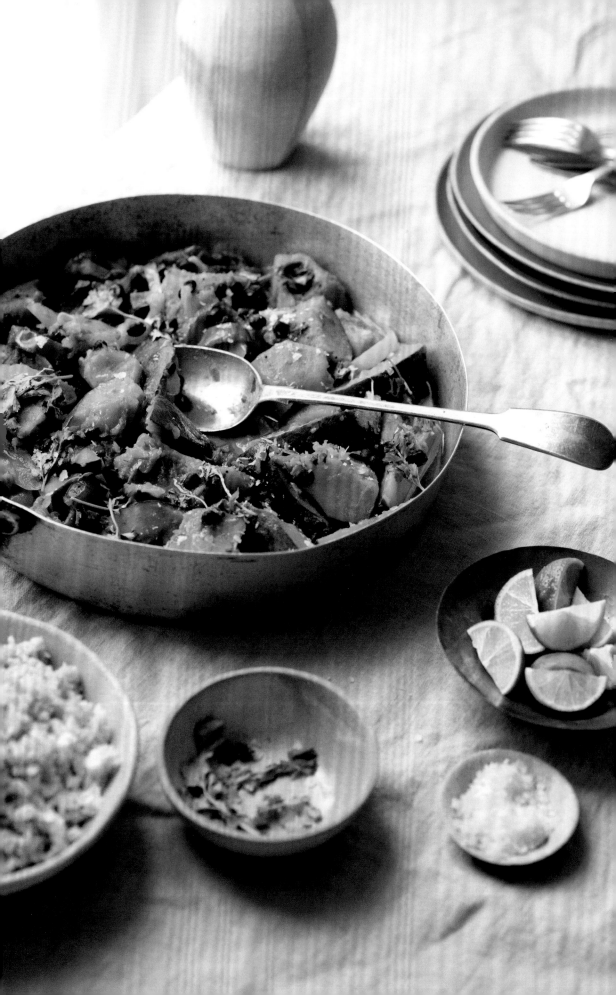

Roasted pumpkin and black rice

Serves 4
467 calories per serving

Roasting rice is a really great way to add a new dimension to a recipe. You boil the rice first and then roast it, which makes it crispy on the outside with a soft, chewy centre. This is a really beautiful dish, with the bright orange pumpkin, black rice and jewel-like green pistachios. The addition of sumac gives a tangy flavour, while the za'atar spice blend adds its own nutty, herby edge.

220g black rice
1 pumpkin
1 tbsp rapeseed oil
1 tbsp ground sumac
Zest of 2 lemons
1 red onion, sliced
A handful of fresh mint, leaves picked
A handful of fresh flat-leaf parsley
100g pistachios

For the dressing
Juice of 1 lemon
1 tbsp olive oil
1 tbsp za'atar (see page 162 or use ready-made)
1 tsp dried chilli flakes
Flaked sea salt and cracked black pepper

1 Preheat the oven to 200°C/Fan 180°C/Gas 6. Line a baking tray with greaseproof paper.

2 Put the rice in a pan with a pinch of salt and cover with three times the amount of water. Bring to the boil, then leave to simmer for 30–35 minutes until the rice is tender and fluffy. Drain in a sieve and rinse under cold water until cooled.

3 Cut the pumpkin in half and remove the seeds and fibres. Slice each half into four or five thin wedges. Spread the pumpkin wedges on the baking tray along with the rice. Drizzle the oil over the pumpkin and sprinkle with the sumac, lemon zest and some salt and pepper. Roast for about 30 minutes until the pumpkin is tender and the rice is crispy.

4 While the pumpkin and rice are in the oven, make the dressing. Whisk together all of the ingredients in a bowl with a pinch each of salt and pepper. Add the sliced red onion and leave to soak for about 20 minutes – the onion will turn a brighter shade of pink.

5 Transfer the pumpkin and rice to a serving platter. Chop the herbs with the pistachios and sprinkle over the top with the pink onion. Drizzle over the dressing.

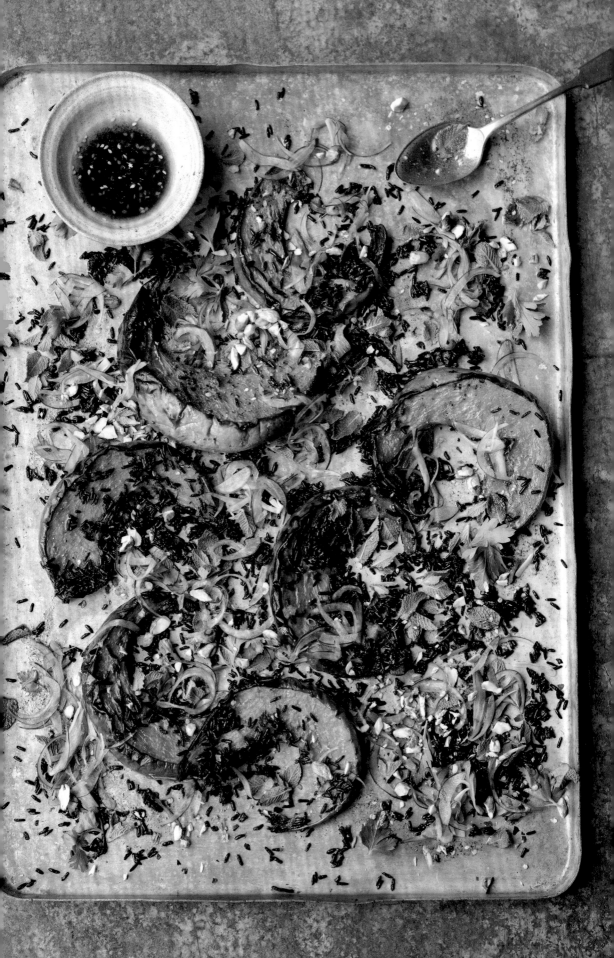

Porridge with pumpkin and salted caramel

Serves 2
610 calories per serving
The pumpkin sauce in this recipe is like a subtly sweet compote, and it's a great addition to your breakfast. With its smooth texture, it is delicious stirred into a bowl of hot porridge, along with some salted date caramel.

½ small pumpkin
2 tbsp maple syrup
1 tsp ground cinnamon
100ml freshly pressed apple juice
150g pitted dates
200g porridge oats
150ml coconut milk
200ml water
Flaked sea salt

1   Preheat the oven to 200°C/Fan 180°C/Gas 6. Line a baking tray with greasproof paper.
2   Peel the pumpkin and remove the seeds and fibres, then cut into 2.5cm pieces. Spread the pieces on the lined baking tray and drizzle over the maple syrup. Roast for 20 minutes until soft. Tip the pumpkin into a saucepan and add the cinnamon and apple juice. Cook over a low heat for 15 minutes, stirring occasionally, until the pumpkin has completely broken down to form a compote. Set aside.
3   To make the salted caramel, put the dates into a bowl, cover with boiling water and leave to soak for 30 minutes. Pour the dates and water into a food processor and blitz until completely smooth. Add a pinch of salt and blitz again.
4   Put the oats into a saucepan and add the coconut milk and water. Bring just to the boil, then simmer for 3–6 minutes, stirring, until the porridge is smooth and creamy.
5   To serve, add a few spoonfuls of pumpkin compote to each bowl of porridge plus some date caramel and a drizzle of extra maple syrup, if you like.

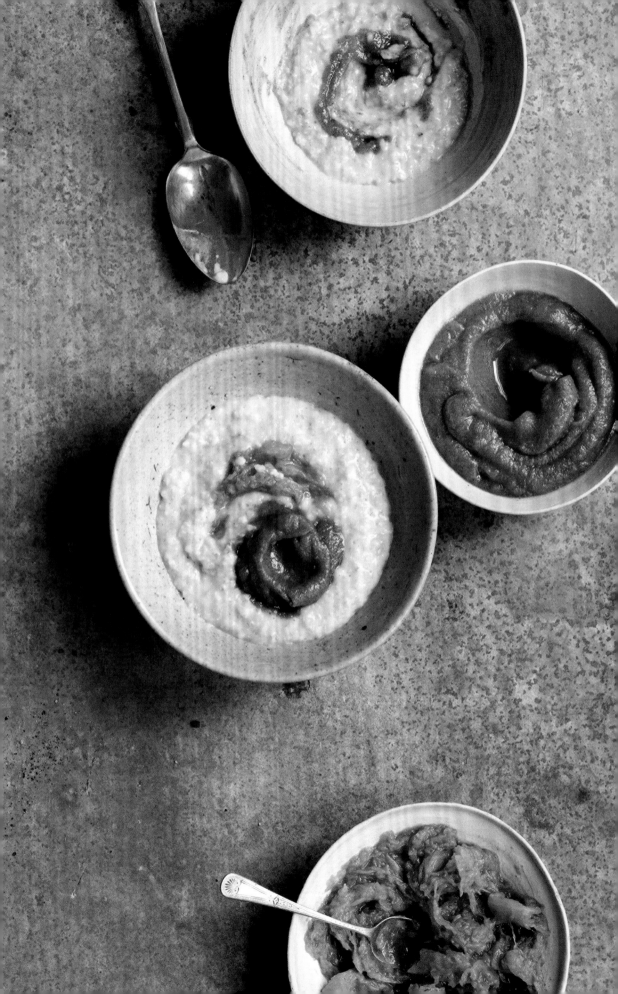

Pumpkin, cherry and almond pie

Serves 4
646 calories per serving

Using pumpkin in sweet dishes has a long history – pumpkins were once stuffed with apples, sugar and spices to serve with savoury foods, and spicy, sweet pumpkin pie is traditional for American Thanksgiving. I love the naturally sweet, smooth texture of this pumpkin filling, which works very well with cherries. The pastry base can be a little fiddly as it doesn't hold together like a regular shortcrust, but it's worth the faff. If the pastry breaks as you line the tin, you can just patch it.

For the pastry
200g porridge oats
150g ground almonds
Grated zest of 1 orange
4 tbsp maple syrup
1 egg
1 tbsp wheat-free flour, plus extra for rolling out and dusting the tin

For the filling
400g pumpkin, peeled, seeded and cut into chunks
4 tbsp rapeseed oil
2 tbsp maple syrup
1 tbsp mixed spice
½ tsp ground cardamom
70g ground almonds
Grated zest of 1 orange
3 eggs
400g fresh cherries, stoned and cut in half

To serve
100g fresh cherries
1 tbsp honey
Coconut yoghurt

1. To make the pastry, put the oats, almonds, orange zest, maple syrup and egg into a large mixing bowl and bring together with your hands to form a dough.

2. Dust your work surface with the tablespoon of flour. Place the dough on the surface and knead into a ball. Wrap in cling film and chill for 30–40 minutes.

3. Preheat the oven to 200°C/Fan 180°C/Gas 6. Dust a 20cm fluted tart tin with flour.

4. Remove the dough from the fridge and roll it out on the lightly floured surface. Place it over the tart tin and gently press over the bottom and into the sides. Trim off the excess and use to patch any holes. Line the pastry case with greaseproof paper and fill with baking beans. Blind bake for 10 minutes. Remove the paper and beans, then set the pastry case aside to cool. Leave the oven on.

5. To make the filling, spread out the pumpkin on a baking tray and roast for about 30 minutes until tender. Leave to cool, then tip into a food processor, add the oil and maple syrup, and blitz until smooth. Add the rest of the filling ingredients, except the cherries, and blitz to combine – the texture should be similar to a sponge cake mixture.

6. Pour the filling into the pastry case. Scatter the cherries evenly over the surface and press them halfway into the mixture so that they are still visible on top. Bake for 25–35 minutes until the filling has set and is lightly golden on top. Allow the pie to cool to room temperature before serving.

7. While the pie is in the oven, put the additional cherries in a pan with the honey and cook on a low heat for a few minutes until the cherries have softened. Allow to cool.

8. To serve, top each piece of pie with coconut yoghurt and some honeyed cherries.

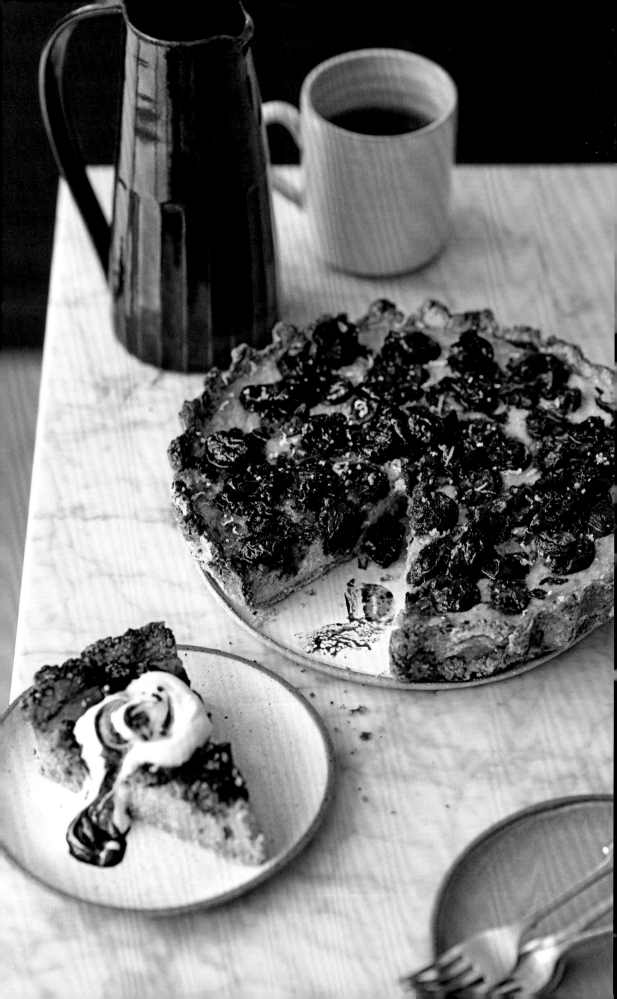

Sweet potato

Steamed, mashed, baked or roasted, sweet potato is one versatile ingredient. At its simplest, you can put a sweet potato on a baking tray, pop it into a moderate oven and return about 40 minutes later to a piping hot lunch. I love to split open a baked sweet potato and top it with some avocado or a dollop of hummus.

The soft orange potatoes originally came from Central and South America, where they have been eaten since time immemorial. In the UK they're at their best from October through to March, and they do lend themselves brilliantly to warming wintry dishes. Sweet potato is the perfect vehicle for herbs and spices, working particularly well in stews and curries. As with most vegetables, there are lots of nutrients in the skin, so I tend to leave this on when cooking and then eating.

Research suggests that in order to increase your uptake of the beta-carotene in sweet potatoes you should eat them alongside a little fat. This is easily done if you serve some avocado with your sweet potato and black rice tortillas (see page 180), or use coconut milk in a sweet potato curry (see page 178).

Nutritional bonus

Often touted as a 'healthier' alternative to the white potato, sweet potatoes are rich in **complex carbohydrates**, **fibre** and **beta-carotene** (which is what gives them their deep orange colour). Beta-carotene is an important nutrient that is converted to **vitamin A** in the body, and as such helps to maintain healthy skin and teeth. Sweet potatoes also provide good amounts of other vitamins and minerals, in particular **vitamin C**.

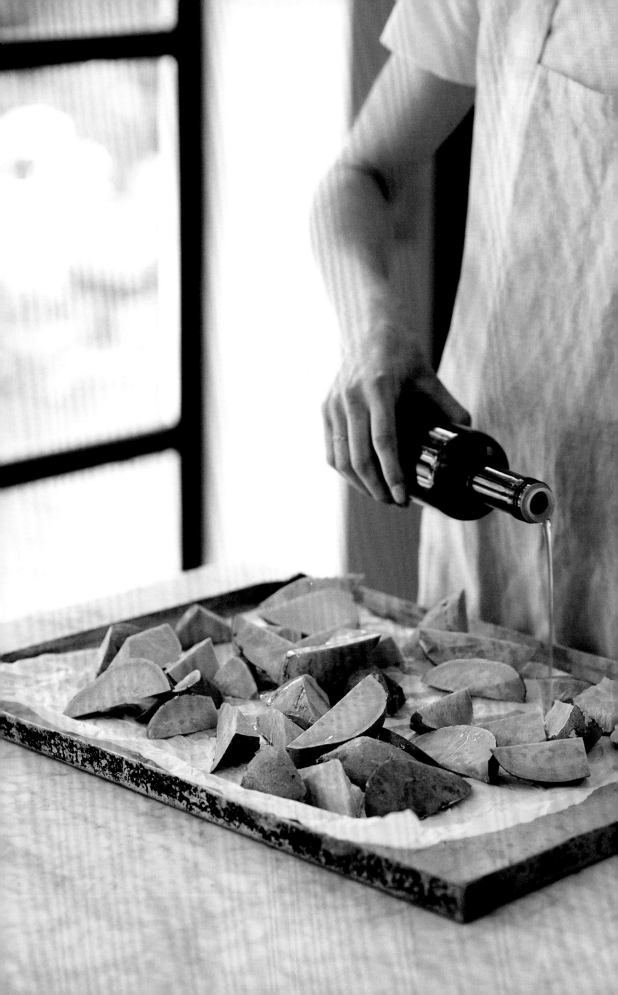

Sweet potato massaman curry

Serves 4
476 calories per serving
A Thai massaman curry should be spicy, sour and nutty. It usually includes fish sauce and peanuts but I have swapped these for tamarind paste and cashew nuts. Roasting the sweet potato once you have tossed it in the spices gives the finished dish an aromatic flavour and lots of texture.

4 sweet potatoes, cut into 2.5cm pieces
400ml coconut milk
150g cashew nuts
1 tbsp tamarind paste
Juice of 3 limes

For the curry paste
2 shallots
2 lemongrass sticks
2 garlic cloves
A thumb-sized piece fresh root ginger
2 tsp dried chilli flakes
1 tsp ground coriander
1 tbsp ground cumin
1 tsp ground cloves
1 tsp ground cardamom
1 tsp flaked sea salt
1 tsp cracked black pepper

To serve
Quinoa
Fresh coriander leaves
Lime wedges

1   Preheat the oven to 200°C/Fan 180°C/Gas 6.
2   To make the curry paste, put the shallots, lemongrass, garlic and fresh ginger in a food processor and blitz to a paste. (You can also pound the ingredients in a pestle and mortar if you have more time.) Transfer to a bowl, add the rest of the paste ingredients and mix well.
3   Add the sweet potatoes to the paste and toss to coat. Spread out on a baking tray and roast for 25–30 minutes until the sweet potatoes are cooked but still firm to touch.
4   Transfer the sweet potatoes to a saucepan and add the coconut milk and half of the cashew nuts. Bring just to the boil, then simmer for 10–15 minutes until the sweet potatoes are very soft. Add the tamarind paste and lime juice and stir to mix.
5   While the curry is simmering, toast the rest of the cashew nuts in a dry frying pan. Chop roughly.
6   Sprinkle the curry with the toasted cashews and serve with quinoa, coriander leaves and lime wedges for squeezing over.

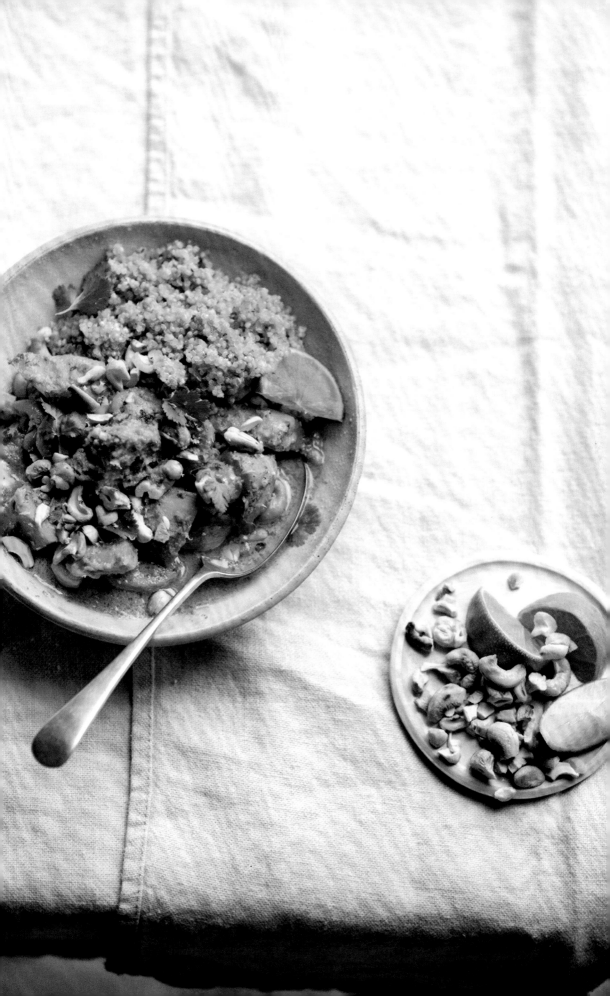

Sweet potato, black rice and chilli tortillas

Serves 4
349 calories per serving
An excellent trick for feeding friends at short notice is always to have a packet of corn tortillas in the cupboard because there is nothing that doesn't taste good folded into a tortilla. Not only are these sweet potato and black rice tortillas quick and easy to make, you can just lay out everything on the table and let your guests help themselves.

4 sweet potatoes (unpeeled)
150g black rice
2 avocados
½ cucumber, peeled, seeded and diced
Zest and juice of 1 lime, plus lime wedges to serve
A small handful of fresh coriander, finely chopped
A pinch of ground cumin
12 small corn tortillas
1 red chilli, seeded and sliced
Flaked sea salt and cracked black pepper
Micro coriander, to garnish

1 Preheat the oven to 200°C/Fan 180°C/Gas 6.
2 Prick the sweet potatoes, place on a baking tray and bake for 40–60 minutes until they are completely soft. Remove from the oven and leave to cool.
3 While the sweet potatoes are baking, put the rice in a pan with a pinch of salt and cover with three times the amount of water. Bring to the boil, then simmer gently for 30–35 minutes until the rice is tender. Drain and keep warm.
4 While the potatoes are cooling, make the avocado salsa. Halve the avocados and scoop out the flesh into a bowl. Mash roughly with a fork. Add the diced cucumber, lime juice and chopped coriander and mix together. Season with salt and pepper to taste.
5 When the sweet potatoes are cool enough to handle, peel off the skin and discard it. Place the flesh in a bowl, add the cumin, lime zest and some salt and pepper, and mash together.
6 Cook the tortillas in a hot ridged griddle/grill pan or frying pan to soften them and slightly brown both sides.
7 Arrange the tortillas on a large serving platter. Top each one with a scoop of rice, a scoop of mashed sweet potato, a dollop of avocado salsa and a few red chilli slices. Garnish with micro coriander and serve, with lime wedges for squeezing over.

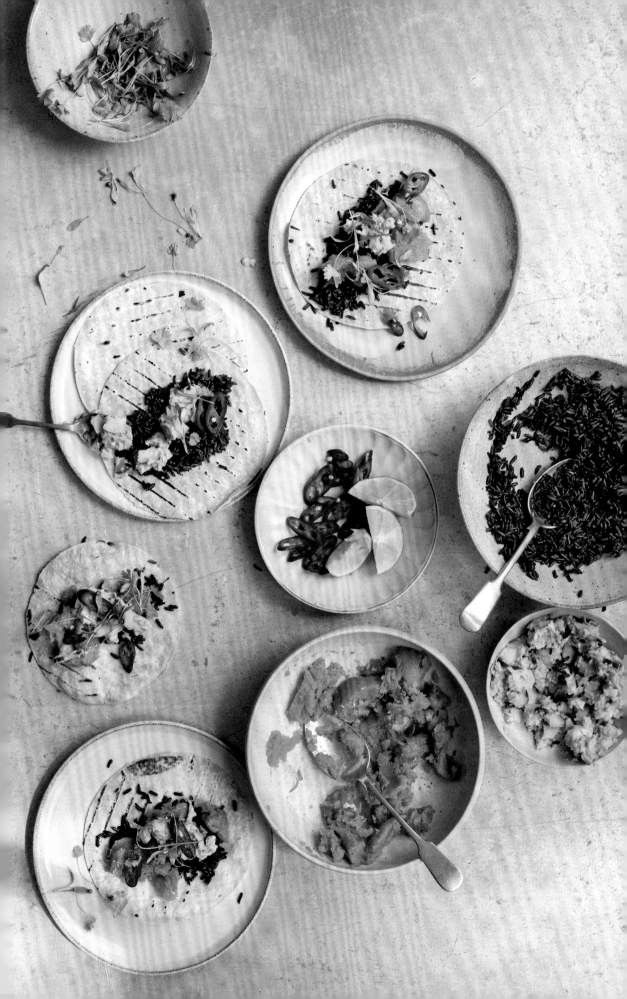

Sweet potato chilli

Serves 4
329 calories per serving
A spicy chilli typically contains meat. My delicious vegetarian version uses sweet potatoes, which are the perfect ingredient to soak up the flavours in the rich tomato sauce. I've stirred in a little cacao powder at the end as it has a miraculous way of adding depth of flavour and bringing out the earthy sweetness of the tomatoes.

2 sweet potatoes, cut into 2cm cubes
1 tsp olive oil, plus extra for frying
200g brown rice
1 onion, diced
2 garlic cloves, finely chopped
1 red pepper, seeded and thinly sliced
½ tsp chilli powder
1 tbsp dried oregano
1 tbsp ground cumin
A pinch of ground cinnamon
200g plum tomatoes, roughly chopped
150ml vegetable stock
1 tbsp cacao powder
A small handful of fresh coriander, roughly chopped
Flaked sea salt

1 Preheat the oven to 200°C/Fan 180°C/Gas 6.
2 Place the sweet potatoes on a baking tray and drizzle over the olive oil. Roast for 30 minutes.
3 Put the rice in a pan with a pinch of salt and cover with three times the amount of water. Bring to the boil, then leave to simmer for 20–25 minutes until the rice is tender and fluffy. Drain and keep warm.
4 While the rice is cooking, heat a little oil in a saucepan and fry the onion and garlic for 10 minutes until the onion is translucent. Add the red pepper, chilli powder, oregano, cumin and cinnamon and stir to coat the onion. Stir in the tomatoes and stock. Add the cooked sweet potatoes and simmer for 15–20 minutes until the cubes are almost falling apart.
5 Stir in the cacao and chopped coriander. Remove from the heat and leave to stand for about 5 minutes before serving with the rice.

Sweet potato wedges

Serves 4
205 calories per serving

This is a simple but unbeatable recipe. You can buy steak seasoning but I like to make my own as it keeps well and has so many uses. The addition of rosemary brings a floral note. The wedges work equally well as an accompaniment to a roast or alongside a big salad.

3 sweet potatoes (unpeeled)
1 tbsp rapeseed oil
1 tsp 'steak' seasoning (see page 132)
2 fresh rosemary sprigs, leaves picked and
    roughly chopped
1 garlic clove, sliced
1 tbsp gluten-free flour
Flaked sea salt and cracked black pepper

1 Preheat the oven to 220°C/Fan 200°C/Gas 7.
2 Cut each sweet potato into six wedges. Put them in a bowl with the oil, steak seasoning, chopped rosemary, garlic, and some salt and pepper. Toss to coat the potato wedges. Dust over the flour and toss the wedges again so that they are lightly covered all over.
3 Spread out the wedges on a baking tray and roast for about 40 minutes until crisp on the outside and soft inside.

Stuffed sweet potatoes

Serves 4
512 calories per serving
I always have sweet potatoes in my vegetable drawer because everyone in my family loves them. If you keep them cool, they will last a good week. This recipe for stuffed sweet potatoes is rich and spicy, with a smooth cashew nut cream on top to offset the heat. Serve with a green salad.

4 sweet potatoes (unpeeled)
2 spring onions, finely chopped
10 cherry tomatoes, cut into quarters
A small handful of fresh coriander, finely chopped
A pinch of ground cumin
2 tbsp nutritional yeast (yeast flakes)

For the dressing
100g cashew nuts
2 tbsp rapeseed oil
100ml water
Zest of 1 lemon
Flaked sea salt and cracked black pepper

To serve
1 avocado, peeled, quartered and sliced
1 red chilli, finely sliced (optional)
Fresh coriander leaves

1 Preheat the oven to 200°C/Fan 180°C/Gas 6. Prick the sweet potatoes, place them on a baking tray and bake for 40–60 minutes until soft throughout. Remove from the oven and allow to cool.

2 When the sweet potatoes are cool enough to handle, cut each one in half lengthways and scoop out most of the flesh into a bowl. Leave the skins open, cut side up, on the baking tray.

3 Mash the sweet potato flesh in the bowl. Add the spring onions, tomatoes, coriander, cumin and some salt and pepper and mix everything together. Spoon the mixture into the sweet potato skins and top each with a sprinkle of nutritional yeast. Bake for 10–15 minutes until slightly golden on top.

4 To make the dressing, put the cashew nuts and oil into a food processor and blitz to a paste. Add the water, lemon zest, and a pinch each of salt and pepper and blitz until smooth.

5 Drizzle the dressing over the potatoes and top with avocado and chilli, if using. Sprinkle with a few coriander leaves and serve.

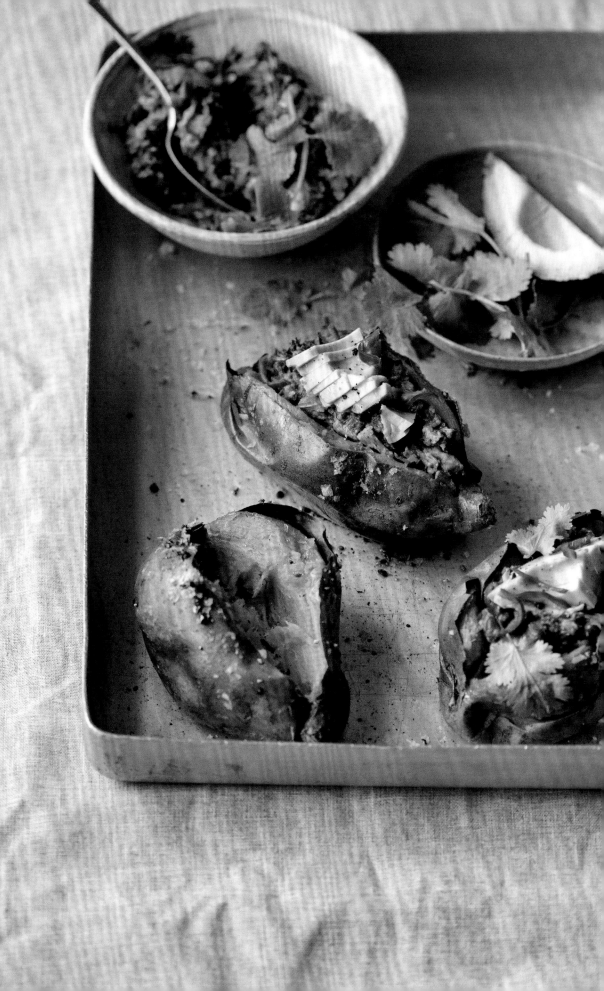

Jerusalem artichoke

Contrary to what you might think, the Jerusalem artichoke is neither from Jerusalem, nor is it a real artichoke. In fact, Jerusalem artichokes originate from North America and belong to the sunflower family.

Best eaten during the winter months, these knobbly tubers are a delight to cook with because below the lumpy surface their flesh has a distinctive nutty, earthy flavour. They work well in a variety of dishes and can be boiled, roasted, braised or sautéed.

There is rarely a need to peel off the skin of a Jerusalem artichoke (which is good as the shape is so irregular) – simply scrub well and remove any particularly hard knobs before you start. The skin becomes very crisp when the vegetables are roasted, which is one of the reasons that Jerusalem artichokes will always appear in any roast dinner of mine, especially teamed with parsnips and baby beetroots (see page 188).

Nutritional bonus

Jerusalem artichokes contain two **prebiotics** called fructo-oligosaccharides (FOS) and inulin, which are thought to play a role in the maintenance of a healthy digestive system. If eaten in excess, though, they can cause a build-up of wind, so it's best to eat Jerusalem artichokes in small amounts or build up your intake gradually. It's worth it.

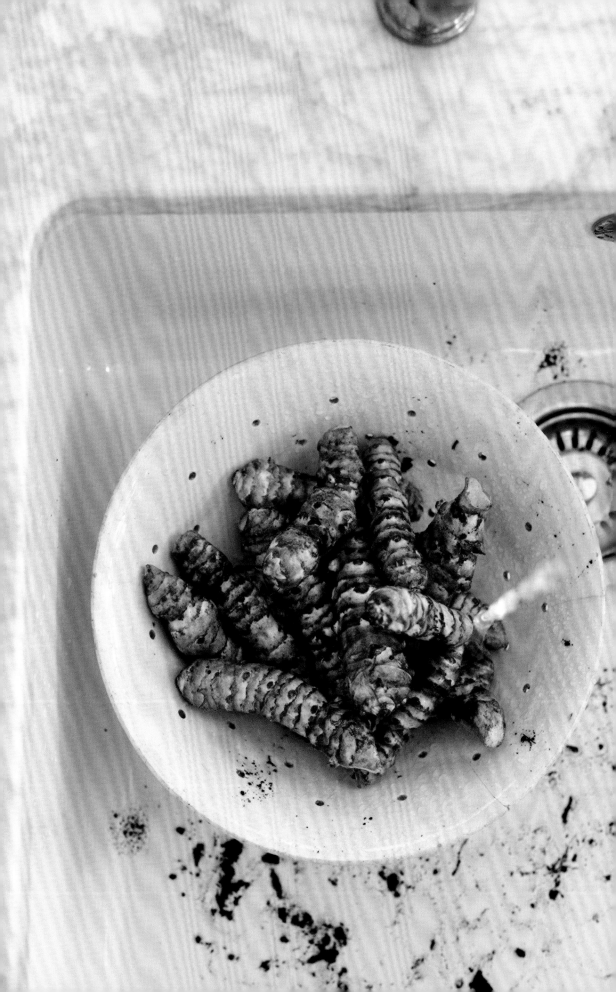

Herb-roasted root vegetables

Serves 4
201 calories per serving
A dish of roasted root vegetables is a wonderful accompaniment to a roast dinner. Crisply roasted Jerusalem artichokes are soft-centred nuggets of pleasure, and here they are teamed with equally delicious parsnips and baby beetroots.

400g Jerusalem artichokes, scrubbed clean
2 parsnips (unpeeled)
400g raw baby beetroots (unpeeled)
Olive oil for drizzling
1 tbsp honey
A small handful of fresh thyme
4 fresh rosemary sprigs
1 tbsp dried tarragon
1 tbsp dried oregano
Flaked sea salt and cracked black pepper

1   Preheat the oven to 200°C/Fan 180°C/Gas 6.
2   Scrub the artichokes and parsnips thoroughly, then cut them into 2cm pieces and place on a baking tray. Scrub the beetroots and add them to the baking tray (if any are particularly large, cut them in half or into quarters so that the vegetables are all roughly the same size).
3   Drizzle a little olive oil and the honey over the vegetables and scatter over the herbs and a good pinch each of salt and pepper. Roast for about 35 minutes until the vegetables are tender but crisp on the outside.

Jerusalem artichoke and shallot soup

Serves 4
122 calories per serving
This is a sublime soup to make during the winter months, so thick and creamy and wonderfully more-ish. I roast the artichokes first as this brings out their nutty, caramel flavour. Leaving the skins on adds even more flavour, so be sure to blitz well for a silky-smooth soup.

400g Jerusalem artichokes, scrubbed clean
4 banana shallots, cut into quarters through the root
2 garlic cloves
4 fresh thyme sprigs, plus extra to garnish
1 tsp rapeseed oil, plus extra for drizzling
500ml vegetable stock
Flaked sea salt and cracked black pepper

1   Preheat the oven to 200°C/Fan 180°C/Gas 6.
2   Roughly chop the artichokes. Place on a baking tray with the shallots, garlic and thyme sprigs. Drizzle over the oil and season with salt and pepper. Roast for 20–25 minutes until soft.
3   Pour the stock into a pan and bring to the boil.
4   Remove the sprigs of thyme from the tray, then tip the artichokes, shallots and garlic into the stock. Lower the heat to a simmer and cook for 10 minutes. Blitz together with a hand blender, or in a food processor, to make a completely smooth soup.
5   Serve hot, garnished with a few thyme leaves, a drizzle of oil and some cracked black pepper.

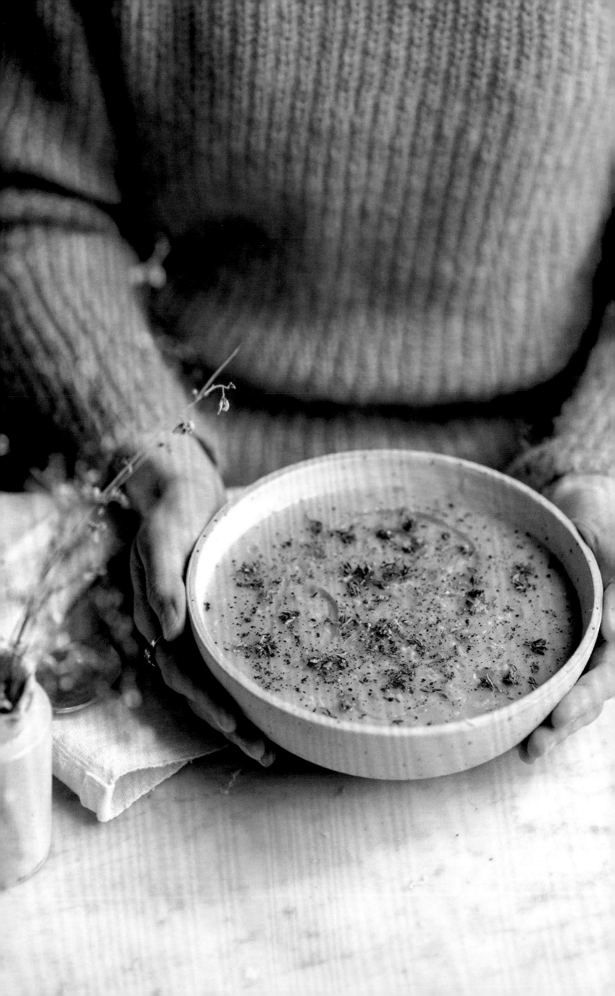

Jerusalem artichoke
polpette with tomato sauce

Serves 4
265 calories per serving
These vegetarian meatballs in a classic tomato
sauce are the epitome of comfort food. Roasted
artichokes give a richly earthy taste to the little
balls, and the chickpeas add lightness to the
texture. I often serve these with wild rice, but the
dish also works well with spaghetti, courgetti or
mashed potato.

200g Jerusalem artichokes, scrubbed clean
    and roughly chopped
Rapeseed oil for drizzling and frying
2 eggs
200g jarred chickpeas (drained weight)
6 tbsp chickpea flour
1 tbsp dried mixed herbs
Zest of 2 lemons
Fresh basil leaves, to garnish

For the tomato sauce
500g cherry tomatoes, cut in half
100ml water
1 garlic clove, chopped
1 celery stick, diced
2 tbsp capers
A pinch of celery salt
½ tsp dried mixed herbs
Flaked sea salt and cracked black pepper

1   Preheat the oven to 200°C/Fan 180°C/Gas 6.
    Spread out the chopped artichokes on a
    roasting tray and drizzle over a little oil. Roast
    for 20–30 minutes until tender. Allow to cool,
    then place in a food processor and blitz well
    until smooth.

2   Transfer the blitzed artichoke to a large mixing
    bowl. Whisk in the eggs. Add the chickpeas,
    flour, mixed herbs, lemon zest and ½ teaspoon
    each of salt and pepper. Mix together well.
    Form into small balls and place on a plate.
    Cover with cling film and chill for 40 minutes.

3   To make the tomato sauce, put all of the
    ingredients into a small saucepan. Bring to
    the boil, then simmer, stirring occasionally, for
    20–30 minutes until the tomatoes have broken
    down and the sauce has thickened.

4   Heat some oil in a frying pan. When it is hot,
    add the artichoke polpette and fry until they
    are golden on all sides. Serve with the tomato
    sauce and garnished with basil.

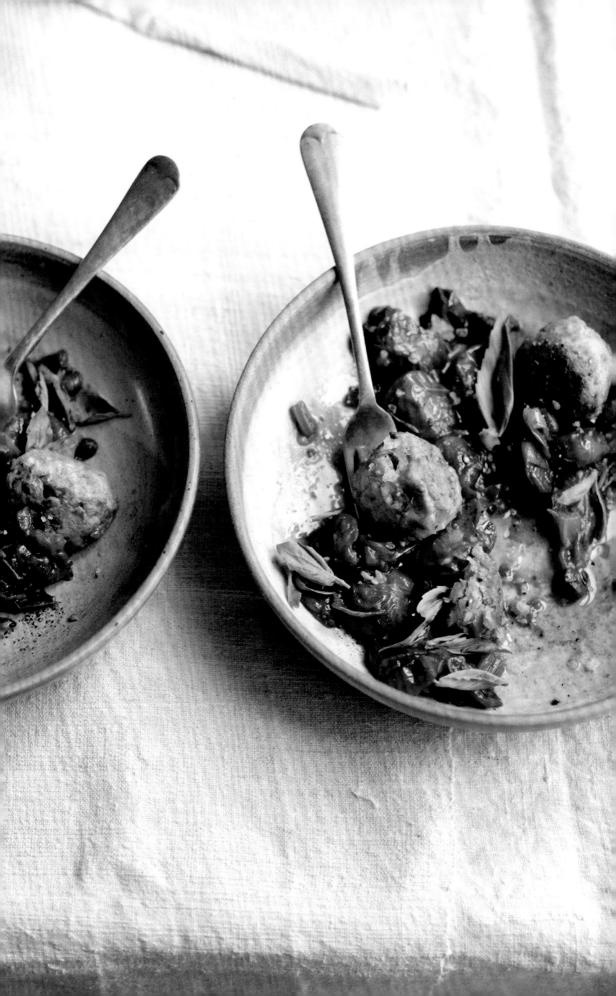

Carrot

You can probably tell from the fronds of the carrot that it is part of the parsley family, meaning that it's related to celery, fennel and parsnips. (It's always useful to know the family tree of a vegetable because relatives tend to work well together in cooking – as proven by the carrot, fennel and celery salad on page 194.)

With carrots, quality is crucial but finding a carrot that tastes as good as it looks can be a difficult task. I insist on buying organic carrots (one of the few organic items in my shopping basket) because mass-produced 'donkey' carrots do not a tasty dish make. I am partial to heritage carrots. These can be difficult to come by in the supermarket but are generally available in good greengrocers and farmer's markets in season. During the months of May to October, nothing can beat the beautiful purple, yellow and pink varieties that crop up.

If I'm making a stew like the one on page 198, I will always hunt down a stubby Chantenay carrot for its good flavour and firm texture. I also love to use carrots in baking as they add a subtle, earthy sweetness. My mini carrot muffins (see page 200), for example, are perfect to enjoy during the afternoon with a cup of tea, as they sit somewhere between a sweet treat and a savoury snack.

Carrots are fairly easy to grow in your garden. They just need a good amount of sunshine and some well-drained fertile soil. Sow the seeds in April for a late-summer crop.

Nutritional bonus

Nutritionally, carrots are a great source of **carotene**, which the body turns into **vitamin A,** and of **fibre**. But the question on everyone's lips is: will eating carrots help you to see in the dark or give you an orange complexion? Only if you eat 100kg a week!

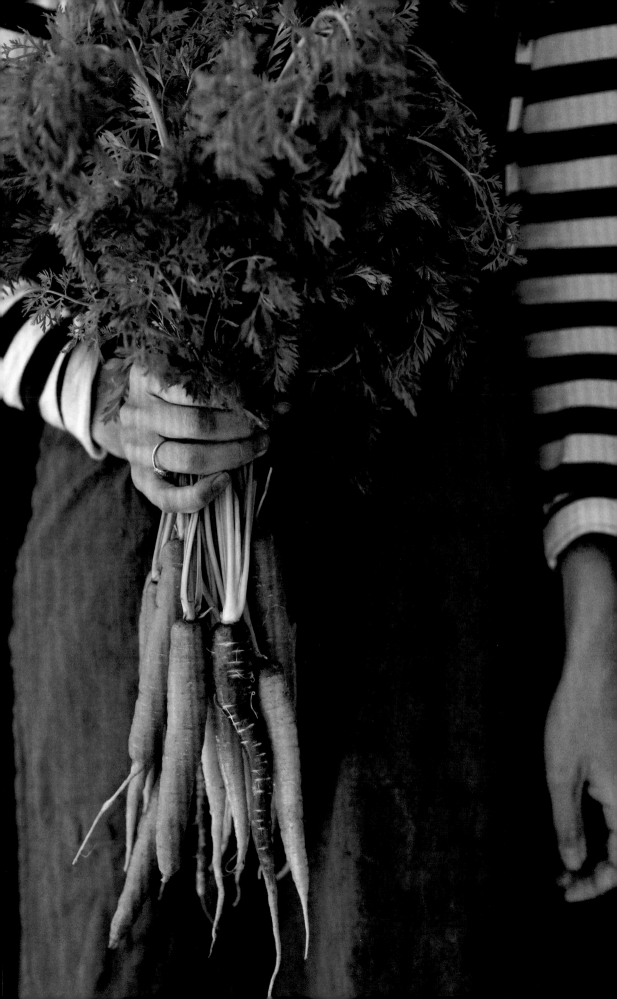

Carrot, fennel and celery salad with vegan mayo

Serves 2
252 calories per serving
This salad is minimalist perfection. The ribbons of carrot mingle with thin slices of fennel and celery in a rich vegan mayonnaise. It is a perfect side dish for frittata or quiche, or you can mix in some rice or chickpeas for a more substantial main dish.

3 large carrots
2 fennel bulbs, fronds removed
2 celery sticks

For the vegan mayo
3 tbsp soya yoghurt
1 tsp English mustard powder
Juice of ½ lemon
2 tbsp rapeseed oil
Flaked sea salt and cracked black pepper

To garnish
Zest of 1 lemon
A small handful of fresh dill, roughly chopped

1 Use a vegetable peeler to shave the carrots into long ribbons. Place them in a large mixing bowl. Using a mandoline, thinly slice the fennel and celery. If you don't have a mandoline just use a sharp knife and cut the vegetables as thinly as possible.
2 To make the vegan mayo, place the soya yoghurt in a small bowl, add the mustard powder and lemon juice, and mix thoroughly. Gradually add the oil while whisking so that it binds with the yoghurt. Season with salt and pepper to taste.
3 Mix the mayo with the vegetables and garnish with lemon zest and fresh dill.

Heritage carrot and black rice salad

Serves 2
555 calories per serving
There are now lots of organic farms in the UK rising to the challenge of producing colourful and delicious heritage carrots. In this salad they look beautiful against a dark background of black rice. The tarragon dressing is bold and full of flavour.

100g black rice
100g Puy lentils
150g rocket
1 tbsp chopped fresh tarragon
1 tbsp capers
Zest of 2 lemons
1 tbsp sunflower seeds, toasted
1 tbsp rapeseed oil, plus extra for frying
300g small heritage carrots, scrubbed
Flaked sea salt and cracked black pepper

1 Put the rice in a pan with a pinch of salt and cover with three times the amount of water. Bring to the boil, then leave to simmer for 30–35 minutes until the rice is tender.
2 At the same time, put the lentils in another pan, cover with three times the amount of water and simmer for 15–20 minutes until cooked but still with a bite.
3 Drain the rice and lentils and leave to cool, then tip into a mixing bowl and set aside.
4 Finely chop the rocket, tarragon and capers together. Put into a small mixing bowl and add the lemon zest, sunflower seeds, oil, and salt and pepper to taste. Mix well. Add half of the herb mixture to the lentils and rice and fold in.
5 Heat a little oil in a frying pan and sauté the carrots until tender, adding a splash of water if the pan gets too hot and the carrots begin to catch.
6 To serve, spoon the rice mixture on to plates, add the carrots and top with the remaining herb mixture.

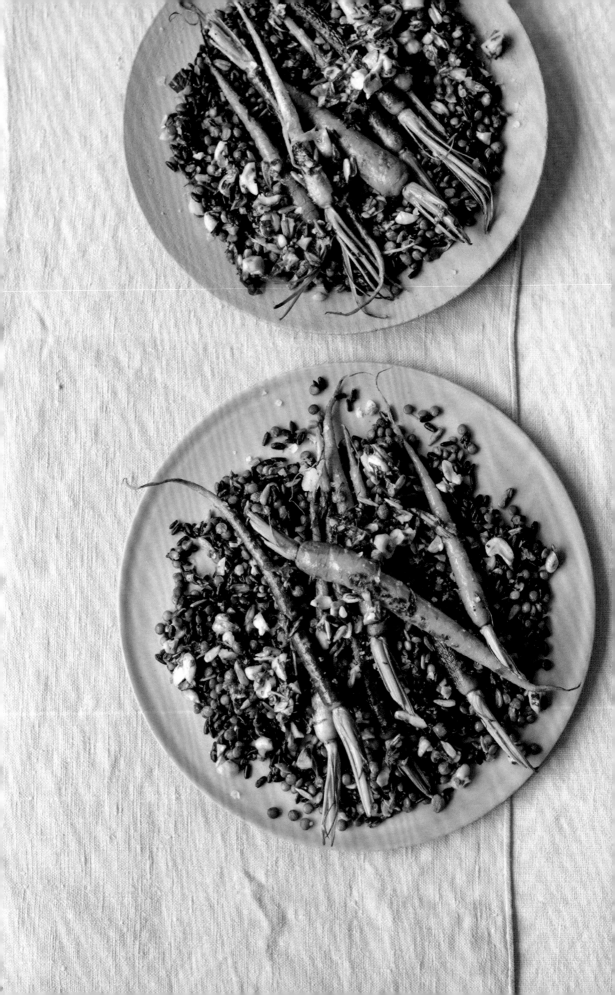

Roasted carrots, buckwheat and pecan salad

Serves 2
705 calories per serving
I am a big fan of preserved lemons and they work particularly well in this warm salad. Sweet carrots, nutty buckwheat, preserved lemon and crunchy pecans make a heavenly combination, remarkably easy to rustle up for lunch or dinner.

150g buckwheat
6 heritage carrots, scrubbed and cut
   lengthways in half
1 garlic clove, chopped
1 tbsp olive oil
1 tbsp honey
Zest of 1 lemon
50g pecans
1 preserved lemon
200ml soya yoghurt
½ tsp ground cumin
Flaked sea salt and cracked black pepper

1. Preheat the oven to 200°C/Fan 180°C/Gas 6. Line a baking tray with greaseproof paper.
2. Put the buckwheat into a pan with a pinch of salt and cover with three times the amount of water. Bring to the boil, then simmer gently for 15–20 minutes until the buckwheat is tender and has become a lighter shade of green. Drain well and set aside.
3. Spread the carrots on the lined baking tray with the garlic. Drizzle the olive oil and honey over the carrots, and sprinkle with the lemon zest and a pinch each of salt and pepper. Roast for 20 minutes. Add the pecans and continue roasting for 8 minutes until the pecans are toasted and the carrots are tender.
4. Put the preserved lemon, soya yoghurt and ground cumin in a small food processor and blitz until smooth.
5. Mix the roasted carrots and pecans with the buckwheat. Drizzle over the preserved lemon dressing to serve.

Carrot, broccoli stalk and barley soup

Serves 2
289 calories per serving

My children love broccoli florets but refuse to eat the stalks, so I often have broccoli stalks hanging around in my vegetable bowl. I have now found a great way to use them up by combining them with carrots in a soup. With its chunky texture and flavoursome broth, it's reminiscent of minestrone – a particular favourite with my husband.

100g pearl barley
3 carrots, roughly chopped
300g broccoli stalks/stems, roughly chopped
1 heaped tsp vegetable bouillon powder
Flaked sea salt and cracked black pepper

1   Rinse the pearl barley in cold running water, then put it into a large pan with three times the amount of water. Bring to the boil and simmer for about 25 minutes until tender. Drain and set aside.

2   Add the carrots and broccoli to a pan of water with a pinch of salt and bring to the boil. Cook until tender but not too soft. Using a spider or slotted spoon, scoop out the vegetables and place them in a food processor; keep the cooking liquid in the pan. Blitz the vegetables until they are finely chopped but not mushy.

3   Return the vegetables to the pan of water and add the pearl barley, vegetable bouillon and a pinch of pepper. Simmer for a few minutes, then serve.

Carrot cassoulet

Serves 4

502 calories per serving

I think carrots should always feature prominently in a cassoulet. In this recipe, I roast carrots with other orange and red vegetables before tipping them into a casserole dish with some stock and haricot beans. The whole lot is then left to simmer away in the oven, developing a lovely depth of flavour before the crispy topping is added. A spinach and watercress salad is the perfect accompaniment for the cassoulet, which offers a maximum of fuzzy comfort on a winter's evening.

1 onion, chopped
3 garlic cloves, chopped
500g carrots (preferably Chantenay), sliced
1 swede, diced
1 red pepper, seeded and sliced
4 sun-dried tomatoes, roughly chopped
3 fresh thyme sprigs
1 bay leaf
2 tbsp olive oil
500g jarred haricot or cannellini beans, drained
400ml vegetable stock
2 slices light rye bread

For the salad (optional)
100g spinach
100g watercress
1 tbsp olive oil
Juice of 1 lemon
Flaked sea salt and cracked black pepper

1 Preheat the oven to 200°C/Fan 180°C/Gas 6.
2 Spread the onion, garlic, carrots, swede, red pepper and sun-dried tomatoes on a baking tray. Add the herbs. Drizzle over half of the oil and season with a little salt and pepper. Place in the oven and roast for 20–25 minutes until the vegetables are slightly browned and are beginning to catch on the ends.
3 Transfer the vegetables to a casserole. Add the haricot beans and vegetable stock and stir to mix. Cover the casserole, place it in the oven and cook for a further 30–35 minutes until all the vegetables are tender.
4 Tear the rye bread into small chunks. Remove the lid from the casserole and scatter the rye bread pieces over the vegetables. Continue to cook in the oven, uncovered, for 10–15 minutes until the bread pieces are crisp.
5 If you wish to make the salad, put the leaves into a bowl, drizzle over the oil and lemon juice, season to taste and toss.

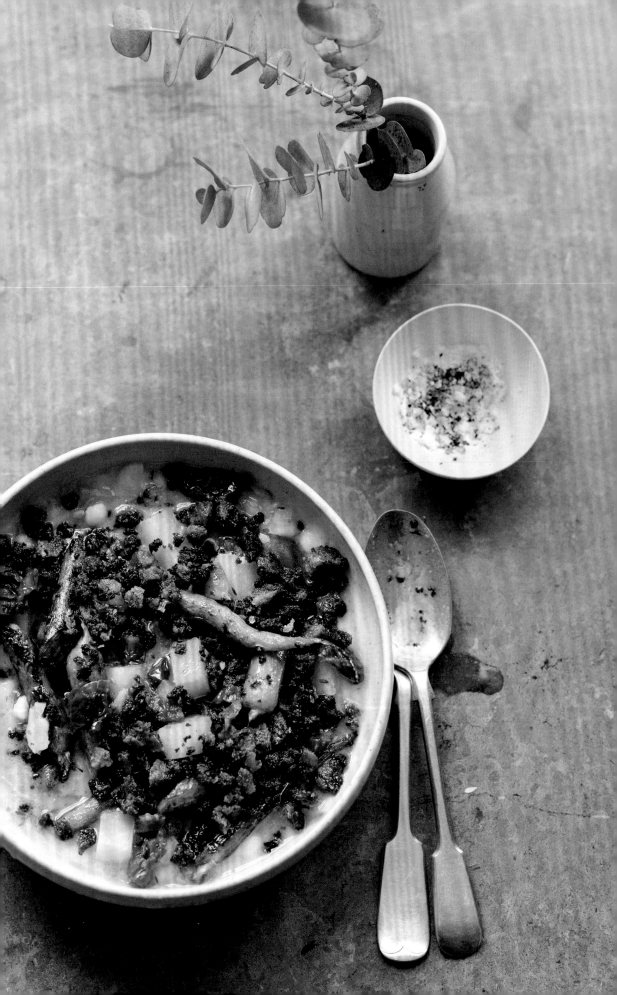

Carrot muffins

Makes 9

232 calories per muffin

These muffins are both sweet and spicy. I use coconut sugar in them, which brings out the sweetness of carrots better than a standard refined sugar. The muffins can be stored in an airtight container, ready to serve for breakfast or as a snack any time over two or three days.

2 eggs
70ml rapeseed oil
1 ripe banana, mashed
2 tbsp honey
2 tbsp unrefined coconut sugar
1 apple, grated
2 carrots, grated
A pinch of flaked sea salt
½ tsp gluten-free bicarbonate of soda
½ tsp ground cinnamon
100g porridge oats
100ml oat milk
2 tbsp gluten-free flour
50g walnuts, chopped

1   Preheat the oven to 200°C/Fan 180°C/Gas 6. Line a 9-hole muffin tin with paper cases.

2   Put the eggs into a large mixing bowl and whisk them together. Add the oil and whisk until the mixture is fluffy. Add the banana, honey and coconut sugar and whisk until smoothly combined. Add the apple, carrots, salt, bicarbonate of soda, cinnamon, oats, oat milk and flour and mix well together with a wooden spoon.

3   Divide the mixture equally among the muffin cases. Sprinkle the walnuts on top. Bake for about 30 minutes until golden and soft to the touch but cooked through (a skewer inserted into the centre of a muffin should come out clean). Remove from the oven and allow to cool in the tin for 10 minutes before transferring the muffins to a wire rack to cool further.

4   Serve warm, or cool completely and keep in an airtight container for up to 2 days.

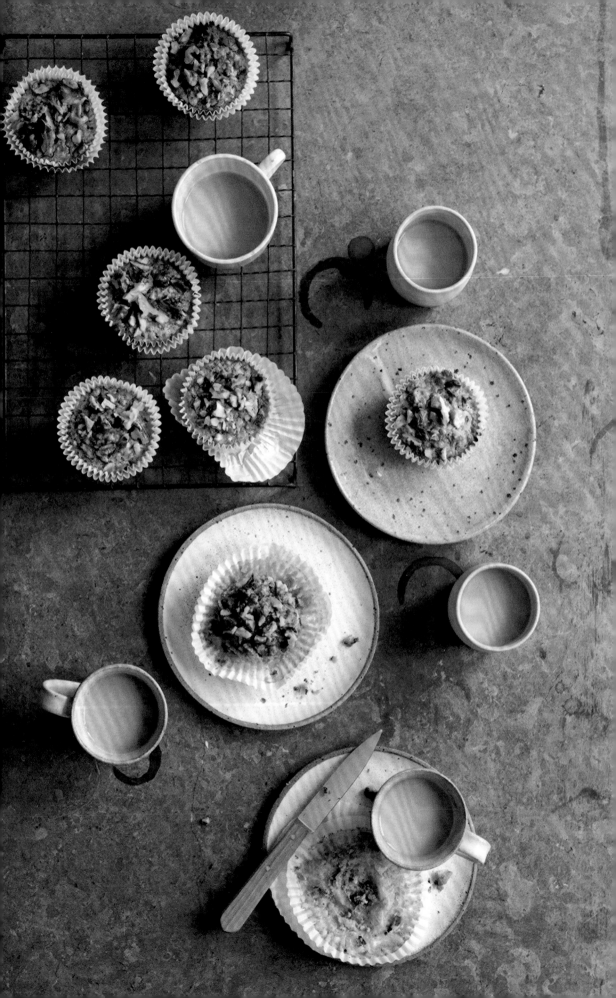

Parsnip

Like their relative the carrot, parsnips are biennial plants (which means they naturally come to fruition every second year). They can be eaten raw, but are more often roasted, sautéed or steamed. Most of us know that we enjoy crispy parsnips with our roast dinner but there are many more possibilities to explore. For example, using grated parsnips instead of potato in a classically savoury dish such as rosti (see page 204) will add a delightful sweetness.

Parsnips are easy to grow since they need very little maintenance, and they can be left in the ground in your vegetable garden until you are ready to cook with them. When selecting parsnips from your greengrocer, go for the small to medium-sized ones, as larger parsnips tend to be more fibrous and less flavourful.

Parsnips are in season between September and March, which is why they are most commonly used in warming, hearty dishes during the colder months.

Nutritional bonus

Parsnips are nutritious vegetables and a particularly good source of soluble **fibre**, which helps to reduce levels of 'bad' cholesterol, as well as supporting a healthy digestive system. Parsnips are also a good source of **folate** and **potassium**.

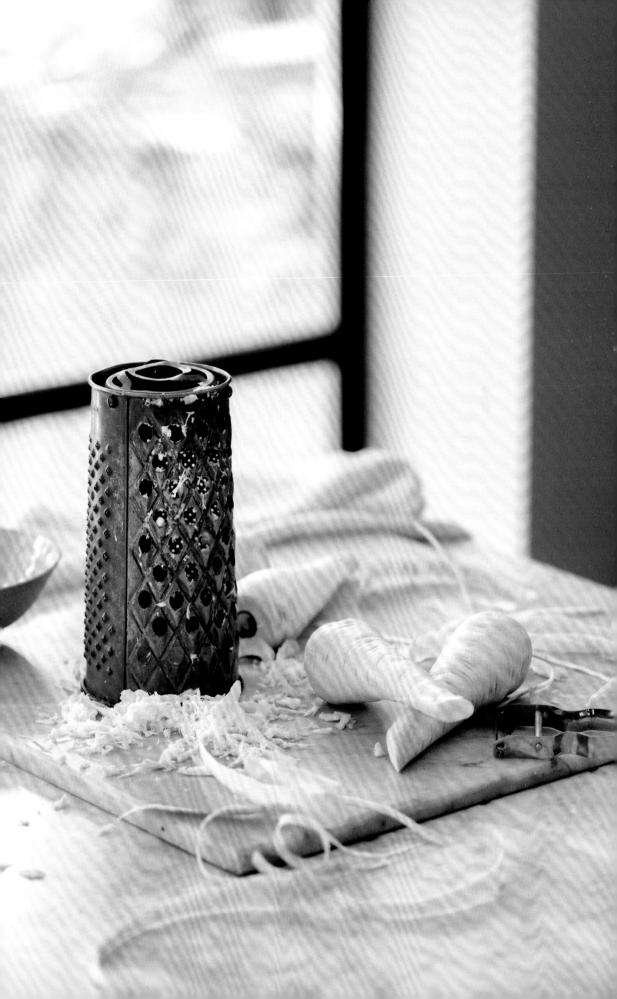

Parsnip rosti with fried egg

Serves 2

371 calories per serving

A rosti is typically made with potato but I find that parsnips work just as well, particularly when the rosti is topped with a tangy dressing and a rich fried egg. The parsnip rosti crisp up beautifully when fried and have a good balance of sweet and savoury flavours.

4 eggs
Fresh flat-leaf parsley leaves, to garnish

For the dressing
2 tbsp capers
1 tsp dried tarragon
Zest of 1 lemon
A small handful of fresh flat-leaf parsley
A drizzle of olive oil

For the rosti
300g parsnips
1 egg, beaten
2 tbsp gluten-free flour
Rapeseed oil for frying
Flaked sea salt and cracked black pepper

1 Put all the ingredients for the dressing on a chopping board and roughly chop them all together to form a coarse mix. Transfer to a bowl and set aside.

2 Grate the parnips on to a thick tea towel. Gather up the edges of the towel and squeeze out any excess liquid from the parsnips – the drier they are, the crisper the rosti will be. Place the grated parsnips in a bowl and add the egg, flour, and a pinch each of salt and pepper. Mix well.

3 Divide the mixture into four equal pieces and shape each portion into a flat patty. Heat a little oil in a non-stick frying pan and fry the patties until crisp and golden on both sides.

4 In another frying pan, fry the eggs in a little oil until cooked the way you like them.

5 To serve, place two rostis on each serving plate, top with a fried egg and spoon over the caper dressing. Garnish with parsley leaves.

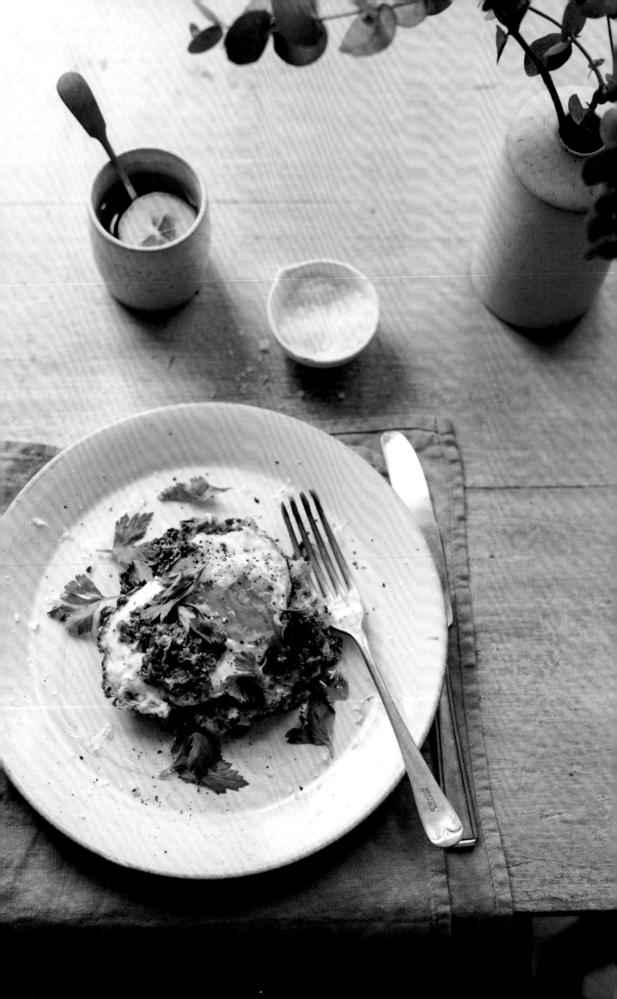

Parsnip rémoulade

Serves 2

401 calories per serving

Celariac rémoulade is a classic French winter salad with a rich, creamy sauce. I've made my version with parsnips rather than celeriac as I find them to be sweeter with a softer texture, and I've left the mayonnaise and cream out of my sauce, insteading whisking oil into mustard until creamy. This makes a lovely sharp, fresh topping for a thick slice of rye bread, along with some crisp lettuce.

2 tbsp Dijon mustard
1 tbsp wholegrain mustard
1 tbsp brown rice vinegar
Juice of 2 lemons
2 tbsp rapeseed oil
4 parsnips
3 fresh tarragon sprigs, chopped
A handful of fresh flat-leaf parsley, chopped
Flaked sea salt and cracked black pepper

To serve
Rye bread
Baby Gem lettuce

1   Whisk together the mustards, vinegar and lemon juice in a bowl, then gradually whisk in the oil to create a thick sauce. Season with a good pinch each of salt and pepper.
2   Coarsely grate the parsnips. Stir them into the sauce. Mix through the tarragon and parsley. Serve with some warm rye bread and Baby Gem lettuce or make open sandwiches.

Honey-roasted parsnips and carrots

Serves 4

320 calories per serving

A perfectly roasted parsnip should be crispy on the outside and fluffy on the inside. Tossing the parsnips in honey before roasting brings out their mellow sweetness and adds a lovely sticky glaze. Serve this as a side dish, or make a meal of it with wild rice and salad.

3 parsnips, scrubbed
4 large heritage carrots, scrubbed
2 tbsp honey
1 tbsp rapeseed oil
2 tbsp tamari
4 fresh thyme sprigs, leaves picked
1 tsp dried oregano
½ tsp dried tarragon
1 tsp dried parsley
100g pistachios, roughly chopped
Juice of 1 lemon

1   Cut each of the parsnips and carrots in half lengthways and then into quarters. Cook in boiling water for 5 minutes. Drain, rinse with cold water and leave to cool.
2   Mix together the honey, oil, tamari and herbs in a bowl. Add the parsnips and carrots. Leave to marinate in the fridge for at least 30 minutes.
3   Preheat the oven to 200°C/Fan 180°C/Gas 6. Line a baking tray with greaseproof paper.
4   Tip the parsnips and carrots, with their marinade, on to the prepared tray and roast for 20–25 minutes until golden. Transfer the roasted vegetables to a platter. Sprinkle with the pistachios and lemon juice.

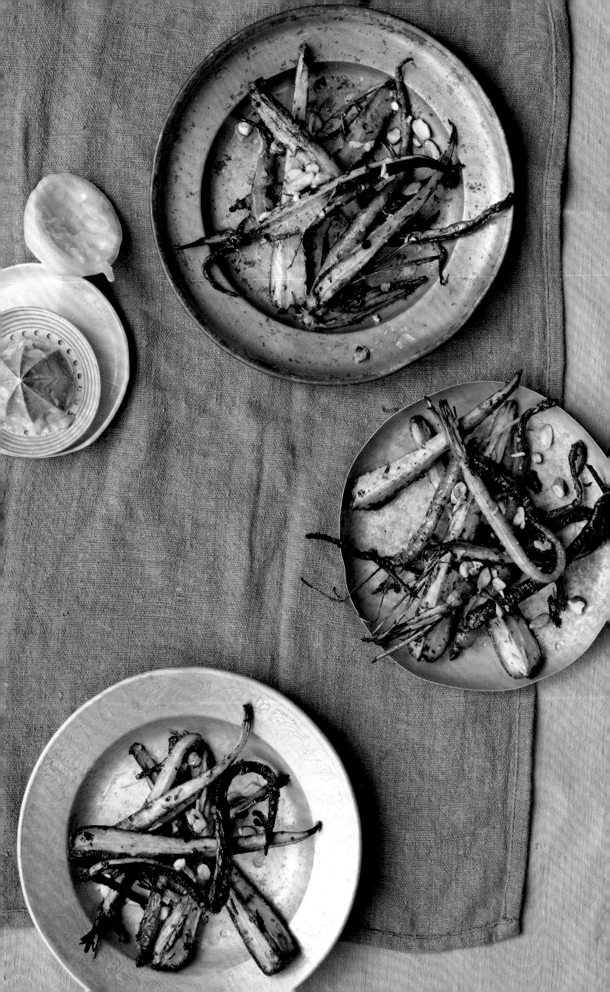

Beetroot

Have you ever made a pickled-beetroot egg? Well, I hadn't even heard of them until recently, when an American friend told me that she had eaten them as a child. To make them you pickle some beetroots for about 2 hours (I like to use a combination of brown rice vinegar and honey). Then you remove the beetroots and put hard-boiled eggs into the pickling liquor in their place. Leave the eggs until they are a bright pink colour. The liquor also gives them a sweet, tangy taste. I now like to make pickled-beetroot eggs with my three-year-old son Fin, who thinks the idea of eating a pink egg is hilarious. (Use the pickled beetroot in a simple salad with some rocket leaves and good mayonnaise, and top it with a pink egg.)

Beetroots come in a rainbow of colours, and in all shapes and sizes. I like to add candy-striped Chioggia beetroot to salads, as its light pink and white rings will make any dish look lovely. Golden beetroot, which has a more subtle flavour than the classic red variety, is great for roasting.

As well as the exciting colour, beetroot has much to commend it in terms of flavour and texture. Whether it's grated for fritters, pickled for a salad, simmered in a curry or blitzed into a pancake batter, there are no limits for the bold, bright beetroot. (I am also a fan of beetroot juice, which adds earthiness to a fruit juice mix, especially one made with celery and apple.)

Nutritional bonus
Beetroot is a great source of **potassium** and **folate**. The leafy tops are nutritious too, containing **calcium** and **iron**, so don't throw them away.

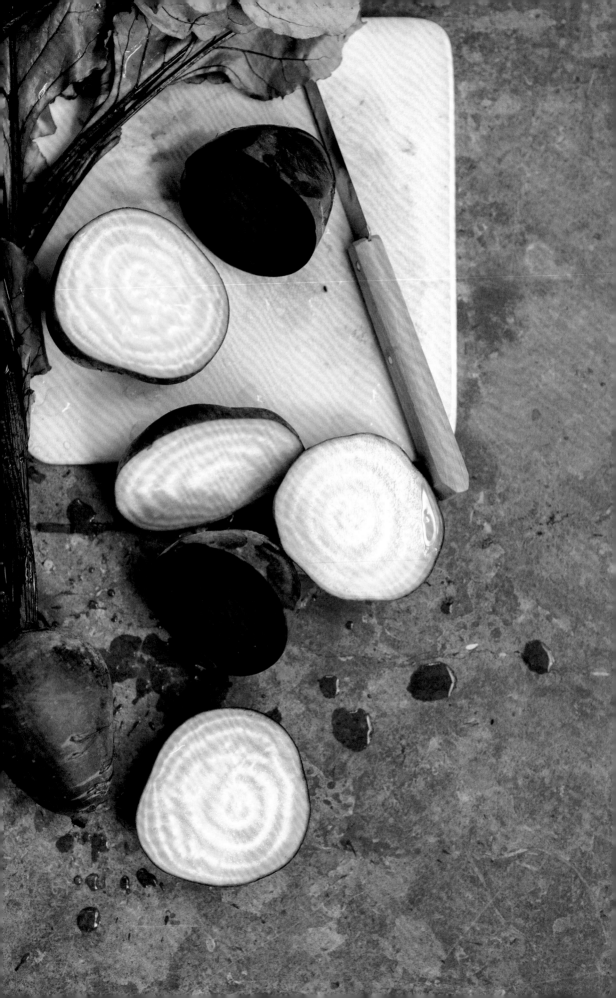

Spiced root vegetable rosti with poached egg

Serves 2
372 calories per serving

Come the weekend, you might want something a bit more inspiring than toast or cereal for breakfast, and I bet it will usually involve an egg. If you like your eggs poached, these spiced root vegetable rostis are the perfect base. They can be made with most root vegetables: here I've used beetroot, potato and carrot, but butternut squash, parsnips and sweet potato are also good.

1 small potato
1 raw beetroot
1 carrot
1 tsp 'steak' seasoning (see page 132)
1 tbsp gluten-free flour
3 eggs
Olive oil for drizzling
1 avocado, peeled and sliced
A handful of fresh coriander, chopped
Flaked sea salt and cracked black pepper

1 Grate the potato, beetroot and carrot. Mix them together in a large mixing bowl, sprinkle generously with salt and leave for 20 minutes.

2 Tip the vegetable mixture on to a thick tea towel. Gather up the edges of the towel and squeeze out all of the excess liquid. Put the vegetables back into the bowl and add the steak seasoning, flour and 1 egg. Mix well. Place in the fridge to chill for 20 minutes.

3 Preheat the oven to 200°C/Fan 180°C/Gas 6.

4 Divide the mixture into six equal balls and place them on a baking tray. Flatten each ball to create a disc about 8cm in diameter. Drizzle with oil. Bake for 20–25 minutes until crisp and golden.

5 Bring a pan of water to the boil, then turn down to a simmer. About 3 minutes before the rostis are ready, poach the remaining eggs: swirl the water around with a wooden spoon to create a well, then drop the first egg into it. Create another well and drop in the second egg. Cook for 2 minutes, then use a slotted spatula to remove the eggs from the water and place on kitchen paper to drain.

6 Place three rostis on each plate and top with a poached egg and sliced avocado. Sprinkle with salt, pepper and coriander.

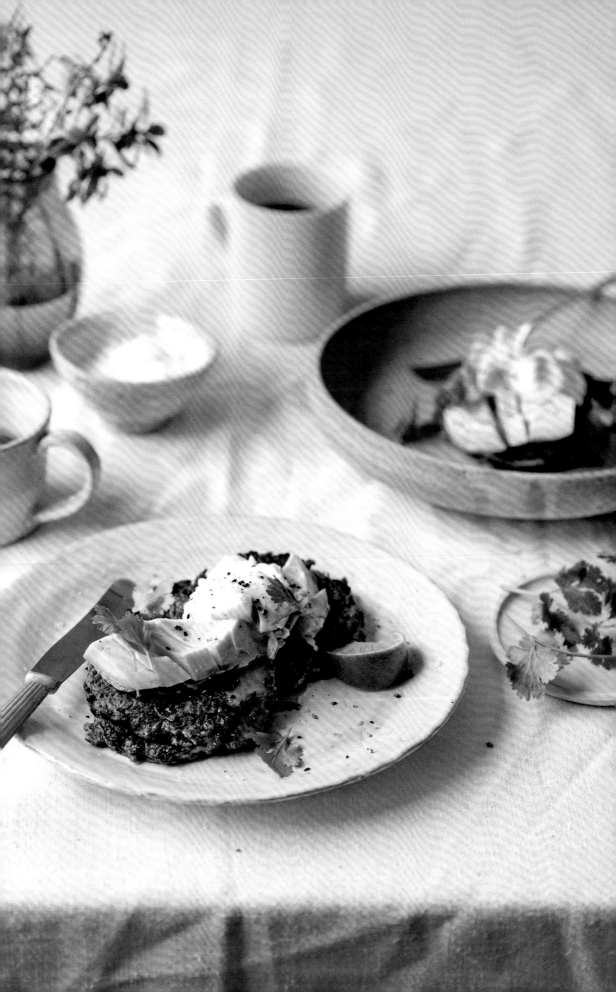

Beetroot crêpes with creamy tarragon mushrooms

Serves 4
272 calories per serving

These crêpes are a fun way to get children to eat vegetables. They'll love the bright red colour of the beetroot batter and can help with whisking it. The filling can be anything you choose – some rocket and a few slices of avocado, or hummus with chopped tomatoes. This mushroom and tarragon filling is an indulgent treat and probably my favourite.

2 large raw beetroots
2 eggs
2 tbsp gluten-free flour
200ml oat milk
1 tbsp sunflower seeds
1 tbsp rapeseed oil

For the filling
Rapeseed oil for frying
200g chestnut mushrooms, sliced
1 tbsp gluten-free flour
200ml oat milk
A small handful of fresh tarragon, leaves picked
  and roughly chopped
Zest of 2 lemons
Flaked sea salt and cracked black pepper

1 To make the batter for the crêpes, grate the beetroots, then place in a food processor and blitz to a smooth paste. Transfer the paste to a bowl and whisk in the eggs. Sift in the flour and whisk together to form a thick paste, then gradually whisk in the oat milk to make a batter that has a consistency similar to single cream. Season with a good pinch of salt. Set aside at room temperature for about 20 minutes.

2 Toast the sunflower seeds in a small dry frying pan until golden. Set aside.

3 To make the filling, heat a little oil in a frying pan and sauté the mushrooms until they are crisp. Add the flour and mix it through the mushrooms on a medium heat. Gradually add the oat milk, whisking it in to create a sauce. Remove from the heat and stir in the tarragon (reserve some for garnish), half the lemon zest, and salt and pepper to taste.

4 To make the crêpes, place a non-stick frying pan on a high heat and add the oil, then ladle in about a quarter of the batter, tipping the pan to create an even coverage on the bottom. When the crêpe is lightly golden on the base, flip it over and cook the other side until golden. Tip the crêpe on to some greaseproof paper, cover with a tea towel and keep warm. Continue to cook the remaining crêpes in the same way.

5 While you are cooking the crêpes, gently reheat the filling. Spoon it on to the crêpes and top with toasted sunflower seeds and the remaining tarragon and lemon zest, then fold over.

Candy beetroot and blood orange salad

Serves 2
606 calories per serving

A salad should always be two things: beautiful to look at and delicious to eat. This salad is just that. The stripes of candy beetroot add a fun element, and their sweet flavour is perfectly matched with tangy blood oranges.

5 raw candy beetroots
2 blood oranges
1 courgette
2 carrots
70g cashew nuts

For the dressing
1 blood orange
2 lemons
1 tbsp ready-made English mustard
1 tbsp rapeseed oil
A small handful of fresh chives, roughly chopped
Flaked sea salt and cracked black pepper

To garnish
1 tbsp snipped fresh chives
2 fresh mint sprigs, leaves picked

1. To make the dressing, squeeze the juice from the orange and lemons into a small mixing bowl, then whisk in the mustard, rapeseed oil, chives, and salt and pepper to taste. Set aside.

2. Cut the beetroots into very fine slices using a mandoline. (Alternatively, you can grate the beetroots; cut them into matchsticks; or slice them as thinly as possible with a sharp knife.) Place the beetroot in a large mixing bowl.

3. Peel the blood oranges, then cut out the segments from the surrounding membrane. Add the orange segments to the beetroot.

4. Using a vegetable peeler, shave the courgette and carrots into long ribbons. Add these to the mixing bowl.

5. Toast the cashew nuts in a small dry frying pan, then add to the bowl. Pour the dressing over and toss everything together. Serve garnished with chives and mint leaves.

Beetroot and shallot fritters

Serves 2
254 calories per serving

These fritters are delicious as a snack or starter, or they can be a part of an indulgent weekend breakfast. To ensure the crispest result, be sure to drain as much liquid from the grated beetroot as possible before mixing it with the rest of the ingredients. Then, as long as you have a good non-stick pan and your oil is hot, you can just ladle in the batter and let the heat work its magic.

3 raw beetroots
3 shallots, sliced
1 tbsp ground cumin
A handful of fresh coriander, finely chopped
1 green chilli, seeded and finely chopped
Zest of 1 lemon
2 eggs
2 tbsp gluten-free flour
1 tsp rapeseed oil
Flaked sea salt and cracked black pepper

To serve
Fresh coriander leaves
Lime or lemon wedges

1 Grate the beetroots on to a thick tea towel. Gather up the edges of the towel and squeeze out any excess liquid from the beetroot. Place the beetroot in a bowl with the shallots, cumin, coriander, green chilli, lemon zest and eggs and mix together well. Add the flour and some salt and pepper and mix again. Leave to stand for 10 minutes.

2 Heat the oil in a large non-stick frying pan. Add spoonfuls of the beetroot mixture to the hot pan, using about a heaped tablespoon for each fritter and cooking only a few at a time. Cook until the fritters are golden on both sides. Sprinkle with salt and pepper, garnish with coriander leaves and serve with lime or lemon wedges for squeezing over.

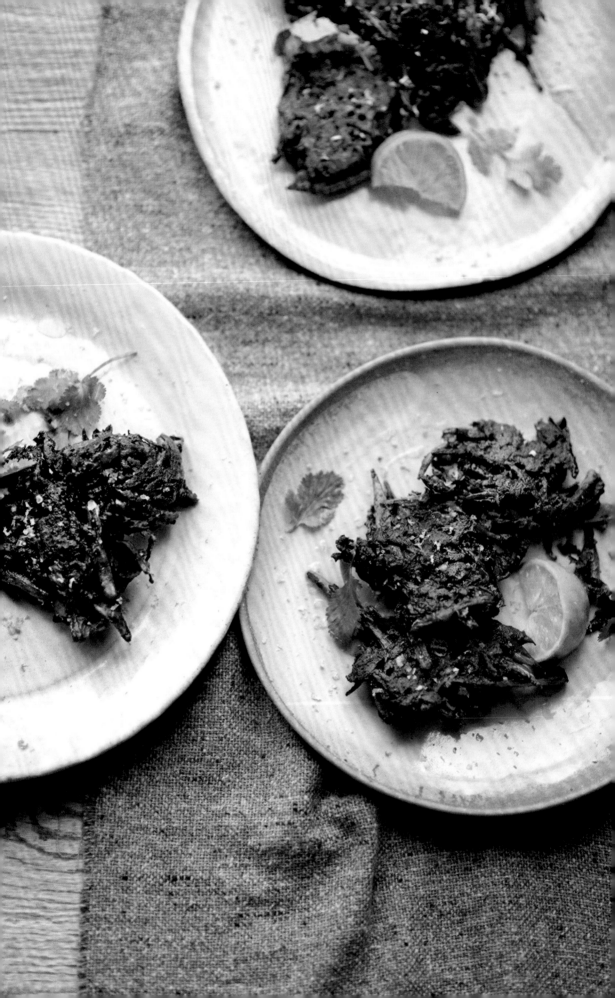

Beetroot and coconut curry

Serves 2
706 calories per serving

I find that beetroot works well with big bold spices as its sweetness brings a good balance, so here I've roasted it with both whole and ground spices, plus ginger and garlic. Adding the spices at the start of cooking the beetroot gives them time to penetrate the vegetable properly.

1 tsp fennel seeds
1 tsp cumin seeds
1 tbsp ground cumin
1 tbsp ground turmeric
1 tbsp sweet paprika
1 tsp crushed cardamom seeds
5 raw beetroots, peeled and quartered
1 onion, diced
1 garlic clove, finely chopped
A thumb-sized piece fresh root ginger, finely
   chopped
Coconut oil for frying
300ml water
2 celery sticks, diced
1 yellow pepper, seeded and sliced
250ml coconut milk
200g brown rice
Lime to serve

To garnish
1 tsp mustard seeds
1 tsp fennel seeds
A handful of fresh curry leaves

1   Preheat the oven to 200°C/Fan 180°C/Gas 6. Line a baking tray with greaseproof paper.
2   Mix together all the spices in a large bowl. Add the beetroot quarters and toss to coat them with the spices, then tip them on to the baking tray. Roast for 30 minutes until the beetroot is almost tender but still firm.
3   Meanwhile, fry the onion, garlic and ginger in a little coconut oil in a saucepan until the onion is browned.
4   Add the roasted beetroot to the saucepan along with the water, celery and yellow pepper. Bring to the boil, then put the lid on the pan and simmer gently for 20–30 minutes until the beetroot is tender. Add the coconut milk, stir well and simmer for a further 5 minutes.
5   While the curry is simmering, put the rice in a saucepan with a pinch of salt and cover with three times the amount of water. Bring to the boil, then simmer gently for 20–25 minutes until the rice is tender and fluffy. Drain.
6   Heat the mustard and fennel seeds with the curry leaves in a little coconut oil in a small frying pan until fragrant. Spoon this mixture on top of the curry and serve with the brown rice and lime to squeeze over.

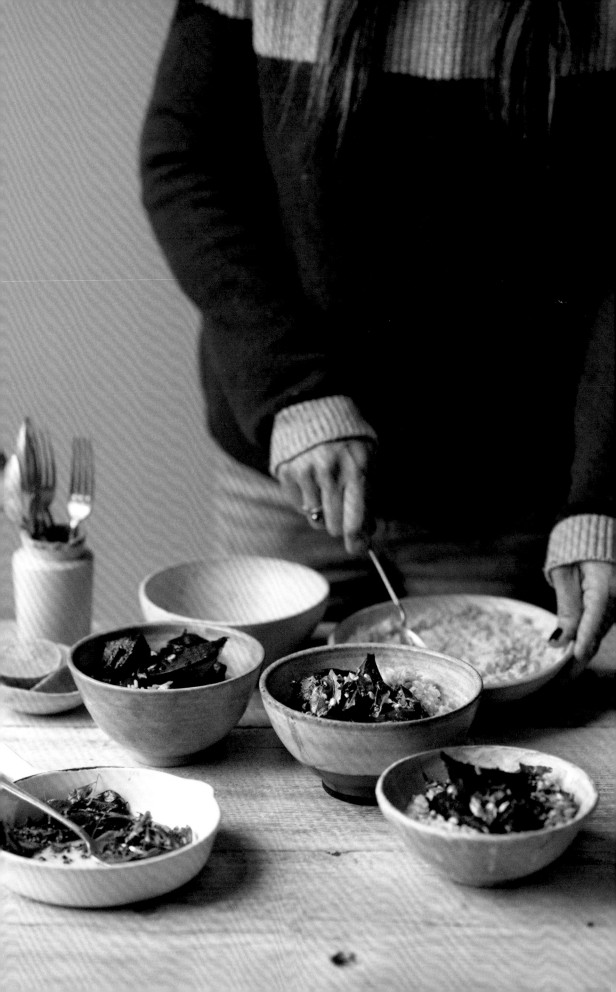

Leek

Leeks are part of the allium family, which means they're related to garlic and onions. Leeks may seem like biddable cousins when they're diced or sliced to be used as the base of a pie, soup or stew, but they come to the fore when left whole or in large pieces to be baked or roasted. Then their buttery, sweet flavour and deliciously soft texture can be truly appreciated.

They are quite easy to cook, but you still have to be alert because an undercooked leek is squeaky and tough, while an overcooked one will be slimy and bland. The secret to success is cooking them until they are golden and soft, but still holding their shape.

If you want to grow your own leeks, it's very simple. Sow the seeds in a pot in the spring before moving the leeks to the vegetable patch a few months later. During the summer months it's important to keep the soil moist, so you'll need to water your leeks at least two or three times a week. You should then get a good crop that will last from autumn all the way through to late winter.

Choosing the best leeks is important, whether in shops or from your garden – smaller is always better, as this means the leeks will have a deeper, sweeter flavour when you cook them.

Nutritional bonus
The most noteworthy benefit of leeks is that they contain plenty of a phytochemical of the flavonoid variety called **kaempferol**, which has been linked to reducing the risk of developing chronic disease.

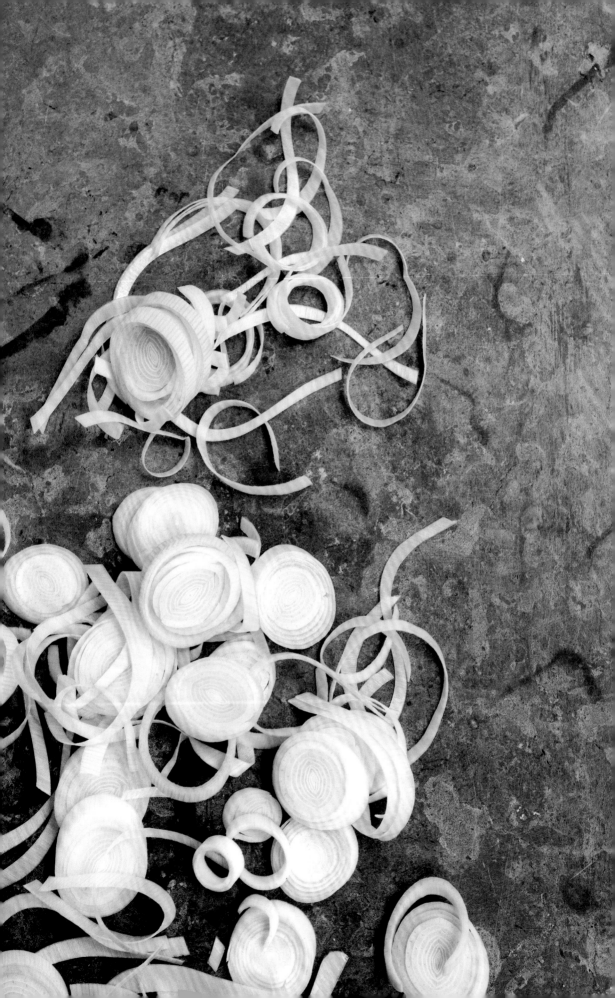

Leeks, peas and capers
on sourdough toast

Serves 1

602 calories per serving

This recipe was given to me by a friend who said it was her favourite evening dish when she was too tired to cook anything complicated. It's a quick recipe that delivers on flavour and satisfaction. The soft leeks, bright little peas and salty capers are all brought together with a good spoonful of Dijon mustard and the refreshing aniseed flavour of tarragon.

Rapeseed oil for frying
2 leeks, diced
100g podded fresh peas (or thawed frozen peas)
1 tbsp capers
1 tsp Dijon mustard
2 fresh tarragon sprigs
2 slices sourdough bread
Flaked sea salt and cracked black pepper

1   Heat a little oil in a frying pan over a medium heat and cook the leeks until they are softened and slightly golden.

2   Add the peas and capers and cook for a few more minutes until the peas are bright green. Stir in the mustard and tarragon and heat through. Remove from the heat and season to taste with salt and pepper.

3   Toast the sourdough bread and spoon the leek mixture on top.

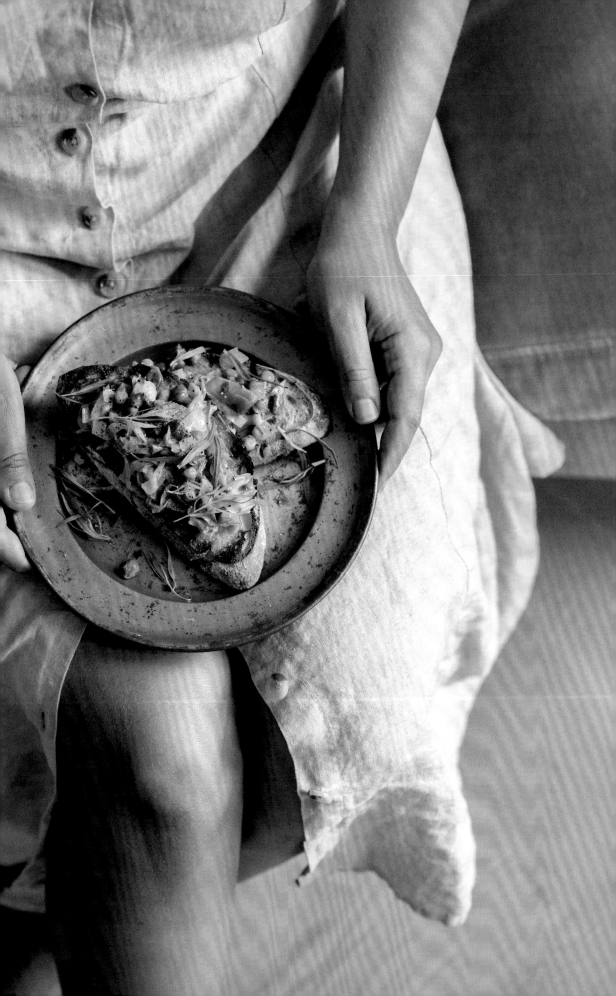

Leek and broccoli bake

Serves 4

327 calories per serving

This leek and broccoli bake is actually my mum's recipe, which I now make whenever I am in need of comfort. The browning of the leeks is important for the texture of the dish. Serve with a green salad.

2 leeks, dark green part trimmed
Rapeseed oil for frying
500g broccoli, cut into small florets
½ cauliflower, cut into small florets
150g gluten-free breadcrumbs

For the sauce
1 tbsp rapeseed oil
2 onions, finely chopped
2 garlic cloves, sliced
4 vine tomatoes, roughly chopped
6 chestnut mushrooms, roughly chopped
1 large courgette, roughly chopped
1 red pepper, seeded and roughly chopped
1 tsp dried mixed herbs
500ml water
Flaked sea salt and cracked black pepper

1   To make the sauce, heat the oil in a saucepan and cook the onions and garlic until softened. Add the tomatoes, mushrooms, courgette, red pepper, mixed herbs, water, and a little salt and pepper. Bring to the boil, then simmer for 20 minutes, stirring occasionally. Transfer to a food processor and blitz until smooth. Set the sauce aside in a clean pan.
2   Preheat the oven to 200°C/Fan 180°C/Gas 6.
3   Cut each leek across into three pieces about 7.5cm long. Heat the oil in a frying pan, add the leek pieces and sauté for about 10 minutes until they are browned on all sides. Add the broccoli and cook for a few minutes until it gets some colour.
4   Tip the leeks and broccoli into a baking dish and add the cauliflower florets. Cover with the sauce and scatter the breadcrumbs on top. Bake for 25–30 minutes until the crumbs are golden and all the vegetables are tender.

Leek, black lentil and caper salad

Serves 2

460 calories per serving

The mix of textures in this salad is what makes it so special – the al dente lentils with the softened leeks and crunchy rocket make for an enjoyable mouthful every time. Capers add a welcome sharp saltiness to complement the sweet leeks.

200g black lentils
1 tsp rapeseed oil
2 leeks, diced
1 courgette, diced
2 tbsp capers
100g sugarsnap peas, sliced in half
A small bunch of radishes, thinly sliced
A small handful of rocket
1 lemon, cut into wedges
Flaked sea salt and cracked black pepper

1   Put the lentils in a saucepan and cover with three times the amount of water. Bring to the boil, then simmer for about 20 minutes until soft. Drain and set aside.
2   Heat the oil in a frying pan and gently cook the leeks until softened. Add the courgette, capers and sugarsnap peas and sauté for about 5 minutes until all the vegetables are tender. Season with salt and pepper to taste.
3   While the vegetables are still warm, add the lentils and gently mix together. Fold in the radishes. Serve with the rocket and lemon wedges to squeeze over.

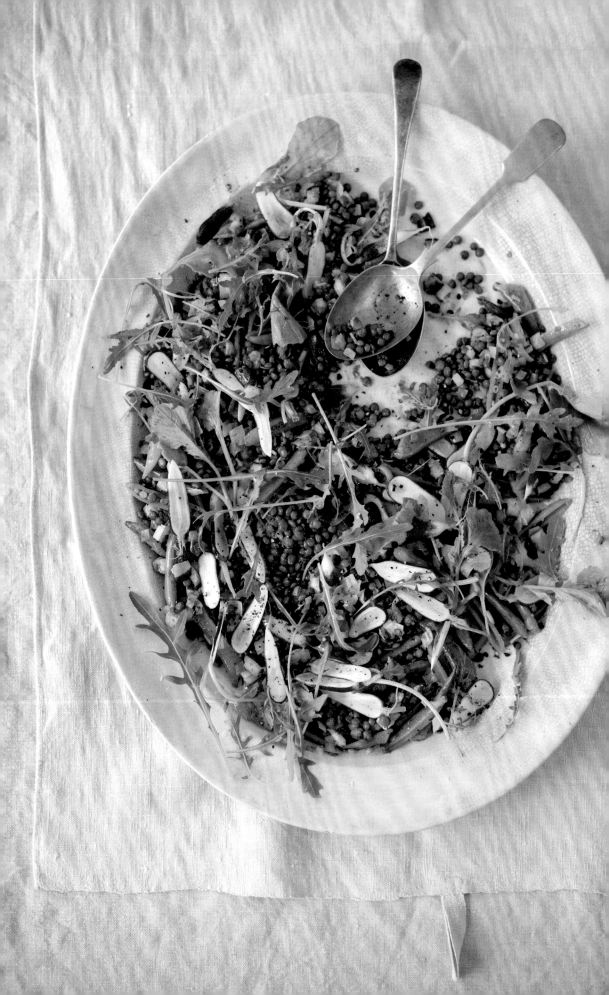

Onion

Onions form the basis of some of the best dishes in the world. I certainly couldn't cook without my artillery of red onions, white (or yellow) onions, spring onions and shallots.

Red onions are perhaps the most versatile of the large varieties, as they are equally good raw or cooked. When raw they offer a welcome crunch, a flash of rich colour and a sweet, mild flavour; cooking makes them even sweeter. I use white onions in Asian-style curries or stews, as they have a stronger flavour and bring a good savoury depth to the finished dish. I tend to use shallots in risottos or soups. The little spring onions are at their best raw and I often include them in salads.

Here is a tip for preparing succulent, sweet shallots that can either be added to a salad or thrown into a pasta dish, elevating either one to a new deliciousness. First, cut the shallots in half, leaving the skin on. Melt a tablespoon of honey with a tablespoon of coconut oil in an ovenproof pan over a medium heat, then place the shallot halves cut side down in the pan and cook until they start to turn brown. Transfer the pan to a 200°C/Fan 180°C/Gas 6 oven and cook for about 30 minutes. Voilà!

Nutritional bonus

As well as being an essential ingredient in most dishes, onions offer a wide range of useful nutrients. Historically they have been used as a medicine to cure colds and flu, although this has not been scientifically proven.

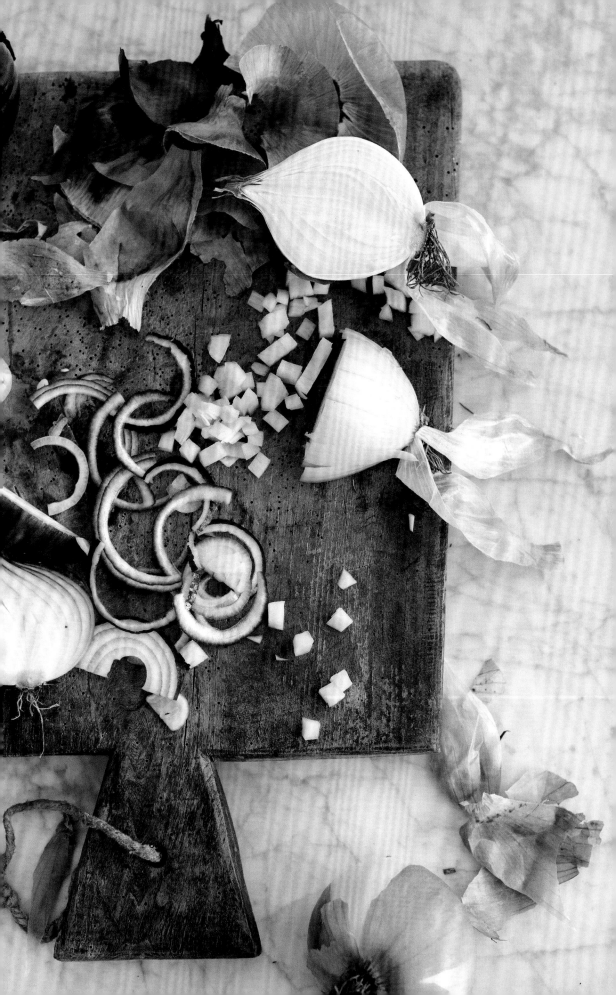

Onion and buckwheat patties with avocado salad

Serves 2

641 calories per serving

The savouriness of browned onion is the key to the tastiness of these patties. They have a lovely crumbly texture inside their crisp crust – be sure to chill them well before frying to ensure golden sides. Teamed with an avocado and sweetcorn salad, they are a perfect weekend lunch or dinner.

100g buckwheat
1 tbsp rapeseed oil, plus extra for frying
1 large onion, finely sliced
200g jarred chickpeas, drained and rinsed
1 egg
2 tbsp buckwheat flour
Zest of 1 lemon
A handful of fresh coriander, roughly chopped

For the salad

1 avocado
100g frozen sweetcorn, thawed
2 spring onions, sliced
100g cherry tomatoes, cut in half
Juice of ½ lemon
A handful of fresh coriander, roughly chopped
Flaked sea salt and cracked black pepper

1. Put the buckwheat in a saucepan with a pinch of salt and cover with three times the amount of water. Bring to the boil, then leave to simmer gently for 15–20 minutes until the buckwheat is tender and has become a lighter shade of green. Drain the buckwheat in a sieve, then cool under cold running water. Leave to drain thoroughly.

2. Heat the oil in a small frying pan over a medium heat and sauté the onion until lightly browned. Tip into a mixing bowl and leave to cool.

3. Put the chickpeas in a mixing bowl and crush roughly with a fork. Add the onion, buckwheat, egg, flour, lemon zest, coriander, and a pinch each of salt and pepper. Bring the mixture together, then chill for 20 minutes.

4. Divide into six equal balls and flatten each one slightly into a patty. Place on a tray lined with greaseproof paper and chill for 10 minutes.

5. Meanwhile, make the salad. Peel the avocado and roughly chop the flesh. Mix with the rest of the salad ingredients in a bowl and season with salt and pepper to taste.

6. When the patties are chilled, heat a little oil in a large frying pan and cook the patties (in batches if necessary) for 3–4 minutes on each side until lightly browned and crispy. Serve hot, with the avocado salad.

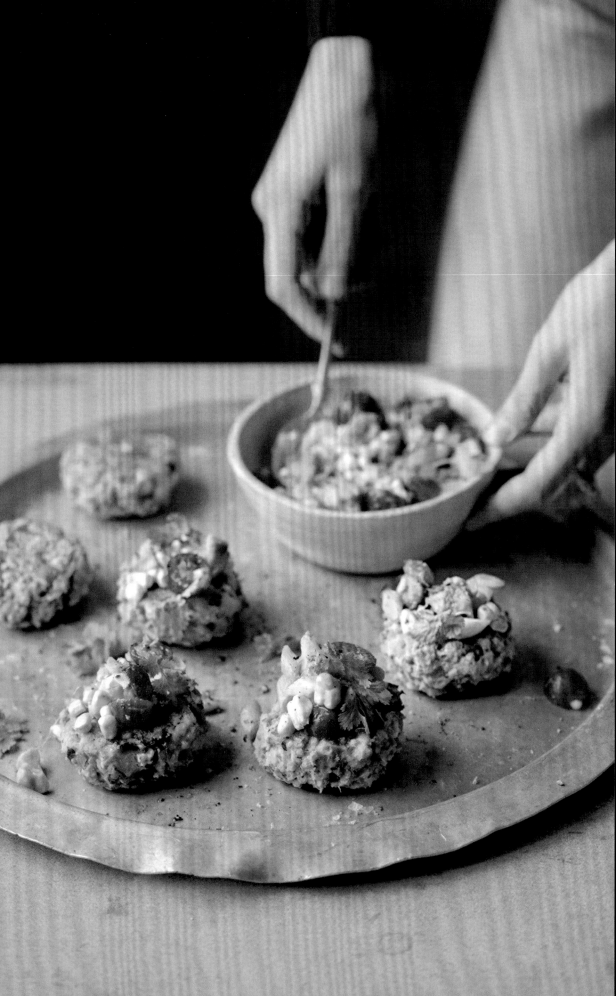

Three-onion 'voké' bowl

Serves 2

601 calories per serving

A poké is a popular Hawaiian salad based on raw fish that usually includes rice or noodles. It is typically flavoured with onions and chilli. In my 'voké' version, onions prepared three ways top the rice in the bowls. The onion and ginger jam is particularly delicious.

200g brown rice
100g radishes, thinly sliced
4 spring onions, sliced
1 green chilli, sliced

For the crispy onions
1 onion, cut into rounds and separated into rings
1 tsp rapeseed oil

For the pickled onions
1 red onion, sliced
Juice of 2 lemons

For the onion and ginger jam
1 tsp rapeseed oil
1 onion, sliced
1 tbsp grated fresh root ginger
2 tbsp honey
1 tsp ground ginger
1 tsp ground coriander
Flaked sea salt and cracked black pepper

1   Preheat the oven to 200°C/Fan 180°C/Gas 6. Line a baking tray with greaseproof paper.
2   For the crispy onions, spread the onion rings on the baking tray and drizzle over the oil. Roast for 20 minutes until crisp. Remove from the oven and set aside.
3   To prepare the pickled onions, heat a little oil in a small frying pan and fry the onion over a medium heat for 10 minutes until softened but not browned. Add the lemon juice and remove from the heat. Leave to cool, then tip into a bowl and place in the fridge to chill. The onions should turn bright pink.
4   For the onion jam, heat the oil in a pan and fry the onion and ginger for 10 minutes until soft. Stir in the honey, ground ginger and ground coriander with a splash of water, then simmer on a low heat for about 20 minutes until the jam is soft and sticky. Add a little more water if it starts to catch. Set aside.
5   Put the rice in a pan with a pinch of salt and cover with three times the amount of water. Bring to the boil, then leave to simmer gently for 20–25 minutes until the rice is tender and fluffy. Drain well.
6   To serve, put a portion of rice into each bowl, then add a spoonful of onion jam, radishes, onions and green chilli. Top with some pickled and crispy onions.

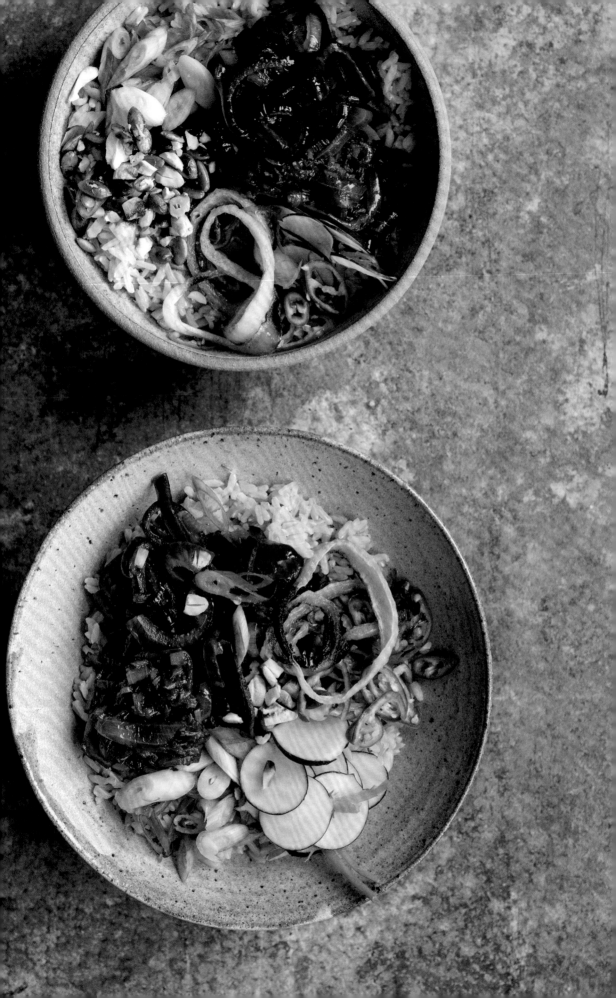

Red onion and blood orange salad with buckwheat

Serves 2
377 calories per serving
Red onions complement sharp-sweet flavours, so teaming them with blood oranges works brilliantly. These two star ingredients are brought together on a bed of herby buckwheat.

6 blood oranges
2 red onions, cut into rounds and separated into rings
Juice of 2 lemons
150g buckwheat
A small handful of fresh coriander, roughly chopped, plus extra to garnish
A small handful of fresh flat-leaf parsley, roughly chopped
A small handful of fresh chives, roughly chopped
1 tsp olive oil
Flaked sea salt and cracked black pepper

1   Peel four of the blood oranges and slice into rounds. Set aside. Squeeze the juice from the fifth orange.
2   Soak the onions in the orange and lemon juices with a pinch each of salt and pepper.
3   Put the buckwheat in a pan with a pinch of salt and cover with three times the amount of water. Bring to the boil, then leave to simmer gently for 15–20 minutes until the buckwheat is tender and has become a lighter shade of green. Drain the buckwheat in a sieve and cool under cold running water. Tip into a bowl and mix through the chopped herbs, oil, and salt and pepper to taste.
4   Spread the buckwheat on a serving plate. Pour the onions, with their soaking juice, over the buckwheat and arrange the sliced blood oranges on top. Garnish with extra coriander. Cut the remaining blood orange into wedges to squeeze over.

Vegetable-fried rice with avocado and a fried egg

Serves 4
508 calories per serving
An onion's deep savouriness and subtle sweetness will add depth to any dish. Here, with the backdrop of fried rice and vetables, onions do exactly that. A fried egg garnish and a sprinkle of shop-bought dried onions makes the dish utterly more-ish.

200g brown rice
Rapeseed oil for frying
4 spring onions, sliced
2 garlic cloves, diced
1 tbsp grated fresh root ginger
A handful of mangetout, sliced lengthways
100g frozen sweetcorn, thawed
4 tbsp tamari
Juice of 2 limes
1 red chilli, thinly sliced
4 eggs
2 avocados, peeled and chopped
4 tbsp dried onions
Flaked sea salt and cracked black pepper

1   Put the rice in a pan with a pinch of salt and cover with three times the amount of water. Bring to the boil, then leave to simmer gently for 20–25 minutes until the rice is tender and fluffy. Drain in a sieve, rinse under cold water and set aside.
2   Heat a little oil in a wok and add the spring onions, garlic and ginger. Stir-fry just until the garlic is golden. Add the mangetout and sweetcorn and stir-fry for a few more minutes until the vegetables are tender but crispy. Add the cooked rice along with half of the tamari, half of the lime juice, ½ teaspoon black pepper and the red chilli. Continue cooking, stirring occasionally, until some of the rice is crisp.
3   Mix together the remaining tamari and lime juice in a small jug.
4   Heat a little oil in a frying pan and fry the eggs sunny side up.
5   Divide the rice among four bowls and top with the avocado, dried onions and fried eggs. Serve with the tamari-lime for drizzling over.

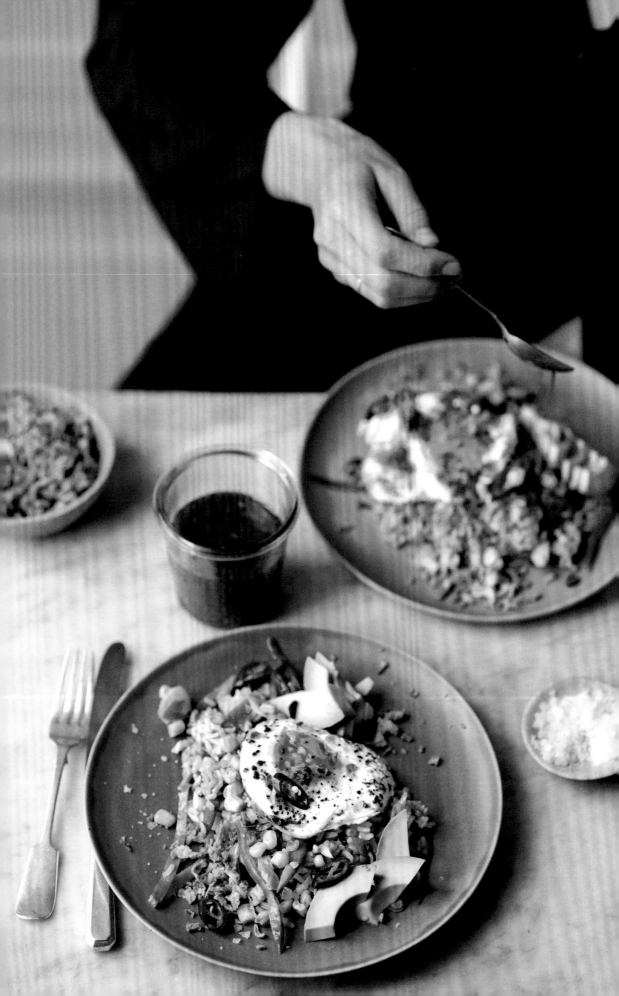

Mushroom

I know, I know… a mushroom is not a vegetable at all, but a fungus. However, mushrooms are so fantastic that they have to be included here. There are over 10,000 types of mushroom. Of the edible kind, you'll probably be most familiar with the cultivated button, chestnut, Portobello, oyster and shiitake mushrooms, plus perhaps a few of the oriental and wild varieties.

While most types of mushroom are available year round, they're usually at their peak in autumn and winter. When shopping, opt for those that are firm and evenly coloured, avoiding any that look damaged or wet.

The first rule in the kitchen is not to wash mushrooms. They are already made up of around 90 per cent water, so washing them could lead to sogginess. Instead, wipe off any dirt with kitchen paper, and then you're ready to sauté, grill or bake your mushrooms. When they are cooked they will have a meaty broth-like flavour. Alternatively, you can simply enjoy them raw in a salad (see page 234).

Nutritional bonus

Not only are mushrooms versatile in the ways you can cook them, they also have numerous health benefits. They are one of the few food sources of **vitamin D** – if they have been grown under ultraviolet light – and are a good source of **B vitamins**. They also contain high levels of **selenium**, known for its antioxidant-fighting, immune-system-boosting properties. In addition, you'll find more **potassium** in a medium-sized Portobello mushroom than in a banana.

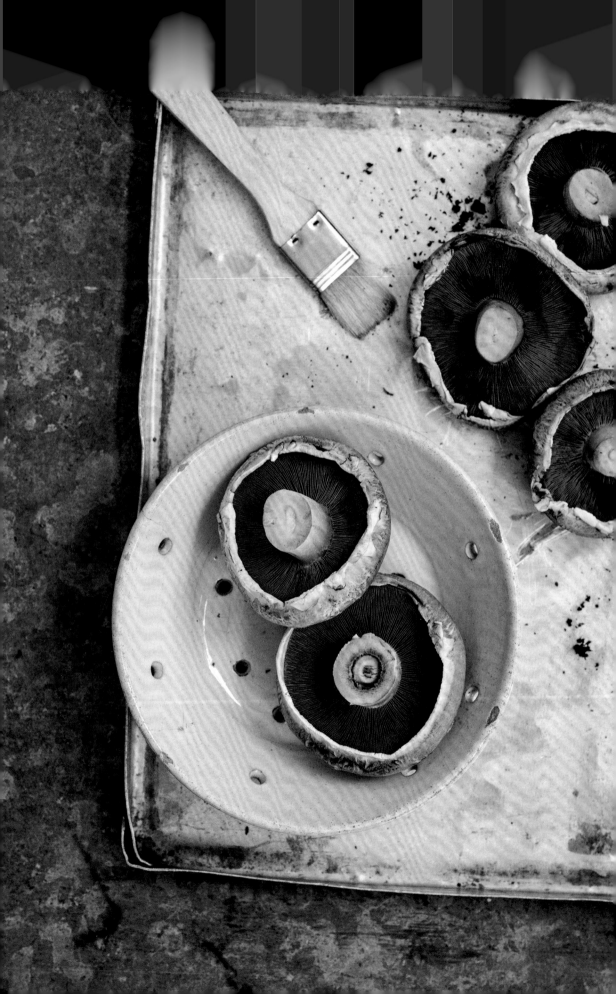

Raw mushroom and sweetcorn salad

Serves 2

264 calories per serving

The smooth, firm texture of raw mushrooms works brilliantly in salads. Here fresh sweetcorn kernels, sweet cherry tomatoes and crunchy seeds provide a great contrast to the mushrooms. This salad is especially good served with poached eggs on toast or on broccoli bread (see page 126).

2 corn on the cob, leaves and silk removed
200g chestnut mushrooms, thinly sliced
100g spinach, finely shredded
100g cherry tomatoes, cut in half
2 spring onions, sliced
A small handful of fresh coriander, roughly chopped
A handful of pumpkin seeds
A handful of sunflower seeds
1 tsp rapeseed oil
Juice of 1 lemon
1 tbsp tamari
Flaked sea salt and cracked black pepper

1   Preheat the grill to medium. Line a baking tray with greaseproof paper.
2   Place the corn on the cob on the baking tray and cook under the grill, turning occasionally, until browned on all sides. Remove from the grill and leave to cool.
3   Put the mushrooms in a salad bowl with the spinach, cherry tomatoes, spring onions and chopped coriander.
4   Toast the pumpkin and sunflower seeds in a small dry frying pan until golden. Add them to the salad bowl.
5   When the corn has cooled and you are able to hold it, use a sharp knife to slice the kernels off the cob. Add to the salad.
6   Drizzle over the oil and add the lemon juice, tamari, and salt and pepper to taste. Mix well.

Oyster mushrooms and avocado on toast

Serves 2

302 calories per serving

This recipe was inspired by my brother Tom, who made it for me in New York, where he lives. There is a strong tradition of brunching in New York and Tom assures me that this is a classic brunch dish. It's a very simple mashed avocado on toast that has been spruced up with some delicious sautéed oyster mushrooms.

If you haven't cooked oyster mushrooms before, be assured that although they might look like oysters they are far easier to prepare. Brush them gently to remove any grit, then feel for the woodier, harder parts of the stalks and trim these off. The mushrooms are then good to go.

150g oyster mushrooms
1 tbsp groundnut oil
1 tsp dried oregano
2 tbsp brown rice vinegar
1 avocado
½ tsp dried chilli flakes
Juice of 1 lemon or lime, plus extra for squeezing
2 slices dark rye bread
A small handful of fresh coriander, leaves picked
Flaked sea salt and cracked black pepper

1   Rinse the mushrooms in cold water to remove any grit. Trim the stems to remove the harder, rubbery ends. Slice larger mushrooms in half or into quarters.
2   Heat the oil in a frying pan over a medium heat and add the mushrooms with the oregano and a pinch each of salt and pepper. Sauté them for 5 minutes. Add the brown rice vinegar and cook, stirring, until it has evaporated. Remove from the heat.
3   Halve the avocado and scoop out the flesh into a bowl. Mash roughly with a fork. Mix in the chilli and lemon or lime juice.
4   Toast the rye bread. Spread the mashed avocado over the toast. Top with the cooked oyster mushrooms and coriander and add a squeeze of lemon or lime.

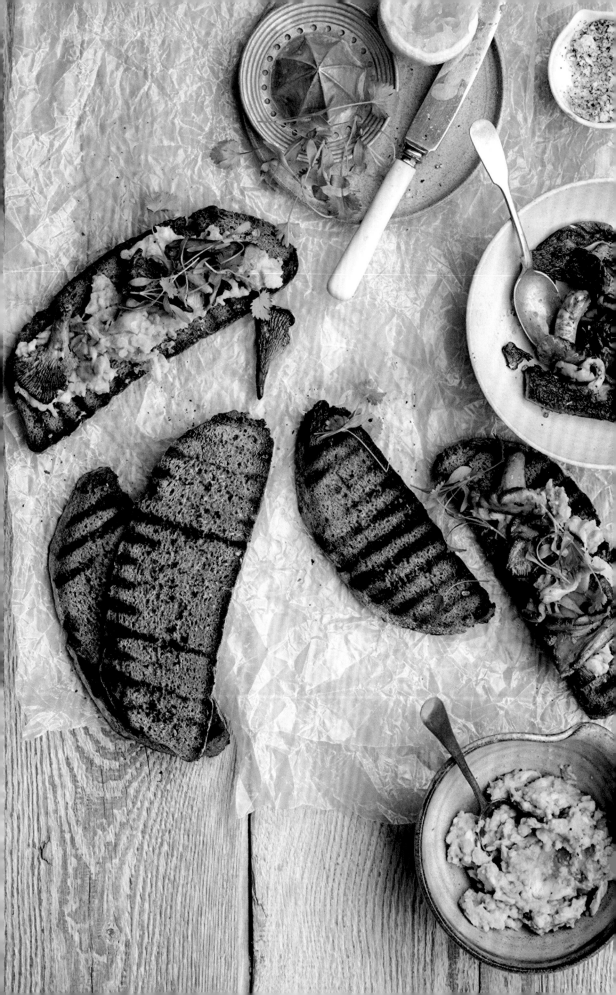

Mushroom burger with salsa verde and beetroot slaw

Serves 4

309 calories per serving

A Portobello mushroom makes a good substitute for a beefburger, especially when it is packed into a bun with a delicious herby salsa and a beetroot and sweetcorn slaw. When you are selecting your mushrooms, buy the largest and thickest ones you can find because they will shrink during cooking.

4 Portobello mushrooms
4 gluten-free burger buns
1 Baby Gem lettuce, leaves separated

For the salsa verde

1 garlic clove
2 tbsp capers
A handful of fresh flat-leaf parsley, leaves picked
A handful of fresh basil, leaves picked
A handful of fresh mint, leaves picked
2 tbsp brown rice vinegar or apple cider vinegar
Zest of 1 lemon
2 tbsp rapeseed oil

For the beetroot slaw

2 raw beetroots
100g frozen sweetcorn, thawed
A handful of fresh mint, leaves picked and roughly chopped
2 tbsp soya yoghurt
Juice of 1 lemon
1 tbsp rapeseed oil, plus extra for drizzling
Flaked sea salt and cracked black pepper

1   To make the salsa verde, finely chop the garlic, capers, parsley, basil and mint together, then transfer to a bowl. Add the brown rice vinegar, lemon zest, oil, and salt and pepper to taste and mix well. Set aside.

2   To make the slaw, peel the beetroots and grate them into a bowl. Mix in the sweetcorn, mint, yoghurt, lemon juice, oil, and salt and pepper to taste. Set aside.

3   Preheat the grill to high.

4   Trim off the mushroom stalks. Arrange the mushrooms, side by side and rounded side up, on a baking tray and drizzle over a little oil. Grill for 5 minutes on each side.

5   Split open the buns and toast under the grill or on a ridged griddle/grill pan.

6   To serve, fill each bun with salsa verde, lettuce leaves, a mushroom and some beetroot slaw.

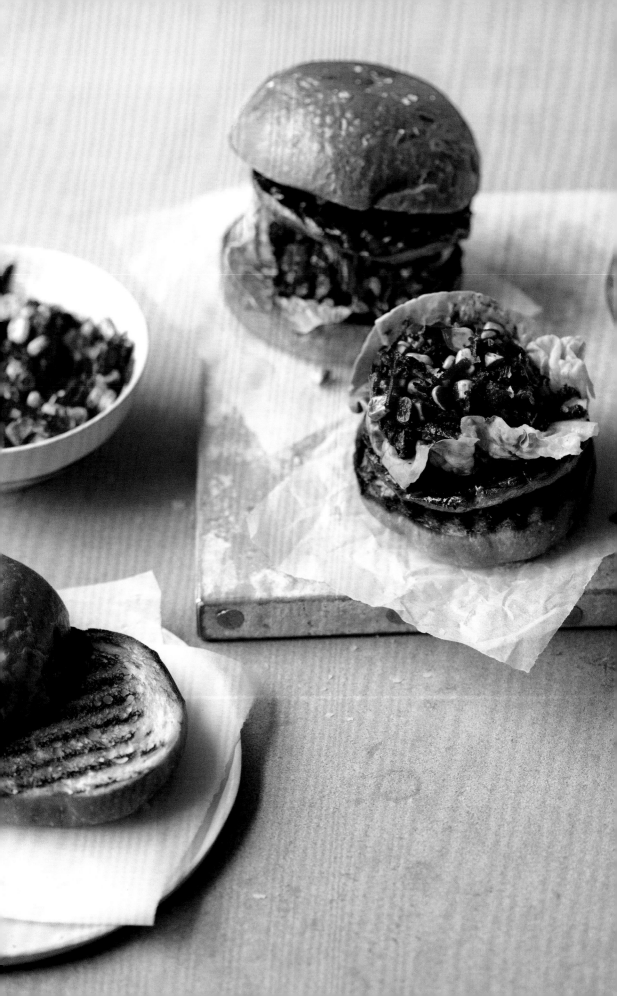

Portobello mushroom, tomato and bean bake with pesto

Serves 4
412 calories per serving
Dishes that need only one baking tray are my kind of recipe. Here Portobello mushrooms are baked on top of a hearty vegetable and bean mixture. A good sprinkle of yeast flakes adds a savoury mouth-watering finish.

Olive oil for frying and drizzling
1 onion, diced
3 garlic cloves, finely chopped
150g cherry tomatoes, cut in half
2 celery sticks, diced
2 carrots, diced
½ small cauliflower, roughly chopped
400g jarred butter beans, drained and rinsed
4 Portobello mushrooms
4 tbsp nutritional yeast (yeast flakes)

For the pesto
100g unsalted cashew nuts
A small handful of fresh basil, leaves picked
2 fresh tarragon sprigs
2 tbsp olive oil
1 garlic clove
Zest of 1 lemon
Flaked sea salt and cracked black pepper

1   Preheat the oven to 200°C/Fan 180°C/Gas 6.
2   Heat a little olive oil in a saucepan and sauté the onion and garlic until softened. Add the tomatoes, celery, carrots and cauliflower and cook, stirring occasionally, until the vegetables are tender. Season with salt and pepper.
3   Tip the vegetables into a roasting tin and mix in the butter beans. Place the mushrooms on top, stalk side up. Add a drizzle of olive oil and scatter the yeast over the top. Bake for about 30 minutes until the mushrooms are cooked and golden.
4   Meanwhile, make the pesto by blitzing all of the ingredients together in a food processor or chopping finely by hand.
5   To serve, spoon the pesto over the vegetable and mushroom bake.

Mushroom curry

Serves 2
682 calories per serving
Mushrooms add a hearty texture to a dish, which you need in a curry. They also have a subtle flavour that lets other flavourings do the talking. Here it is coconut, tomatoes, and fragrant cardamom and cloves that give this curry its distinctive fresh, floral taste.

Rapeseed oil for frying
1 onion, diced
1 garlic clove, finely chopped
1 tbsp grated fresh root ginger
250g chestnut mushrooms, larger ones
    cut in half
1 tbsp curry powder
4 cardamom pods
2 cloves
4 large tomatoes, roughly chopped
1 red pepper, seeded and sliced
200ml coconut milk
Juice of 1 lime
250g brown rice
Flaked sea salt and cracked black pepper

1   Heat a little oil in a sauté pan or saucepan over a medium heat and cook the onion, garlic and ginger until the onion has softened.
2   Heat a little oil in a frying pan and fry the mushrooms until slightly browned. Stir the mushrooms into the onion mixture along with the curry powder, cardamom pods and cloves. Cook gently for 1 minute.
3   Add the chopped tomatoes and red pepper and bring to a simmer. Cook for 10 minutes. Stir in the coconut milk and lime juice, and season with salt and pepper to taste. Simmer gently for a further 5 minutes to heat through.
4   While the curry is cooking, put the rice in a pan with a pinch of salt and cover with three times the amount of water. Bring to the boil, then simmer for 20–25 minutes until the rice is tender and fluffy. Drain.
5   Remove the cloves and cardamom from the curry. Leave to stand for 10 minutes before serving with the brown rice.

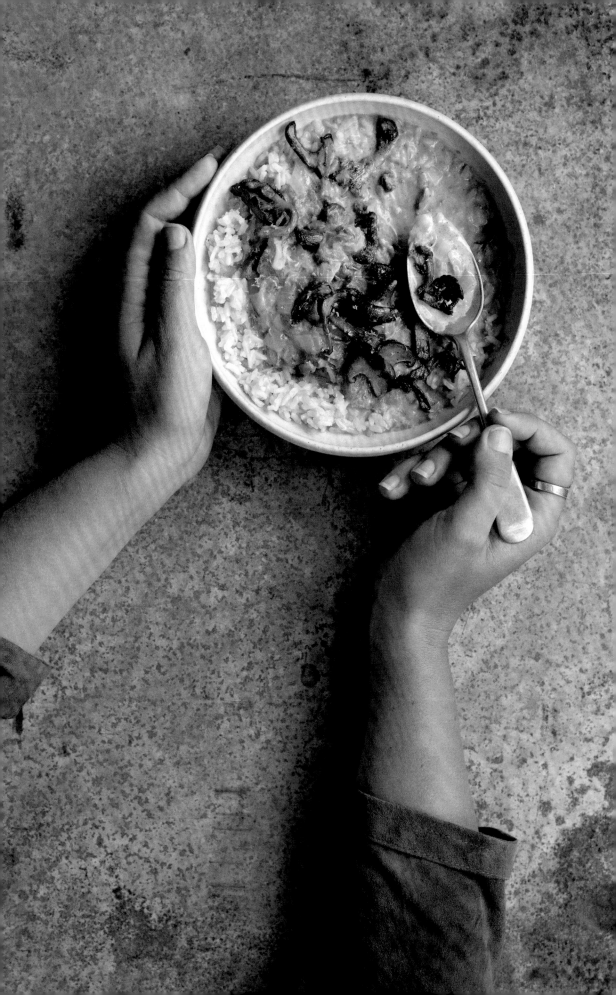

Aubergine

The aubergine is up there in the top three of my list of vegetables because its tender loveliness takes so well to such a wide variety of flavours, from Provençal herbs to bold spices, or the smoky, sharp tastes that are so beloved in Middle Eastern cooking.

Cooked badly, however, aubergine falls into my Room 101. The key is to make sure you cook your aubergines through but avoid going further and overcooking them.

Do not fear the softness of a well-cooked aubergine, however! Baking and roasting can both take the vegetable to the perfect texture. The spicy aubergine fritters on page 248, coated in batter and fried in a little oil, are also quite wonderful, and I would defy anyone not to like them.

There are many different varieties of aubergine. We are most used to the big, bulbous, deep-purple type, but in Asian cusine they use smaller, rounder varieties. These are harder to come by in the UK but are worth looking out for if you are making a curry, as they have a shorter cooking time and tend to be slightly firmer than purple aubergines.

The process of what the French call *dégorger* (sprinkling aubergine with salt to draw out excess moisture before cooking) isn't always necessary. The general rule of thumb is that if you are adding aubergine to a sauce, or roasting or baking it, there is no need to salt it first, but if you are frying aubergine in oil, it is best to do so. This will prevent it from soaking up the oil like a sponge.

Nutritional bonus

Aubergines are deep purple in colour because they contain a phytochemical called **nasunin**, an antioxidant that has been linked to the protection of lipids that help the brain to function, and also to lowering so-called 'bad' cholesterol. Aubergines are packed with a whole range of other nutrients and are low in fat, so they should surely be included in the 'superveg' category. In fact, perhaps the majority of vegetables should be given that status!

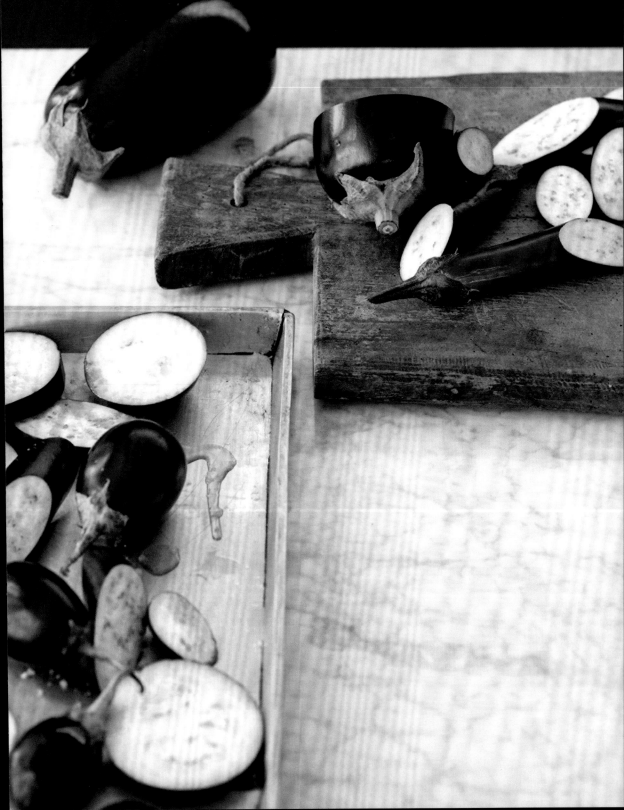

Baked aubergine with preserved lemon yoghurt

Serves 4
214 calories per serving
Baking aubergine with honey and tamari gives it
a lovely salty, sweet stickiness that is incredibly
more-ish. The freshness of the lemony saffron
yoghurt adds to the fragrant complexity of this
Middle Eastern-inspired dish. It is perfect for
a dinner party, as part of a big feast, or simply
served as a weekday supper with some rice
and a green salad.

2 large aubergines, cut into 1cm rounds
2 tbsp tamari
1 tbsp honey
1 tbsp toasted sesame oil
2 preserved lemons, roughly chopped
3 pinches of saffron threads
200ml soya yoghurt
Flaked sea salt and cracked black pepper

To garnish
A small bunch of fresh coriander, finely chopped
2 sprigs of fresh mint, leaves picked and chopped
1 red chilli, sliced
2 tbsp cashew nuts, toasted and chopped

1 Preheat the oven to 200°C/Fan 180°C/Gas 6.
   Line a baking tray with greaseproof paper.
2 Spread the aubergine rounds on the baking
   tray. Whisk together the tamari, honey and
   sesame oil in a bowl and pour evenly over the
   aubergine. Bake for 20–25 minutes until soft
   and golden.
3 Meanwhile, put the preserved lemons, saffron,
   yoghurt, and a pinch each of salt and pepper
   in a food processor and blitz until the yoghurt
   has turned a deep yellow and is smooth.
4 Place the aubergine rounds on a large serving
   dish. Drizzle over the saffron yoghurt dressing
   and garnish with the coriander, mint, chilli and
   toasted cashews.

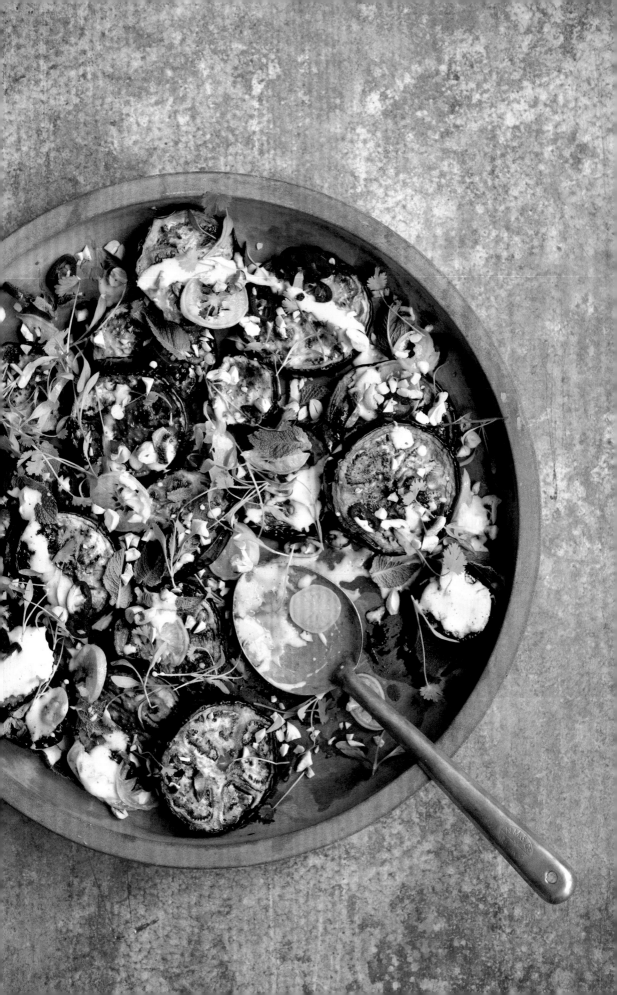

Aubergine and artichoke caponata

Serves 4
165 calories per serving
Caponata is a Sicilian dish of stewed vegetables, and, like all classic recipes, the question of what makes the right combination is quite subjective. I prefer a tangy tomatoey caponata, and think it should also include aubergines, onions, capers and basil. If you start with this happy group of ingredients, you really cannot go wrong. Here I've added artichoke hearts too.

2 aubergines, cut into 2cm chunks
Olive oil for drizzling and frying
1 tbsp dried oregano
150g jarred artichoke hearts packed in oil,
    drained and cut in half
2 garlic cloves, chopped
4 large plum tomatoes, roughly chopped
400g tinned chopped tomatoes
2 celery sticks, finely diced
1 tbsp capers
2 tbsp black olives, roughly chopped
1 tsp honey
Juice of 1 lemon
50ml water
Flaked sea salt and cracked black pepper

To garnish
A small handful of fresh chives, finely chopped
A few fresh basil sprigs

1   Preheat the oven to 220°C/Fan 200°C/Gas 7. Line a baking tray with baking paper.
2   Place the aubergine chunks on the baking tray and drizzle over 1 teaspoon olive oil. Sprinkle with the oregano and a pinch each of salt and pepper. Roast for 15 minutes, then add the artichoke hearts to the tray. Roast for another 15 minutes or so until the aubergine is golden and tender.
3   Meanwhile, make the tomato sauce. Heat 1 tablespoon olive oil in a saucepan and cook the garlic until golden. Add both the fresh and tinned tomatoes, celery, capers, black olives, honey, lemon juice and water. Season with salt and pepper. Simmer, stirring occasionally, for 15 minutes until the tomatoes are completely soft and broken down.
4   When the vegetables are roasted, add them to the tomato sauce and mix well. Check the seasoning before serving, garnished with chopped chives and basil leaves.

Indian-style aubergine stacks

Serves 2
537 calories per serving
Here crisp, golden rounds of aubergine are topped with a mung bean and tomato curry, plus a fresh mint and coriander chutney. Coconut yoghurt offers a cooling contrast. I have long been a fan of mung beans; they are a good alternative to lentils, with a subtly sweet but equally earthy, well-rounded flavour.

100g dried green mung beans
Rapeseed oil for frying
2 onions, diced
3 garlic cloves, finely chopped
3 tbsp grated fresh root ginger
½ tsp ground cumin
½ tsp ground turmeric
2 plum tomatoes, chopped
2 tbsp gluten-free flour
2 aubergines, cut into 1cm rounds
Garam masala to finish

For the chutney
A small handful of fresh mint, leaves picked
A small handful of fresh coriander, roughly
    chopped
1 green chilli, roughly chopped
1 tsp grated fresh root ginger
1 garlic clove
1 tbsp honey
Juice of 1 lemon

For the yoghurt
3 tbsp coconut yoghurt
A small handful of fresh coriander, finely
    chopped
Flaked sea salt and cracked black pepper

1   To make the chutney, put all the ingredients in a small food processor with a pinch each of salt and pepper. Blitz until the ingredients make a coarse-textured mixture. Add some water to loosen if necessary. Set aside.

2   Mix together the coconut yoghurt, chopped coriander and a pinch of salt. Set aside.

3   Put the mung beans in a pan and cover with three times the amount of water. Bring to the boil, then simmer gently for 40–50 minutes until the beans are tender. Drain and set aside.

4   Heat a little oil in a saucepan, add the onions, garlic and ginger, and cook for 10 minutes until the onions are softened. Stir in the cumin and turmeric and cook for a further minute, then add the tomatoes and cooked mung beans and stir to mix. Cook for 10–15 minutes until the tomatoes are completely soft. Season to taste.

5   While the mung bean and tomato mixture is cooking, spread out the flour on a plate and lightly dust the aubergine slices on both sides. Heat 1 teaspoon oil in a non-stick frying pan and fry the aubergine slices until golden on both sides and cooked through.

6   To serve, place the aubergine slices on a large plate and top with the mung bean mixture, chutney and yoghurt. Finish with a sprinkle of garam masala.

Aubergine, artichoke and garden pesto salad

Serves 2

558 calories per serving

A rich, herby garden pesto brings this very classic Italian combination to life, perfect for a sharing supper. For a more substantial dish, mix in some freshly cooked pasta. (The delicious pesto could also be drizzled over blanched French beans for a side dish or starter.) As with all simple salads, quality is of the utmost importance, so buy juicy tomatoes, good-quality artichoke hearts and a plump aubergine.

1 aubergine, cut into 2cm chunks
1 tsp olive oil
200g jarred artichoke hearts packed in oil
4 sun-dried tomatoes, roughly chopped
60g pitted black olives, roughly chopped
4 heirloom tomatoes, cut into quarters
10 fresh basil sprigs
100g fresh flat-leaf parsley
A small handful of fresh chives
50g spinach
100g frozen peas, thawed
2 tbsp cashew nuts
Zest of 2 lemons
Flaked sea salt and cracked black pepper

1   Preheat the oven to 200°C/Fan 180°C/Gas 6. Line a baking tray with baking paper. Place the aubergine on the tray, drizzle with the olive oil and sprinkle with a pinch each of salt and pepper. Roast for 20–25 minutes until tender. Remove from the oven and allow to cool to room temperature.

2   Meanwhile, drain the artichokes, keeping 2 tablespoons of the oil from the jar. Cut the artichokes into quarters and put into a large mixing bowl. Add the sun-dried tomatoes, olives and fresh tomatoes.

3   To make the pesto, put half of the basil and all of the parsley and chives into a food processor. Add the spinach, peas, cashew nuts, lemon zest, 2 tablespoons oil from the artichokes, and some salt and pepper. Blitz to a coarse-textured paste.

4   To serve, transfer the aubergine and artichoke mixture to a salad dish, drizzle over the pesto and top with the remaining basil leaves.

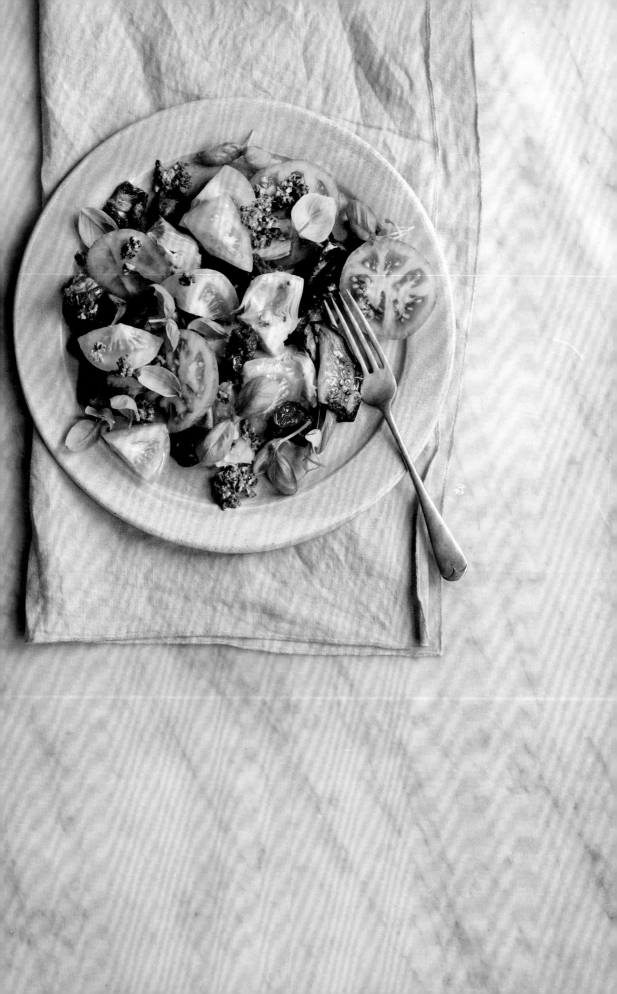

Spiced aubergine fritters with coconut tzatziki

Serves 2

536 calories per serving

The most wonderful thing about frittering any vegetable is the tension between goodness and indulgence. I defy anyone not to love these fritters. If you use a good-quality non-stick pan, you will not need a lot of oil to create a crispy result. The coconut tzatziki is quite divine, and calms the kick of the green chilli in the fritters.

2 large aubergines
3 eggs
100ml brown rice milk
2 tbsp gluten-free flour, plus extra for dusting
1 tsp smoked paprika
Zest of 1 lime
1 green chilli, diced
Rapeseed oil for frying

For the tzatziki
200g soya yoghurt
200g coconut yoghurt
1 cucumber, peeled, seeded and grated
A handful of fresh mint, leaves picked and finely chopped, plus extra to garnish
A handful of fresh coriander, finely chopped, plus extra to garnish
Flaked sea salt and cracked black pepper

1 Cut the aubergine into 1cm rounds. Place on kitchen paper and sprinkle with salt, then leave to drain for 30 minutes.

2 Meanwhile, make the batter. Whisk the eggs in a bowl with the rice milk, flour, smoked paprika, 1 teaspoon salt and a pinch of pepper. Add the lime zest and green chilli. Set aside until the aubergine is ready.

3 Make the tzatziki by mixing all the ingredients together. Set aside.

4 Spread some extra flour on a plate and lightly dust each aubergine slice on both sides. Place a medium frying pan on a high heat and add 1 tablespoon oil. When the oil is hot, dip three or four aubergine slices in the batter and put them straight into the pan. Fry until golden on both sides. Remove from the pan and place on kitchen paper to drain. Repeat until all the aubergine has been battered and fried.

5 Serve the fritters hot, each topped with a dollop of tzatziki and extra fresh mint and coriander.

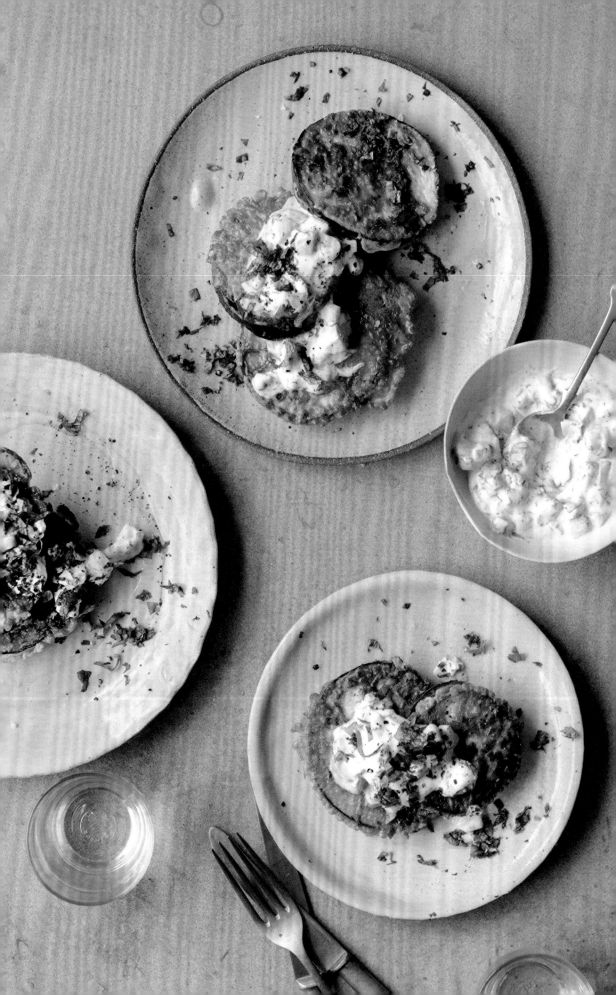

Aubergine fritter burgers

Serves 4

314 calories per serving

It's my opinion that the accompaniments to a burger are what really make it. Here pickled onions add acidity and richness; the tzatziki is fresh and creamy; and the salsa is tangy and vibrant. The aubergine fritters themselves are the perfect balance of crispy and soft. All this comes together in a nice bun with some crunchy lettuce and sliced tomato. The burgers are great for feeding a crowd, as they are filling and utterly more-ish (I always make a few extra for seconds). You can prepare everything in advance so that before serving you only need to fry the fritters and pop them in the buns.

1 aubergine

4 eggs

3 tbsp gluten-free flour

4 gluten-free burger buns

Baby Gem lettuce leaves

2 beef tomatoes, sliced

For the pickled onions

Rapeseed oil for frying

1 red onion, sliced

Juice of 1 lemon

1 tsp honey

For the mustard tzatziki

3 tbsp coconut yoghurt

2 fresh mint sprigs, leaves picked and finely chopped

1 tbsp ready-made English mustard

For the salsa

2 gherkins, diced

2 tbsp capers

1 tbsp brown rice vinegar

1 large beef tomato, finely chopped

A small handful of fresh coriander, finely chopped

Flaked sea salt and cracked black pepper

1. To make the pickled onions, heat a little oil in a frying pan and gently cook the onion until soft (make sure it does not brown). Tip into a bowl and mix in the lemon juice, honey and a pinch of salt. Leave to cool.

2. To make the tzatziki, mix all the ingredients together with a pinch of salt in another bowl. Keep in the fridge until you are ready to serve.

3. To make the salsa, mix all the ingredients in a bowl and leave at room temperature until ready to serve.

4. Cut the aubergine into 1.5cm rounds. Place on some kitchen paper and sprinkle with salt. Leave to drain for about 1 hour.

5. About 20 minutes before you want to cook the aubergine, make the batter. Put the eggs, flour, and a pinch each of salt and pepper into a bowl and mix together until smooth. Add the aubergine rounds to the batter and set aside until you are ready to cook.

6. Preheat the oven to 200°C/Fan 180°C/Gas 6. Line a baking tray with greaseproof paper. Heat some oil in a frying pan. When hot, fry the aubergine fritters until golden on both sides. Transfer them to the baking tray and place in the oven to cook for 20 minutes until soft.

7. Meanwhile, split open the buns and place some tzatziki, a slice of tomato and some lettuce on each base.

8. Place an aubergine fritter in each bun and top with salsa and pickled onion. Pop the top on the bun and enjoy.

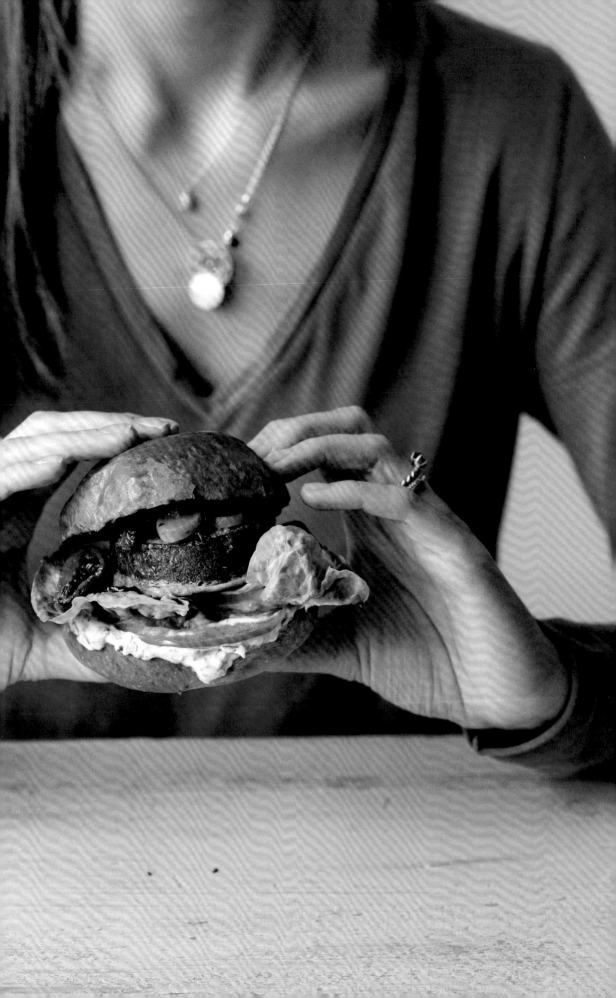

Pepper

Peppers are fruits disguised as vegetables and they are part of the extensive nightshade family, which includes many poisonous cousins. You'll never find those on your plates though! There is a wide variety of peppers out there, but the type most familiar are bell, or sweet, peppers.

Red, yellow and orange peppers all start out green, which is why a green pepper will sometimes have flecks of these bright colours near the stem. Some peppers are harvested when still green, while others are picked once they have ripened to yellow, orange or red.

When you're at the greengrocers, choose firm peppers with taut skin, and pick out the heaviest ones – the heavier they are, the more likely it is that they will be sweet and crisp. In the UK peppers are in season in late summer, from June to September.

Once you get your peppers back to your kitchen, you can slice them thinly and pop them into a salad; use them to scoop up dips; roast them whole or cut up; or throw them into soups and stews. Peppers are always a delicious and colourful ingredient to add to a recipe.

Nutritional bonus

All peppers have a good amount of **vitamin C**. Red peppers in particular provide double the recommended daily intake of this vitamin in just 100g. Peppers also contain **vitamin A**, essential for a healthy immune system, as well as promoting healthy eyes and skin.

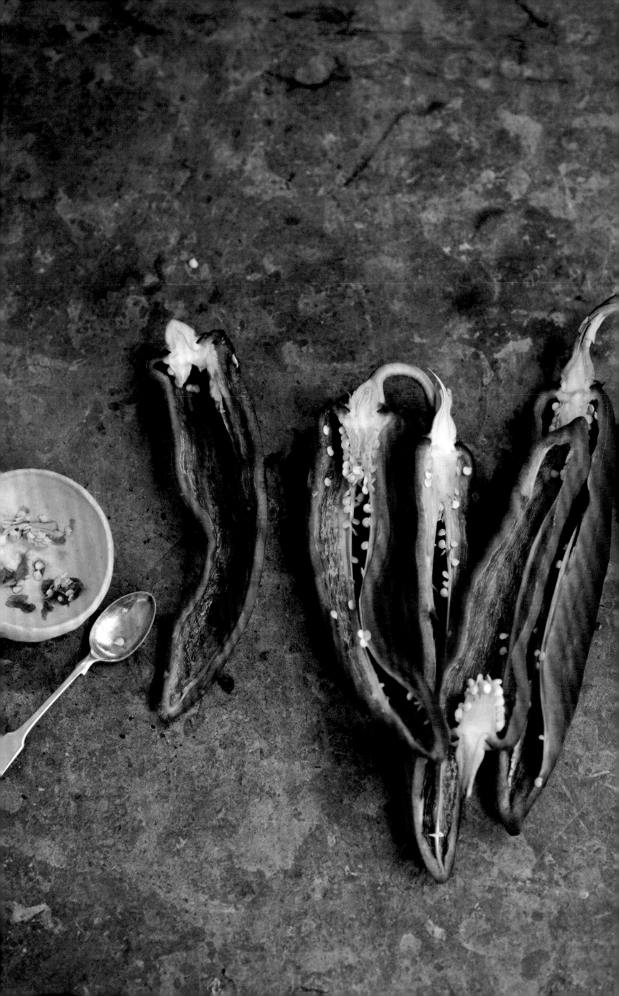

Spanish-style padrón peppers

Serves 2
110 calories per serving
A typical tapas dish from Galicia in Spain, padrón peppers quickly fried in oil make a great canapé or snack. I could happily polish off a whole bowl of them. The key is to cook them until they are slightly charred – it is the balance of the deep smoky flavour, bitter green pepper and sea salt that makes them so more-ish.

1 tbsp rapeseed oil
200g padrón peppers
Flaked sea salt

1   Heat the oil in a frying pan. When the oil is very hot, add the peppers and cook, stirring often, until they have blistered and charred all over.
2   Serve immediately with a good pinch of salt.

Pepper and black bean salad with avocado dressing

Serves 4
241 calories per serving
In this salad I have used three colours: sweet red, fresh green and mellow yellow. They look lovely against the backdrop of shiny black beans. The zingy avocado dressing adds creaminess, and the dish is finished with hard-boiled egg.

4 eggs
1 tbsp smoked paprika
400g tinned black beans, drained and rinsed
1 red pepper, seeded and finely sliced
1 green pepper, seeded and finely sliced
1 yellow pepper, seeded and finely sliced
1 red onion, finely sliced
1 red chilli, finely sliced
A small handful of fresh coriander, roughly chopped

For the dressing
2 avocados
Juice of 3 limes, plus lime wedges to serve
1 tbsp tamari
1 tsp toasted sesame oil
Flaked sea salt and cracked black pepper

1   To make the dressing, halve the avocados and scoop out the flesh into a food processor. Add the rest of the dressing ingredients, with a pinch of pepper, and blitz until smooth. Add water to loosen if the dressing is too thick – it should be the consistency of single cream.
2   Bring a pan of water to the boil on a medium heat. Put the eggs into the water and boil gently for 6 minutes (soft-boiled). Lift out the eggs and rinse them under cold water to cool, then peel off the shells. Roll the eggs in the paprika on a plate so that they are covered. Cut the eggs in half and set aside.
3   Put the beans, peppers and onion in a large bowl and toss to mix. Drizzle the dressing over the salad and sprinkle with the chilli and fresh coriander. Top with the eggs and serve with lime wedges to squeeze over.

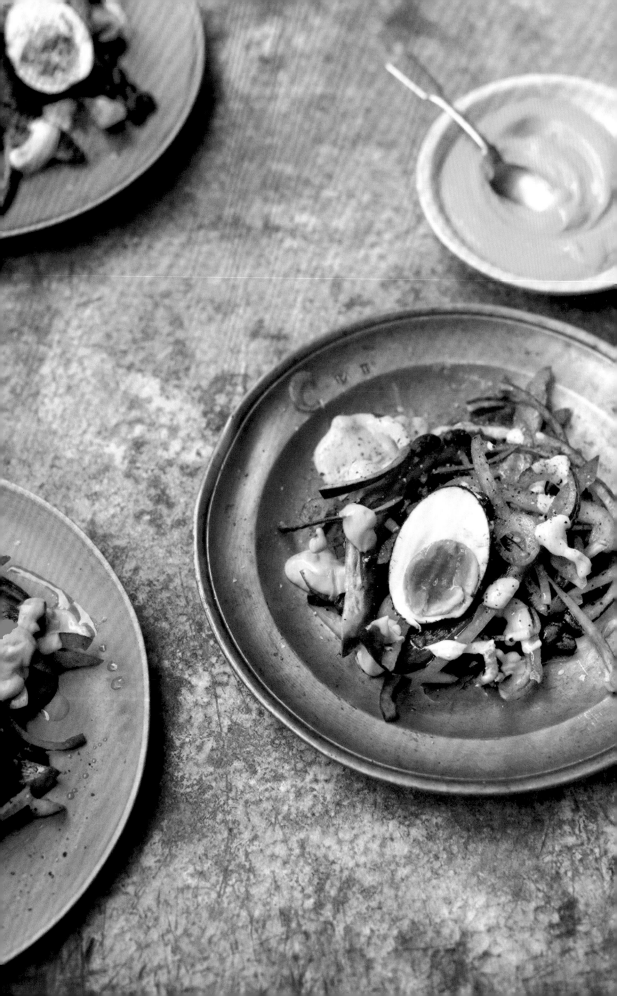

Smoky pepper and sweet potato chilli

Serves 4
313 calories per serving

I often cook a vegetarian chilli at the weekend, and this is one of my favourites. I add almond butter and cacao powder to the tomato base, as these bring a lovely richness to the dish. The peppers and sweet potatoes soak up all of the smoky paprika and chilli spices to create a dish that is both warming and nourishing.

1 tbsp rapeseed oil
2 onions, sliced
100g chestnut mushrooms, roughly chopped
1 tbsp cumin seeds
1 tbsp smoked paprika
1 tbsp cacao powder
1 tbsp almond butter
1 green chilli, sliced
2 sweet potatoes, cut into small chunks
1 red pepper, seeded and diced
1 green pepper, seeded and diced
200g vine tomatoes, roughly chopped
2 tbsp tomato paste
2 Baby Gem lettuces
200g coconut yoghurt
Fresh coriander, roughly chopped
Flaked sea salt and cracked black pepper

1   Heat the oil in a large saucepan and cook the onions and mushrooms until lightly browned. Add the cumin seeds, paprika, cacao powder and almond butter and stir to mix. Cook for a few more minutes so that the onions and mushrooms absorb all the spices, then add the chilli, sweet potatoes, peppers, tomatoes, tomato paste, and some salt and pepper.

2   Cook over a medium heat, stirring occasionally, for 25–30 minutes until the sweet potato is soft. If the chilli starts to catch, stir in a little water to loosen. Serve with Baby Gem lettuce, coconut yoghurt and fresh coriander.

Smooth pepper soup
with sun-dried tomatoes

Serves 4
113 calories per serving
Sundays tend to be big breakfast and big lunch days, so by the evening we all want something light but really delicious that is easy to make. This pepper and sun-dried tomato soup is perfect. It's also a great way to use up any leftover bits and bobs from the weekend cooking. I like to serve it with rye bread or broccoli bread (see page 126).

1 litre water
½ onion, finely diced
1 garlic clove, roughly sliced
1 red pepper, seeded and roughly chopped
1 yellow pepper, seeded and roughly chopped
½ cauliflower, roughly chopped
250g broccoli, roughly chopped
5 sun-dried tomatoes, roughly chopped
1 tsp dried mixed herbs
½ tsp ground coriander
Flaked sea salt and cracked black pepper

1 Pour the water into a saucepan set over a high heat and add all the remaining ingredients with a pinch each of salt and pepper. Bring to the boil, then simmer for 20 minutes until all the vegetables are tender.
2 In batches, blitz the vegetables in a food processor until smooth. Reheat the soup before serving, if necessary.

Stuffed Romano peppers

Serves 4

275 calories per serving

Romano peppers are great for stuffing and baking – their long, narrow shape means the mixture you stuff them with will cook evenly. Here I've used a zesty black rice mixture that has a lovely coarse texture. This is a good weekday supper, as it is easy to make but still feels special.

4 Romano peppers
Olive oil for drizzling and frying
100g black rice
3 spring onions, sliced
2 garlic cloves, chopped
2 tbsp grated fresh root ginger
1 small courgette, diced
¼ cauliflower, cut into small florets
2 vine tomatoes, roughly chopped
3 fresh thyme sprigs
Zest of 1 lemon
2 tbsp tamari
450ml water
100g gluten-free breadcrumbs
Fresh flat-leaf parsley, to garnish

To serve

½ cucumber, peeled, seeded and diced
4 vine tomatoes, sliced
1 Baby Gem lettuce, roughly chopped
Flaked sea salt and cracked black pepper

1 Preheat the oven to 200°C/Fan 180°C/Gas 6.
2 Cut the peppers in half lengthways, through the stalk (keep this attached). Scoop out ribs and seeds. Lay the pepper halves, cut side up, on a baking tray and drizzle over a little olive oil. Season with salt and pepper. Roast for about 20 minutes.
3 Meanwhile, make the stuffing. Put the rice in a pan with a pinch of salt and cover with three times the amount of water. Bring to the boil, then simmer for 30–35 minutes until the rice is tender and fluffy. Drain and set aside.
4 Heat a little olive oil in a frying pan set over a medium heat. Add the spring onions, garlic and ginger, and cook until softened. Add the courgette, cauliflower, chopped tomatoes, thyme, lemon zest, tamari and 200ml of the water. Simmer until the liquid has evaporated, then stir in the rice with the remaining 250ml water. Continue to cook until all the liquid has been absorbed by the rice.
5 Spoon the mixture into the pepper halves and cover evenly with the breadcrumbs. Bake for 15–20 minutes until the crumbs are golden.
6 Serve with a simple cucumber, tomato and Baby Gem salad.

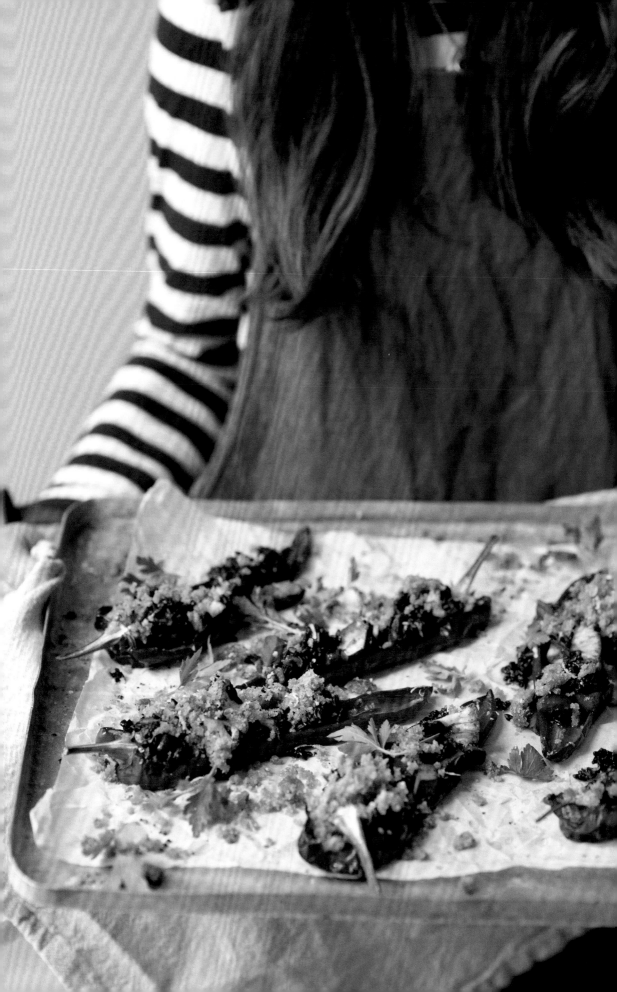

Tomato

The Italian name for a tomato is 'pomodoro', which literally translates as 'golden apple' – it's a word that dates back centuries to a time when tomatoes were generally more of a yellowish colour. The ancient Aztecs, who are thought to have been the first to cultivate the tomato, called it 'tomatl' or 'plump thing with a navel'. Quite accurate, I'd say – we all know that plumpness is the most important thing about a tomato's appearance!

Tomatoes are technically a fruit, as they contains seeds, but we could not do without them in savoury cooking. As shown in the Thai som tam salad on page 264 (one of my all-time favourite recipes) and the Indian tomato and coconut curry on page 269, tomatoes make a fantastic base for a broad range of dishes.

There are hundreds of varieties of tomatoes, from little cherry toms to big beef ones. They vary in colour from deep crimson to yellow or orange. There's even a variety (called 'Black Cherry') that is deep purple with reddish-brown flecks. Whenever I can get hold of them, I like to use heirloom (or heritage) tomatoes in my cooking because their colour and flavour are so good.

If you have a sunny spot in your garden, do think about reserving it for tomatoes. They are easy to grow from seed. Just start them off indoors in a pot on your windowsill, then move the young tomato plants outside in the late spring. The tomatoes will ripen deliciously over the summer.

Nutritional bonus

Tomatoes are a rich source of **lycopene**, a phytochemical that has been linked to reducing the risk of heart disease and other chronic health conditions. Cooking actually increases this nutrient, which is the perfect excuse to make a good tomato sauce (I can highly recommend the recipe on page 266).

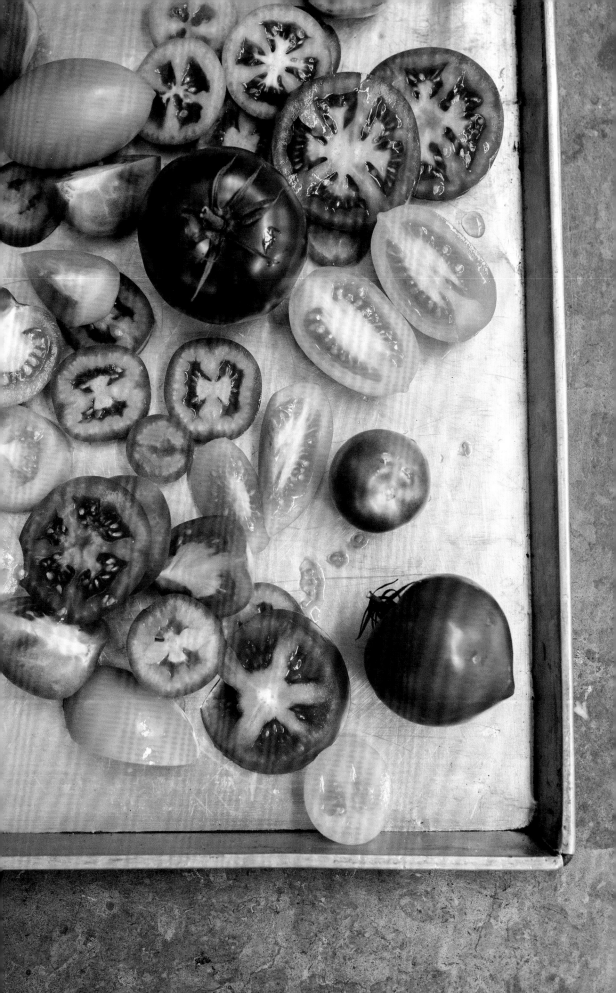

Panzanella

Serves 4
234 calories per serving
The key to this Tuscan bread-based salad is to use the juiciest, sweetest ripe tomatoes at room temperature. Capers and basil are good friends of the tomato, complementing its sweetness.

4 slices of thick-cut rye bread
200g cherry tomatoes, cut in half
200g heirloom tomatoes, roughly chopped
2 tbsp capers
½ red onion, thinly sliced
2 tbsp extra virgin olive oil
2 handfuls of fresh basil leaves
Flaked sea salt and cracked black pepper

1   Tear the bread into big pieces directly into a dry frying pan set on a medium heat. Cook, stirring, until the bread is crisp on all sides, then tip into a bowl.
2   Add the tomatoes, capers, onion, and a pinch each of salt and pepper to the bread pieces and combine well with your hands. Drizzle the olive oil over the salad. Tip on to a platter, add a scattering of basil leaves and serve.

Tomato and onion salad

Serves 2
87 calories per serving
For serving alongside a curry or almost any hot dish, my go-to quick salad is tomato and onion with a salty honey and lemon dressing. This salad is also delicious simply wrapped in a flatbread.

2 ripe beef tomatoes
1 red or white onion
1 tsp honey
Zest and juice of 1 lemon
Flaked sea salt

1   Thinly slice the tomatoes and onion into rounds. Separate the onion into rings. Layer with the tomatoes on a plate.
2   Drizzle over the honey, sprinkle with the lemon zest and squeeze over the lemon juice. Finish with a sprinkle of salt. Leave to marinate for at least 30 minutes before serving.

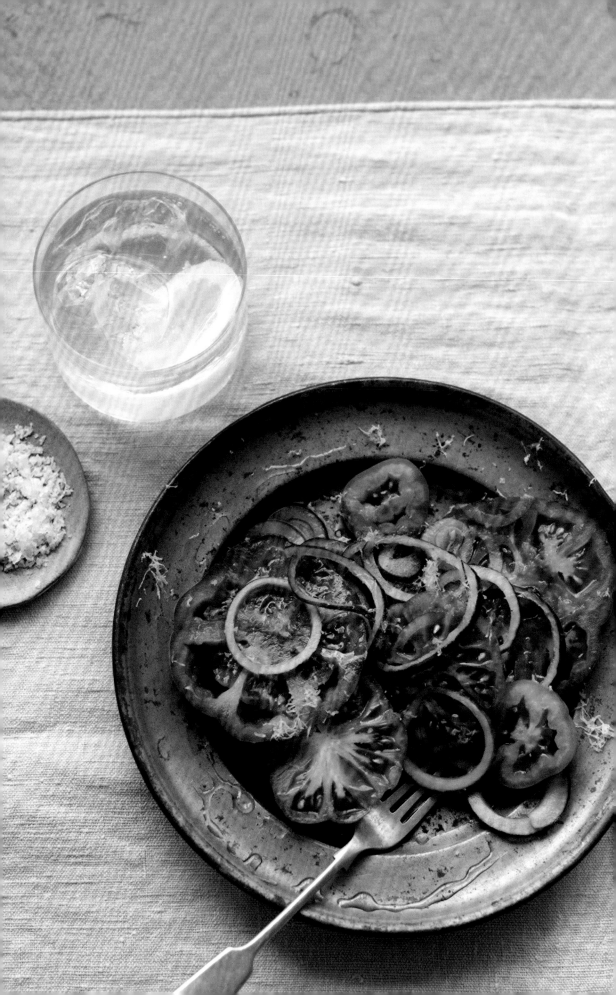

Som tam salad

Serves 2

186 calories per serving

This is inspired by a classic Thai green papaya salad called som tam, which means 'made in a mortar'. The dish is all about the sauce, which should taste sweet, sour, hot and salty. My version achieves that with seven ingredients: garlic, fresh ginger, honey, red chilli, lime juice, tamari and tamarind. Tomatoes always feature in a som tam as they contribute to the balance of sharp and sweet flavours, as well as adding a soft texture. I squeeze the cherry tomatoes into the dish to release their juices, which then run into the sauce.

2 garlic cloves
A thumb-sized piece fresh root ginger, grated
1 red chilli, chopped
2 tbsp honey
Juice of 3 limes
2 tbsp tamari
1 tbsp tamarind paste
100g fine green beans
1 green papaya
150g cherry tomatoes

To garnish
70g peanuts
A small handful of fresh coriander
A small handful of fresh mint, leaves picked

1 Put the garlic in a mortar and pound to a paste. Add the ginger and pound again to combine with the garlic and form a slightly chunkier paste. Add the red chilli, honey, lime juice, tamari and tamarind and pound them together. (It's important to pound the ingredients in stages like this so that everything is broken down well.)

2 Drop the green beans into a pan of boiling water and blanch for 1–2 minutes. Drain and rinse under cold water. Set aside.

3 Peel the papaya, cut it in half and scoop out the central seeds and fibres. Cut the flesh into matchsticks.

4 Squeeze each tomato between your thumb and forefinger over a bowl (this is the best way to get all the juice from them and means that they will soak up the flavours from the sauce too). Place the tomatoes in the bowl. Pour the garlic mixture into the bowl and add the green beans and papaya. Mix together.

5 Toast the peanuts in a small dry frying pan until golden. Roughly chop them.

6 Garnish the salad with the peanuts and fresh coriander and mint leaves.

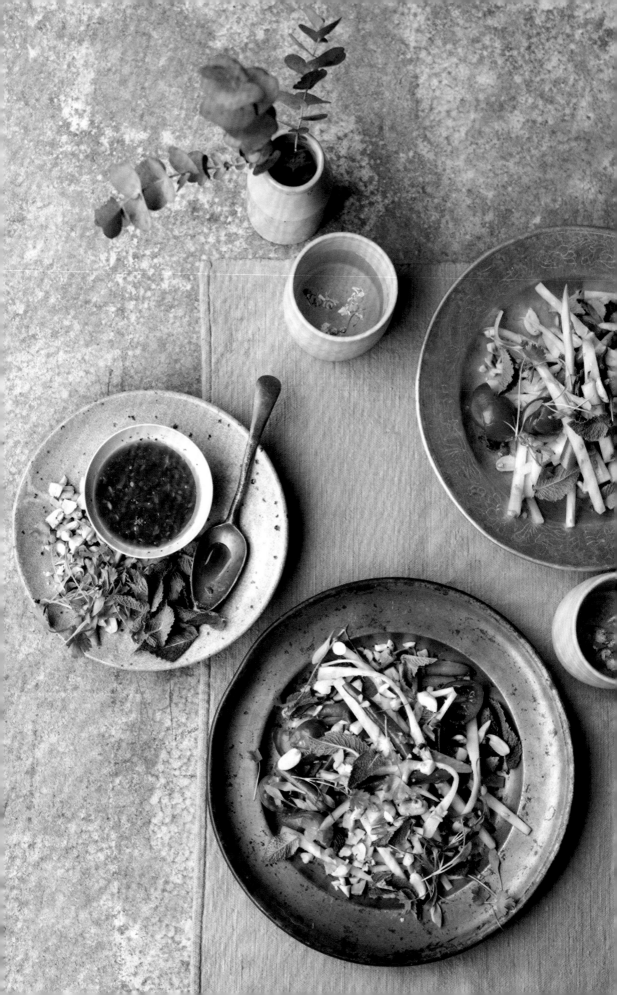

Ed's tomato sauce and pasta

Serves 4

407 calories per serving

My husband's father is Italian and, with a name like De Stefano, one would hope that a good tomato sauce was in his genes. It turns out it is. The key? Patience (something that I lack and he has in abundance, thank goodness!). The sauce is best if you can just let the tomatoes soften and cook down in their own time.

Olive oil for frying
1 red onion, finely chopped
3 garlic cloves, finely chopped
2 tbsp capers
4 sun-dried tomatoes, roughly chopped
4 large beef tomatoes, roughly chopped
100ml water
100g cherry tomatoes
1 tsp honey
½ tsp dried mixed herbs
300g gluten-free pasta (linguine or rigatoni)
Flaked sea salt and cracked black pepper
Fresh basil leaves, to garnish

1   Heat a little oil in a saucepan, add the onion and garlic with the capers, and cook for about 10 minutes until softened. Add the sun-dried tomatoes, the beef tomatoes and water and stir to mix. Cover the pan and leave to cook over a low heat for about 30 minutes until the beef tomatoes have completely softened.

2   Add the cherry tomatoes along with the honey, mixed herbs and a good pinch of black pepper. Stir in. Cover the pan again and cook gently for a further 20 minutes.

3   Cook the pasta according to the instructions on the packet (add a good pinch of salt to the cooking water). Drain, keeping back a ladleful of the water. Mix the tomato sauce through the pasta along with the reserved cooking water. Sprinkle with fresh basil and serve.

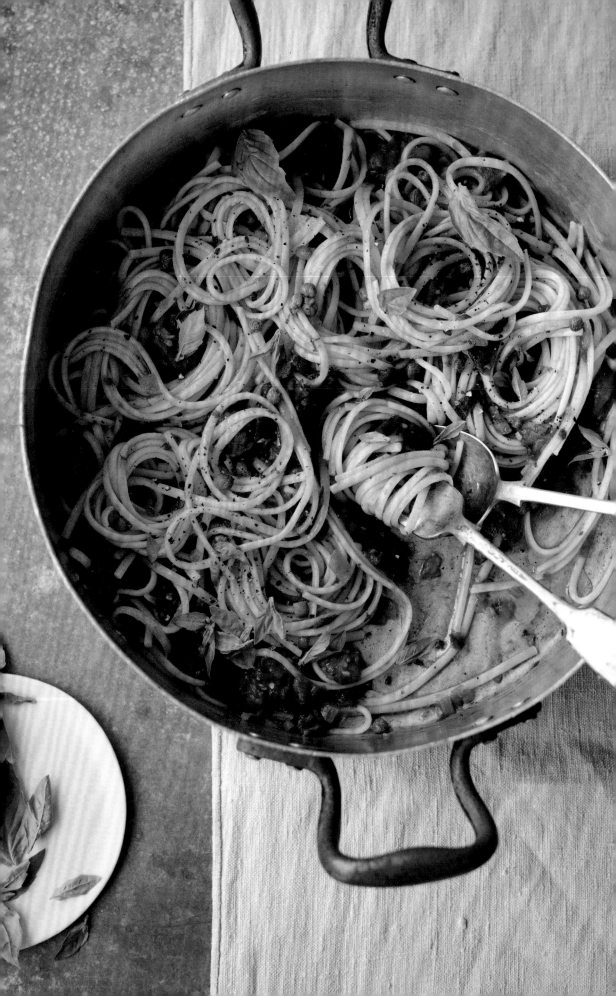

Mac and Tom

Serves 4

246 calories per serving

Creating a dairy-free cheese sauce sounds like an impossible task but in fact this recipe is quite easy and the result is a light, delicious sauce that everyone will enjoy. It's important to use a whisk when mixing the sauce as it can be prone to lumps – whisking will ensure that the texture is thick and creamy. I love the finished macaroni cheese with the bright red cherry tomatoes.

200g gluten-free macaroni
1 tbsp coconut oil
2 tbsp gluten-free flour
200ml oat milk
4 tbsp nutritional yeast (yeast flakes)
1 tbsp onion powder
1 tsp dried mixed herbs
100g cherry tomatoes, cut in half
4 tbsp gluten-free breadcrumbs
Flaked sea salt and cracked black pepper

1 Preheat the oven to 200°C/Fan 180°C/Gas 6.
2 Cook the macaroni according to the packet instructions (be sure to add a good pinch of salt to the cooking water). Drain well and tip into a baking dish.
3 Heat the coconut oil in a saucepan and stir in the flour to make a paste. Gradually add the milk, whisking constantly, and cook, whisking, until thickened. Add half of the nutritional yeast, the onion powder, mixed herbs, and a pinch each of salt and pepper and mix well. Pour this sauce over the macaroni and fold together.
4 Scatter the halved cherry tomatoes over the macaroni. Mix the remaining nutritional yeast with the breadcrumbs and sprinkle evenly over the top. Bake for 20–30 minutes until golden. Serve hot, with a green salad.

Tomato curry

Serves 4

326 calories per serving

This aromatic tomato and coconut curry is a real treat. Everything in the dish adds to the happy marriage of tastes and textures – the acidity in the tomatoes balances the creaminess of the coconut milk and the tempered spices add a punchy finish. I find that curry leaves, a staple of South Indian cooking, add a delicious nutty aroma.

200g black rice
1 tbsp rapeseed oil
3 onions, diced
2 garlic cloves, finely chopped
1 tbsp grated fresh root ginger
300ml water
300g vine tomatoes
1 tsp ground cumin
1 tsp ground ginger
1 tsp garam masala
½ tsp ground turmeric
100ml coconut milk
Flaked sea salt

For tempering
1 tbsp rapeseed oil
1 green chilli, sliced
1 tsp mustard seeds
5 fresh curry leaves

1   Put the rice in a saucepan with a pinch of salt and cover with three times the amount of water. Bring to the boil, then leave to simmer for 30–35 minutes until the rice is tender. Drain and set aside.

2   Heat the oil in a saucepan over a medium heat, add half of the diced onions and cook until translucent. Add the garlic and ginger and cook for a few more minutes until the garlic is golden. Pour in the water and bring to the boil. Add the tomatoes along with the ground spices and the coconut milk. Mix well. Reduce to a simmer and cook for 10 minutes until the tomatoes are soft.

3   To make the tempering mixture, heat the oil in a small frying pan and add the rest of the onions along with the chilli, mustard seeds and curry leaves. Sauté for about 5 minutes.

4   Serve the curry with the black rice and the tempering mixture poured over.

Red lentils and cherry tomatoes

Serves 2
696 calories per serving

This is a great sharing dish, easy to double up for a dinner party. I like to serve the lentil mixture in a big shallow dish topped with the roasted tomatoes, and chickpea flatbreads for dipping.

100g red lentils
Rapeseed oil for frying and drizzling
1 onion, finely chopped
2 garlic cloves, finely chopped
A thumb-sized piece fresh root ginger, finely
   chopped
1 tsp cumin seeds
1 tsp mustard seeds
1 carrot, finely diced
2 vine tomatoes, roughly chopped
100ml water
200g cherry tomatoes on the vine
1 tbsp tahini
Juice of 1 lemon
1 tbsp pumpkin seeds
Flaked sea salt and cracked black pepper
Chickpea flatbreads (see page 86), made
   without the spinach and egg, to serve

1 Preheat the oven to 200°C/Fan 180°C/Gas 6.
2 Put the lentils in a pan with cold water to cover generously. Bring to the boil, then simmer for 12–14 minutes until the lentils are cooked. Drain and set aside.
3 Heat a little oil in a saucepan and sauté the onion, garlic and ginger until softened. Add the cumin seeds with most of the mustard seeds and cook for 1–2 minutes until fragrant. Add the carrot, chopped tomatoes and water and stir to mix. Turn the heat to low and cook for 30 minutes until the carrot is soft.
4 Meanwhile, spread out the cherry tomatoes on a baking tray and drizzle over a little oil. Season with some salt and pepper. Roast for 12–15 minutes until softened.
5 Tip the carrot and tomato mixture into a food processor and add the lentils, tahini, lemon juice and a pinch each of salt and pepper. Blitz until smooth. Pour back into the pan and warm through gently.
6 Toast the pumpkin seeds in a small dry frying pan until golden.
7 Spoon the lentil mixture on to a plate and top with the pumpkins seeds, remaining mustard seeds and roasted cherry tomatoes. Serve with chickpea flatbreads.

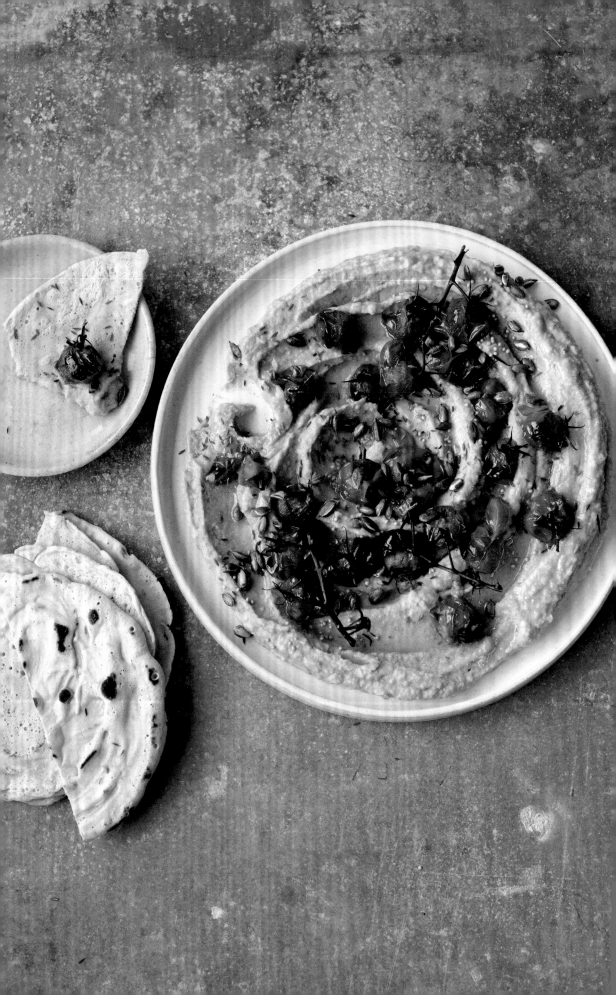

Courgette

The *Oxford English Dictionary* defines a courgette as 'the immature fruit of a vegetable marrow'. In other words, once they get past a certain size, courgettes no longer exist – they have developed into marrows.

Courgettes are harvested when they are 15–20cm long. When buying them you want to go for firm, smaller ones with an unblemished skin. Dark green courgettes are, of course, the most familiar in the UK, but you can also find white and yellow varieties with other shapes at some greengrocers and farmer's markets.

If you are growing courgettes in your garden, you know that they can become something of a nuisance because, well, they are just so easy to grow! They flourish and then infringe on the space of other crops. Courgettes just love a warm sunny day, so in the British summer – on those happy days when the sun does decide to come out at last – they can grow from flower to full-sized fruit in just hours!

When you cook courgettes, take care not to let them get mushy. Whether griddled, baked, roasted or sautéed, if you cook them with care they will show a beautiful, tender side. Or you can enjoy them raw, spiralising them into noodles called courgetti, as in the recipe on page 276).

Nutritional bonus

Courgettes have a lot to offer when added to a vegetable dish: they have a high water content to make you feel full and they are low in calories. They're also a good source of **potassium.**

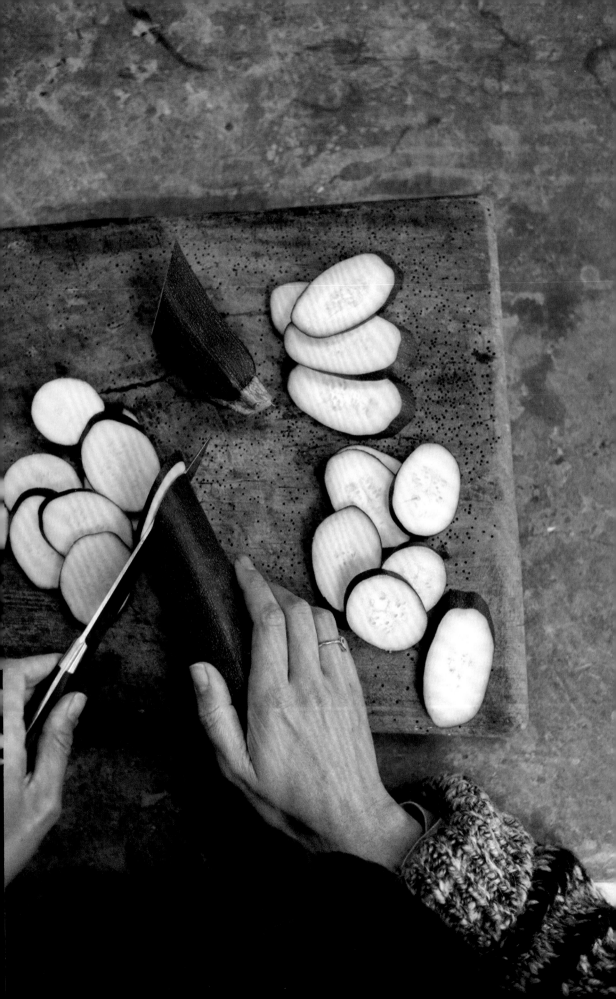

Roasted vegetable tabbouleh

Serves 2
552 calories per serving
Roasting courgettes is one of the best ways to cook them, as it reduces the amount of water they contain and gives them a firmer texture. A tabbouleh is typically made with tomatoes and herbs flecked with bulgar wheat, but I have opted for a wheat-free grain – buckwheat. Instead of tomatoes, I have loaded the tabbouleh with roasted vegetables, which makes for a more substantial dish.

1 aubergine, cut in half lengthways
2 courgettes, cut in half lengthways
1 red onion, cut into wedges
2 Portobello mushrooms, stalks removed
2 tsp rapeseed oil
150g buckwheat
A handful of fresh flat-leaf parsley,
   leaves picked
A handful of fresh coriander
A handful of fresh mint, leaves picked
1 cucumber
Juice of 1 lemon
A handful of flaked almonds
2 garlic cloves, sliced
Flaked sea salt and cracked black pepper

1 Place the aubergine, courgettes, onion and mushrooms on a tray. Drizzle over 1 teaspoon oil. Set aside until you are ready to griddle them.

2 Put the buckwheat in a pan with a pinch of salt and cover with three times the amount of water. Bring to the boil, then leave to simmer gently for 15–20 minutes until the buckwheat is tender and has become a lighter shade of green. Drain in a sieve and rinse under cold water to cool, then leave to drain thoroughly.

3 Finely chop the parsley, coriander and mint together. Cut the cucumber in half lengthways and remove the seeds. Slice each half into four long strips, then cut into small cubes. Mix the herbs and cucumber with the buckwheat in a large mixing bowl. Add the lemon juice and season with salt and pepper.

4 Set a ridged griddle/grill pan over a high heat. When the pan is hot, place the aubergine, courgettes, onion and mushrooms in it and griddle for a few minutes on each side until they are charred and tender. Transfer all the vegetables to a chopping board, season with salt and pepper, and chop roughly.

5 Heat a small frying pan, add the rest of the oil and lightly toast the flaked almonds with the sliced garlic.

6 To serve, put the buckwheat salad into a large dish, top with the griddled vegetables and scatter the flaked almonds and garlic over all.

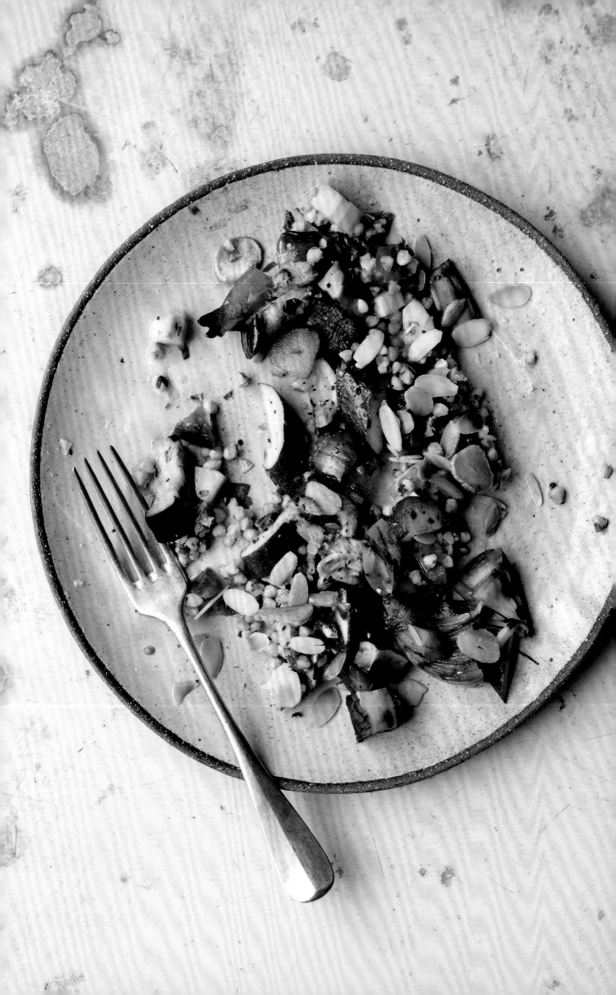

Stuffed courgettes with tapenade

Serves 2
570 calories per serving

There are several different varieties of courgette, yet we usually find only the standard long green ones at the greengrocer. When courgettes are in season in the summer, I try to find the small round variety, which is great for stuffing. Here I've used quinoa mixed with tapenade, a rich black olive and caper mixture.

150g quinoa
4 small round courgettes
1 tsp olive oil

For the tapenade
200g pitted black olives
1 garlic clove
2 tbsp capers
A small handful of fresh basil
1 tbsp olive oil
Flaked sea salt and cracked black pepper

1   Preheat the oven to 200°C/Fan 180°C/Gas 6.
2   To make the tapenade, put all the ingredients in a food processor and blitz to a coarse paste. You can also hand-chop this but everything must be very fine so that the flavours blend together. Season with salt and pepper to taste.
3   Put the quinoa in a pan with a pinch of salt and cover with three times the amount of water. Bring to the boil, then leave to simmer gently for 10–12 minutes until it is cooked and the tail has separated from the seed. Drain in a sieve. Mix with the tapenade.
4   Slice the top off each courgette. Score the central flesh with a small sharp knife, leaving enough flesh around the sides to keep the courgette in shape, then carefully scoop out the scored flesh and discard.
5   Place the courgettes on a baking tray and drizzle with the olive oil. Roast for 20 minutes. Remove from the oven and fill with the quinoa and tapenade mixture. Return to the oven and cook for 20–25 minutes. Serve immediately.

Malaysian laksa and courgetti

Serves 2
249 calories per serving

The kitchen manager at Detox Kitchen is a lovely person named Rohit. We are all very fond of him, not only because of his unshakeable chirpiness but also because he is an amazing chef. When I first tasted a laksa he made, he had only been working with us for a few weeks but I knew right away that I had to make sure he could never leave. This is my version of Rohit's laksa. The Malaysian soup typically has a rich, tangy coconut broth on a base of rice noodles. I've replaced the noodles with courgetti, which makes the dish lighter while still being indulgent.

4 courgettes
1 lemongrass stick
1 red onion, cut into quarters
1 red pepper, seeded and chopped
1 tbsp grated fresh root ginger
1 garlic clove, diced
1 red chilli, seeded and roughly chopped
200ml water
2 tbsp tamari
1 tbsp toasted sesame oil
Juice of 2 limes, plus lime wedges to serve
200ml coconut milk

1   Use a julienne peeler/cutter or spiraliser to make courgetti (courgette noodles).
2   Bash the lemongrass with a rolling pin, then roughly chop. Put it into a food processor along with the onion, red pepper, ginger, garlic and chilli and blitz to a paste. Transfer the paste to a saucepan and add the water, tamari, sesame oil and lime juice. Cook over a medium heat for 10–15 minutes. Stir in the coconut milk and simmer for a further 20 minutes. Pour the broth into a jug.
3   Divide the courgetti among the bowls and pour in the broth. Serve with lime wedges for squeezing over.

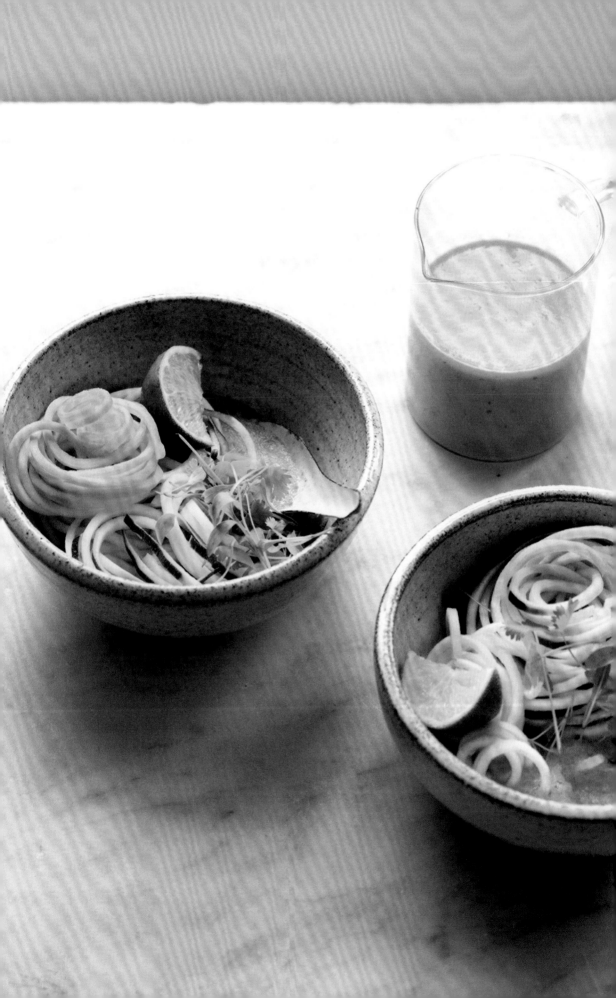

The ultimate vegetable curry

Serves 4
226 calories per serving

I have spent a lot of time in India, and it has stolen my heart in many ways. I love the tea plantations in Kerala, which are so breathtaking and dream-like. Indian cuisine has inspired a great deal of my cooking, particularly the cuisine of Kerala where the use of coconuts is prevalent, as there is such an abundance of them in the south. I've called this the 'ultimate' curry for two reasons: first, because it is jam-packed with vegetables (seven to be precise); and second, because the freshly made curry powder is so fragrant.

Coconut oil for frying
1 onion, chopped
2 garlic cloves, chopped
2 tbsp grated fresh root ginger
1 tbsp tomato paste
4 vine tomatoes, roughly chopped
½ cauliflower, cut into florets
200g baby corn, cut in half lengthways
1 red pepper, seeded and cut into small chunks
1 courgette, diced
300ml coconut milk
A small handful of fresh coriander, roughly chopped
1 tbsp honey
Zest of 2 limes, plus lime wedges to serve
1 tsp mustard seeds
10 fresh curry leaves
Flaked sea salt and cracked black pepper
Black or brown rice to serve

For the curry powder
2 tbsp cumin seeds
1 tbsp fennel seeds
1 tsp coriander seeds
3 cardamom pods
1 tsp ground cinnamon
1 tsp ground ginger
½ tsp ground turmeric

1   To make the curry powder, put the cumin, fennel and coriander seeds in a dry frying pan. Lightly crush the cardamom pods to open them and add their seeds to the pan. Toast the seed mixture for a few minutes, tossing constantly, until fragrant. Tip into a spice grinder or a mortar and grind to a powder. Mix in the ground cinnamon, ginger and turmeric.

2   Heat 1 teaspoon oil in a large saucepan set over a medium heat. Add the onion, garlic and ginger and cook for about 10 minutes until the onion is translucent. Add the curry powder and cook for a few minutes, stirring constantly so the spices do not catch (if they do, they will taste bitter). The key is to keep the spices moving so that they gradually cook in the oil. You can add a splash of water if necessary.

3   Stir in the tomato paste and fresh tomatoes and cover with water. Leave to simmer for about 20 minutes until the tomatoes have completely broken down.

4   Add the cauliflower, baby corn, red pepper and courgette along with 100ml more water. Simmer for 15 minutes until the vegetables are tender but still have a crunch. Stir in the coconut milk and simmer for a further 5 minutes. Finally, stir in the coriander, honey and lime zest. Remove from the heat and leave to stand for 5 minutes.

5   Meanwhile, heat a little oil in a small frying pan and cook the mustard seeds and curry leaves for a few minutes until fragrant.

6   Pour the mustard seeds and curry leaves over the curry and serve with brown or black rice and lime wedges for squeezing over.

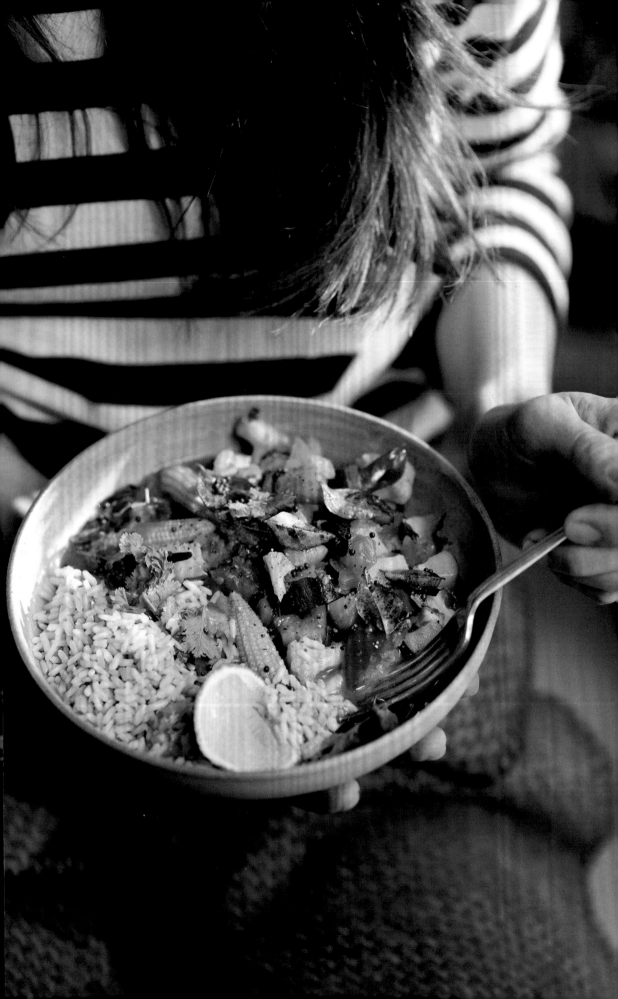

Courgette loaf cake

Cuts into 8 slices
436 calories per slice

This recipe for a courgette cake is pretty much foolproof. I've suggested a sweet icing to make it into a teatime offering, but you could leave it plain. It's then delicious sliced, toasted and spread with nut butter.

Coconut oil for greasing
3 eggs
100ml rapeseed oil
70g coconut sugar
300g courgettes, grated
250g gluten-free flour
1 tsp ground cinnamon
½ tsp grated nutmeg
½ tsp gluten-free baking powder
1 vanilla pod, split open and seeds scraped out
100g pecans, roughly chopped
2 tbsp sultanas

For the icing
200g coconut yoghurt
Zest and juice of 1 lime
1 tbsp maple syrup
1 tsp vanilla paste

1   Preheat the oven to 200°C/Fan 180°C/Gas 6. Grease a small loaf tin.
2   Crack the eggs into a large mixing bowl and whisk in the rapeseed oil and coconut sugar until light and fluffy. Add the courgettes and mix thoroughly. Sift in the flour along with the cinnamon, nutmeg and baking powder and fold through using a large metal spoon. Add the vanilla seeds, chopped pecans and sultanas and incorporate thoroughly.
3   Tip the mixture into the prepared loaf tin. Bake for 35–40 minutes until golden and soft to the touch but cooked through (a skewer should come out clean). Allow to cool.
4   To make the icing, put all the ingredients into a large mixing bowl and whisk together. Chill for 20 minutes to firm up.
5   Remove the cooled cake from the tin. Pour the icing over the cake and cut into slices.

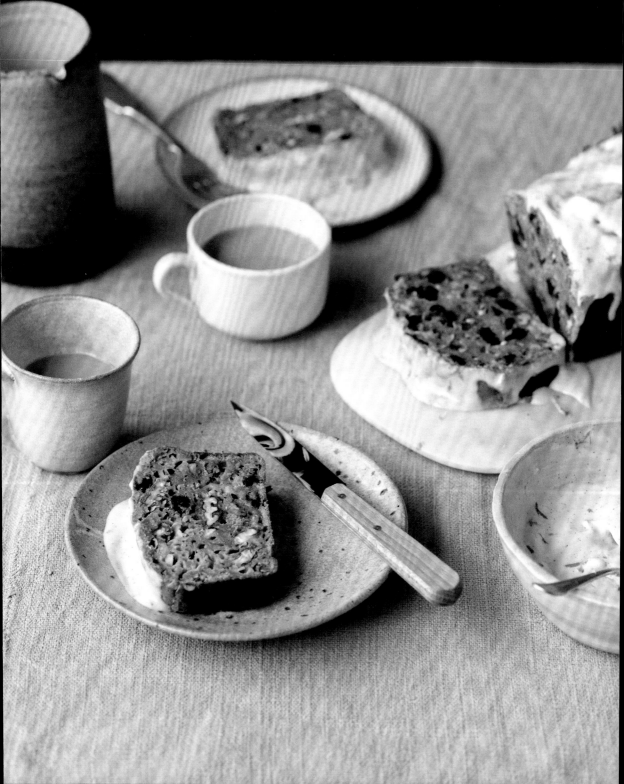

Marrow

The marrow is a tiger-striped beast of a vegetable. It's literally the fully grown version of a courgette, and as part of the cucurbit family is also related to melon, cucumber, pumpkin and butternut squash.

Marrows are a wonderful bonus for the thrifty cook because for their size they are cheap. In addition they are the perfect vehicle for bold flavours. They work brilliantly in curries and stews, and are perfect for stuffing and baking, as they are large enough to take a good amount of filling and porous enough to soak up all the lovely cooking juices.

Take your time when choosing your marrow in the shop. If you want to end up with a dish that actually tastes of something, go for the smallest marrow you can find – about 20cm in length. Once marrows are over a certain size they become bitter and watery, and are of no use at all –except perhaps winning a horticultural competition.

Nutritional bonus
Marrows are wonderfully low in calories and, like courgettes, have a high water content. They are a source of **vitamin C** and **carotene**, which work together to help your immune system.

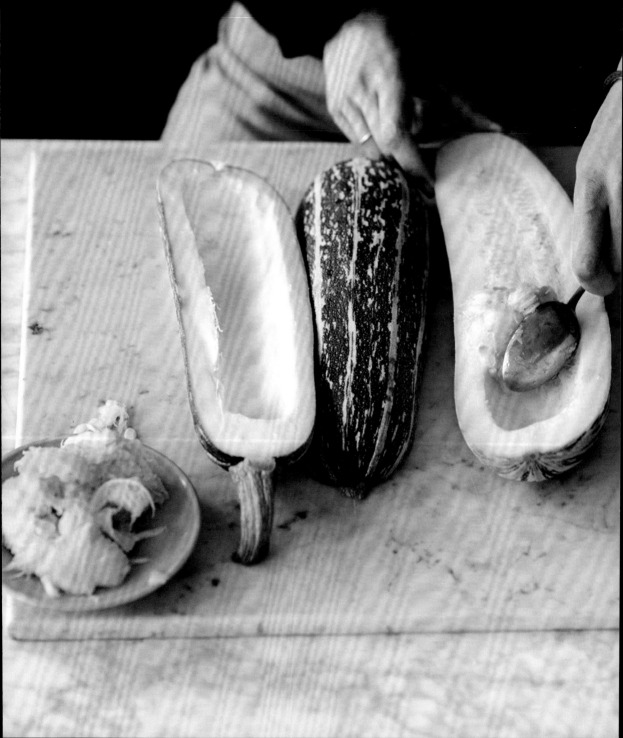

Marrow and aubergine masala

Serves 4
420 calories per serving

Marrow is great at soaking up flavours, which is why it is the perfect vegetable for a curry, along with aubergine. In this recipe, after the marrow has been simmering in the spicy tomato sauce, it almost disappears into the liquid to create a wonderful thick, soft texture.

1 small marrow, about 800g
1 aubergine
1 tbsp rapeseed oil
2 onions, diced
1 garlic clove, finely chopped
1 tbsp grated fresh root ginger
½ tsp mustard seeds
3 fresh curry leaves
1 tsp ground cumin
1 tsp ground fennel
2 cloves
2 cardamom pods
½ tsp ground turmeric
1 tbsp tamarind paste
200g tomatoes, roughly chopped
200ml water
200g brown rice or wild rice
200ml coconut milk
Juice of 2 limes
A small handful of fresh coriander, roughly
    chopped

For the coconut raita
200g coconut yoghurt
1 onion, finely chopped
A small handful of fresh mint, leaves picked
    and finely chopped
1 tsp honey
Flaked sea salt and cracked black pepper

1 Trim the ends off the marrow, then cut it in half lengthways and scoop out all of the seeds and soft flesh in the middle. Sprinkle the cut surfaces with salt and turn over on some kitchen paper to drain for 20 minutes. Rinse off the salt.

2 Cut the marrow halves across into 1cm half-moons and then in half again. Cut the aubergine in half lengthways. Cut across into 1cm half-moons and then in half again. Set the marrow and aubergine aside.

3 To make the coconut raita, mix together all the ingredients in a serving bowl. Cover and set aside in the fridge.

4 Heat the oil in a pan over a medium heat and gently sauté the onions, garlic and ginger until softened. Add the mustard seeds and curry leaves and sauté for a few more minutes until the leaves are fragrant. Add the remaining spices, including the tamarind paste, and a pinch each of salt and pepper. Cook, stirring constantly to make sure the spices don't catch and burn, for 1–2 minutes. Stir in the tomatoes and water, then leave to cook for 30 minutes.

5 Add the marrow and aubergine to the sauce and mix in. Put the lid on the pan and cook for a further 20 minutes until the marrow is soft.

6 Meanwhile, put the rice in a saucepan with a pinch of salt and cover with three times the amount of water. Bring to the boil, then simmer until the rice is tender – brown rice will take 20–25 minutes and wild rice 30–35 minutes. Drain well.

7 Stir the coconut milk, lime juice and chopped coriander into the marrow and aubergine masala and simmer for a few more minutes. Serve with the rice and coconut raita.

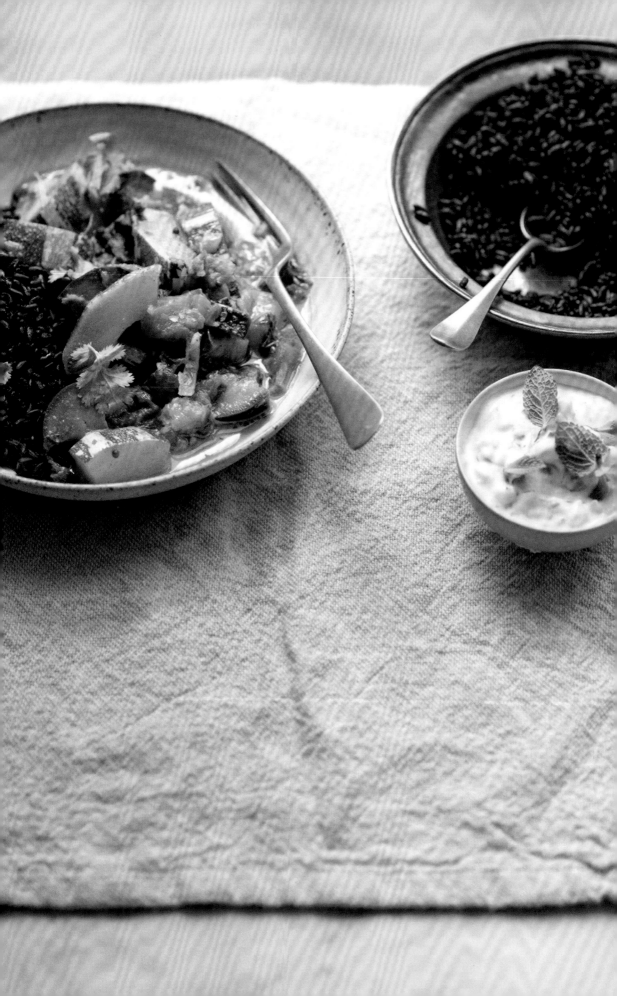

Marrow and bean stew

Serves 4
349 calories per serving
You can add any extra vegetables to this stew, depending on what you have on the day. The key ingredient is the marrow, which will absorb the herbal flavours and bring the whole dish together.

1 small marrow
Rapeseed oil for frying
1 large onion, diced
3 garlic cloves, chopped
250g tomatoes, roughly chopped
1 tbsp tomato paste
A small handful of fresh flat-leaf parsley, finely chopped, plus extra to garnish
3 fresh thyme sprigs
500ml vegetable stock
2 bay leaves
200g fine green beans
200g jarred butter beans, drained and rinsed
240g brown rice
Flaked sea salt and cracked black pepper

1   Peel the marrow and cut in half lengthways. Scoop out the seeds and soft centre with a spoon, then cut the halves across into 2cm half-moons. Place them on some kitchen paper, sprinkle with 1 tablespoon salt and leave to drain for about 20 minutes. Pat dry.
2   Heat a little oil in a large saucepan set over a medium heat and sauté the onion and garlic for about 10 minutes until translucent. Add the chopped tomatoes, tomato paste, parsley and thyme. Reduce the heat and cook, stirring occasionally, for about 10 minutes until the tomatoes are soft.
3   Pour in the stock and add the bay leaves. Bring to the boil, then simmer for 15 minutes until about half of the liquid has evaporated. Add the marrow, green beans and butter beans and stir in. Put the lid on the pan and simmer for 20–25 minutes.
4   Meanwhile, put the rice in a saucepan with a pinch of salt and cover with three times the amount of water. Bring to the boil, then leave to simmer gently for 20–25 minutes until the rice is tender and fluffy. Drain.
5   Serve the stew with the rice and sprinkled with chopped parsley.

Stuffed marrow

Serves 4
415 calories per serving
For the classic Spanish dish on which this is based, the marrow is stuffed with minced beef. I've replaced the beef with brown lentils, which give the stuffing a firm and slightly chewy texture. The herbs and spices add a Moroccan twist.

250g brown or Puy lentils
3 fresh mint sprigs, leaves picked and chopped
A small handful of fresh coriander, roughly chopped
10 fresh chives, finely chopped
1 tsp dried oregano
1 tsp za'atar (see page162 or use ready-made)
Zest of 2 lemons
1 tbsp olive oil
1 medium marrow

For the onion mixture
1 red onion, finely diced
3 garlic cloves, finely chopped
2 tbsp pine nuts
1 tbsp olive oil
Flaked sea salt and cracked black pepper

1   Put the lentils in a saucepan and cover with three times the amount of water. Bring to the boil, then simmer gently for about 20 minutes until the lentils are tender. Drain and place in a mixing bowl. Add the chopped fresh herbs, dried oregano, za'atar, lemon zest, oil, and 1 teaspoon each salt and pepper.
2   Preheat the oven to 200°C/Fan 180°C/Gas 6. Line a baking tray with greaseproof paper.
3   Cut the marrow in half lengthways and scoop out the seeds and soft centre with a spoon. Place the halves cut side up on the baking tray. Roast for about 30 minutes until softened and lightly golden on top. Fill the marrow halves with the lentil mixture.
4   Put all the ingredients for the onion mixture in a bowl, add a pinch each of salt and pepper, and mix together. Spoon on top of the lentils. Bake the stuffed marrow for 30 minutes until the onion topping is crispy.
5   Cut the stuffed marrow halves across into 4cm slices to serve.

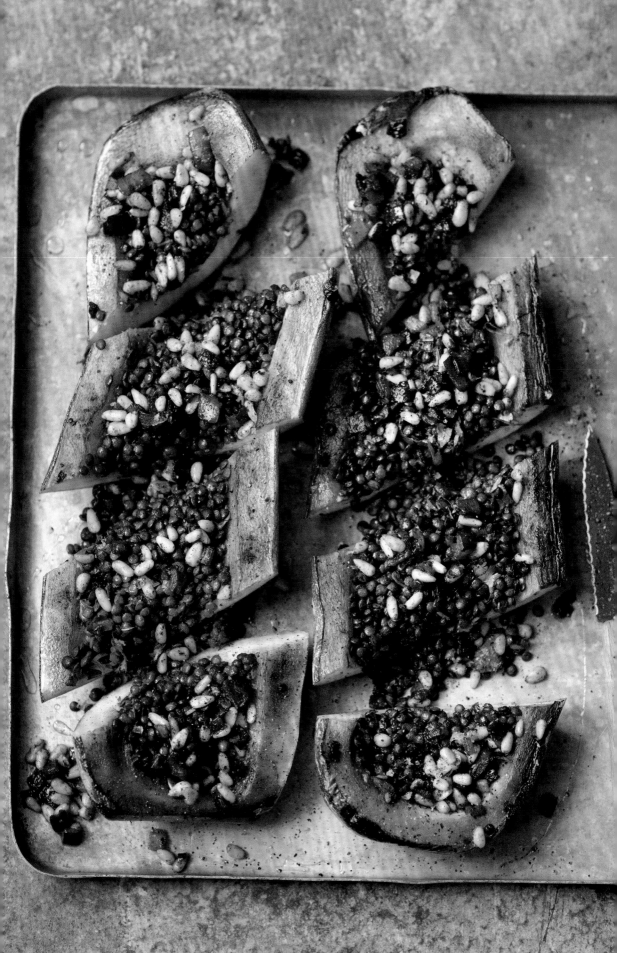

Sweetcorn

Fresh corn on the cob is one of nature's simplest and purest pleasures. When I was small we had special little skewers to spike into the ends of a cooked corn on the cob, so that we could hold it as we devoured it.

If you want sweetcorn kernels, you can slice them off in strips. I very rarely buy tinned sweetcorn, as it just isn't the same as the crunchy, succulent fresh stuff. Frozen sweetcorn, though, does make an acceptable substitute when fresh sweetcorn is not available.

Corn on the cob doesn't have to be boiled – you can grill or griddle it. Sweetcorn kernels can be blended into a soup or added to a mixture that is shaped into little polpette or 'burgers' (see pages 290 and 294). A little chilli and lime will enhance the sweet, nutty taste – the mango and sweetcorn salad on page 292 is a lovely example of this combination.

There is nothing more enchanting than seeing sweetcorn growing in abundance. The plants do like a lot of space and can be difficult to grow in a small garden, but you could always buy a ready-grown sweetcorn plant and pop it into your vegetable patch in May for a good crop later in the summer or the following year.

When choosing corn on the cob in the shops, peel back any green leaves so you can examine the kernels: they should be tightly packed and plump, bright yellow and shiny, not pale or wrinkled.

Nutritional bonus
Made up predominantly of carbohydrate, sweetcorn is one of the higher calorie vegetables, containing about 86 calories per 100g (as a comparison, cauliflower has 23 calories per 100g). But sweetcorn is still a relatively low-calorie option. It offers helpful amounts of **vitamin B3** (niacin) as well as dietary **fibre** and **folate**.

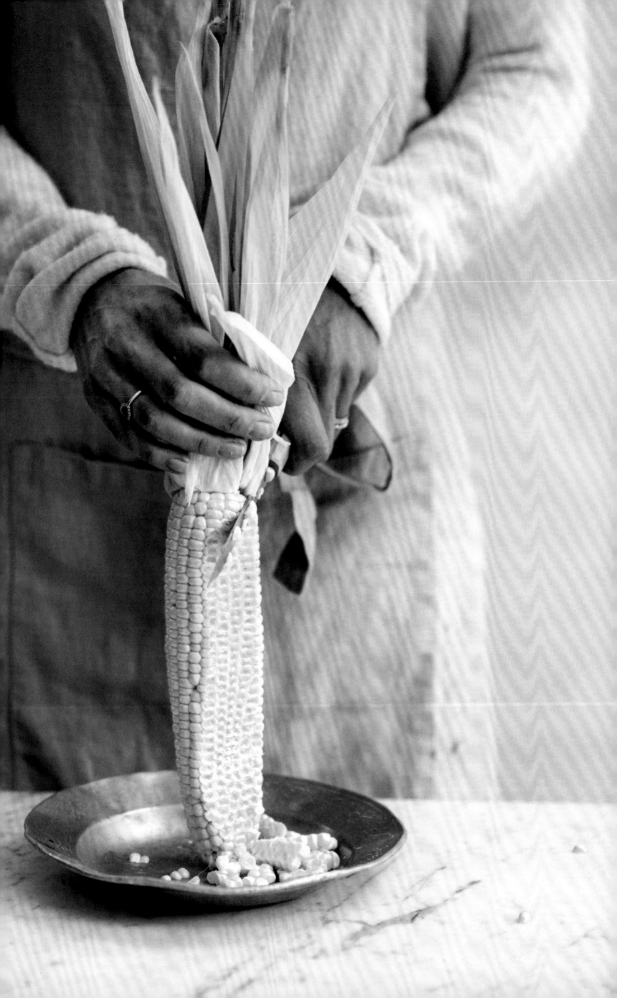

Grilled corn on the cob with herb dressing

Serves 2
232 calories per serving
When we were small, corn on the cob was always such a treat for me and my brothers, and we all had our own way of eating it. I liked to bite off the kernels in a row, rotating the cob as each row was devoured. This recipe is a grown-up version of that childhood treat, served with a delicious fresh herb and garlic dressing.

4 corn on the cob, leaves and silk removed
1 tsp rapeseed oil

For the herb dressing
A few fresh tarragon sprigs
A small handful of fresh flat-leaf parsley
10 fresh chives
2 garlic cloves, chopped
1 tbsp olive oil
Flaked sea salt and cracked black pepper

1 Preheat the grill to high and line a baking tray with greaseproof paper.
2 Place the corn on the cob on the baking tray, drizzle over the oil and season with some salt and pepper. Cook under the grill until the corn is golden and slightly charred all over, turning a little every 5 minutes or so for an even cook.
3 Meanwhile, make the herb dressing. Put all the herbs and garlic on a chopping board and finely chop them together with the olive oil and a pinch of salt. Transfer to a bowl.
4 Remove the corn from the grill and allow to cool for a few minutes before spooning over the herb dressing to serve.

Sweetcorn and kohlrabi chowder

Serves 4
137 calories per serving
Sweetcorn chowder usually contains potatoes but I have substituted kohlrabi – I think it adds freshness, and its bitterness perfectly balances the sweetness of the corn. Instead of cream, I've used coconut milk, which creates a similar texture but with a lightness that makes this the perfect late-summer soup.

1 tbsp rapeseed oil, plus extra for drizzling
2 onions, finely chopped
1 garlic clove, finely chopped
1 tbsp grated fresh root ginger
3 corn on the cob, leaves and silk removed
200ml vegetable stock
1 kohlrabi, peeled and diced
200ml coconut milk
1 tsp sweet paprika
Flaked sea salt and cracked black pepper

1 Heat the oil in a saucepan set over a medium heat and cook the onions, garlic and ginger for about 10 minutes until the onions are soft.
2 Meanwhile, use a sharp knife to shave the sweetcorn kernels off the cob (run the knife close to the cob to remove whole kernels). Add the sweetcorn kernels to the saucepan and cook for a few more minutes.
3 Remove half of the mixture from the pan and set aside. Add the stock and kohlrabi to the pan and simmer for about 10 minutes until the kohlrabi is soft. Stir in the coconut milk and simmer for a further 2 minutes. Using a hand blender (or in a food processor), blitz the mixture until smooth.
4 Return the sweetcorn and onion mix you set aside and stir back into the puréed soup in the pan. Season with salt and pepper to taste. Heat through.
5 Ladle the soup into bowls and add a sprinkle of paprika, an extra drizzle of oil, and some salt and pepper. Serve hot.

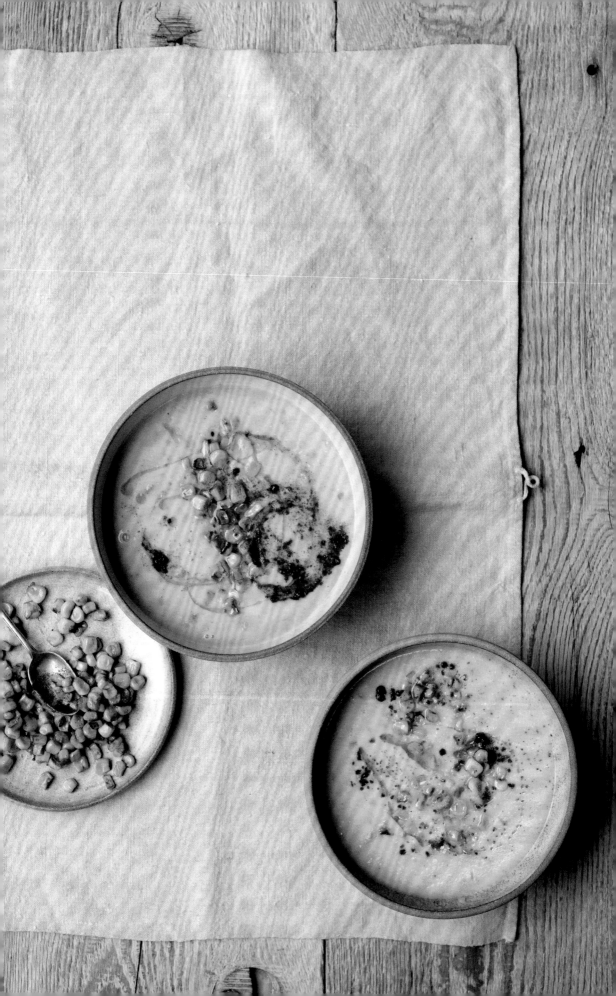

Charred sweetcorn and mango salad

Serves 2
113 calories per serving

Charring fresh sweetcorn into a state of smoky sweetness is one of the best ways to cook it. Adding mango and fresh coriander as well as cherry tomatoes gives this simple summer salad a lovely tropical flavour and colour. Serve as a side dish, or with some black rice and green salad.

1 mango
100g cherry tomatoes, cut in half
2 spring onions, sliced
A small handful of fresh coriander, roughly chopped
2 corn on the cob, leaves and silk removed
Flaked sea salt and cracked black pepper

1 Peel the mango and cut the flesh off the stone. Dice the flesh. Put it into a bowl and add the cherry tomatoes, spring onions, coriander, and salt and pepper to taste.

2 Heat a ridged griddle/grill pan over a high heat. Place the corn on the cob on the pan and cook until tender and charred all over. Remove from the pan and leave for about 5 minutes until cool enough to handle, then use a sharp knife to slice off the kernels (keep the knife close to the cob so that you cut whole kernels). Add the sweetcorn kernels to the mango salad and mix gently together.

Golden sweetcorn patties

Serves 4

407 calories per serving

I love a dish that will appeal to all generations –
it makes for a much more harmonious mealtime.
These sweetcorn patties are just that. Everyone
loves them; they are quick to make; and they can
be served just as easily in a bun or with a big
wholesome salad.

400g jarred chickpeas, drained and rinsed
200g frozen sweetcorn, thawed
A big handful of fresh coriander
A handful of fresh dill
½ tsp ground cumin
½ tsp smoked paprika
Zest of 1 lemon
2 tbsp chickpea flour
Rapeseed oil for frying
Flaked sea salt and cracked black pepper
4 gluten-free burger buns (optional)

1   Put the chickpeas, sweetcorn, herbs, spices
    and lemon zest in a food processor and pulse
    to a coarse texture. You should still be able to
    see whole kernels of sweetcorn. Season with
    salt and pepper.

2   Dust the flour over a plate. Scoop out a quarter
    of the sweetcorn mixture and mould it into
    a ball, then place it on the floured plate. Press
    to flatten slightly into a patty. Do this with the
    rest of the mixture to create four patties. Chill
    to firm them up.

3   Heat a little oil in a frying pan and fry the
    patties for 5–7 minutes on each side until
    golden and heated through.

4   Serve either in buns or with my Best Barbecue
    Slaw (see page 116).

Sweetcorn polpette

Serves 2

618 calories per serving

Here is my vegetarian version of the Italian meatballs called 'polpette'. Chickpeas give them a soft texture, and sweetcorn adds satisfying bulk. With an abundance of herbs and spices, these make for very delicious eating. Meatballs are typically served with a tomato sauce and spaghetti. I've lightened up this version by using courgetti instead.

3 yellow courgettes
Fresh basil leaves, to garnish

For the polpette

200g frozen sweetcorn, thawed
400g jarred chickpeas, drained and rinsed
2 garlic cloves, finely chopped
1 tsp dried oregano
1 tsp dried basil
1 tsp ground fennel
1 tsp ground cumin
1 red onion, finely diced
2 tbsp porridge oats
2 tbsp gluten-free flour
Zest of 1 lemon
1 tsp honey
1 tbsp rapeseed oil, plus extra for drizzling

For the tomato sauce

1 tbsp rapeseed oil, plus extra for drizzling
1 onion, diced
2 garlic cloves, finely chopped
150g cherry tomatoes
Flaked sea salt and cracked black pepper

1. Preheat the oven to 200°C/Fan 180°C/Gas 6. Line a baking tray with greaseproof paper.
2. To make the polpette, put all of the ingredients in a food processor and blitz until the mixture is well mixed. Season with a good pinch of salt. Form the mixture into balls about the size of a 50-pence piece. Lay these polpette on the baking tray. Chill for about 15 minutes.
3. Remove the polpette from the fridge, drizzle over some oil and bake for 20–25 minutes until golden and firm.
4. While the polpette are in the oven, make the tomato sauce. Heat the oil in a small frying pan and cook the onion until translucent. Add the garlic and tomatoes, reduce to a low heat and cook, stirring occasionally, until the tomatoes have completely broken down to form a sauce. Add a little water if the sauce begins to catch. Season with salt and pepper to taste.
5. Use a julienne peeler/cutter or spiraliser to make courgetti (courgette noodles).
6. Serve the courgetti with the tomato sauce and polpette on top, garnished with a scattering of basil leaves.

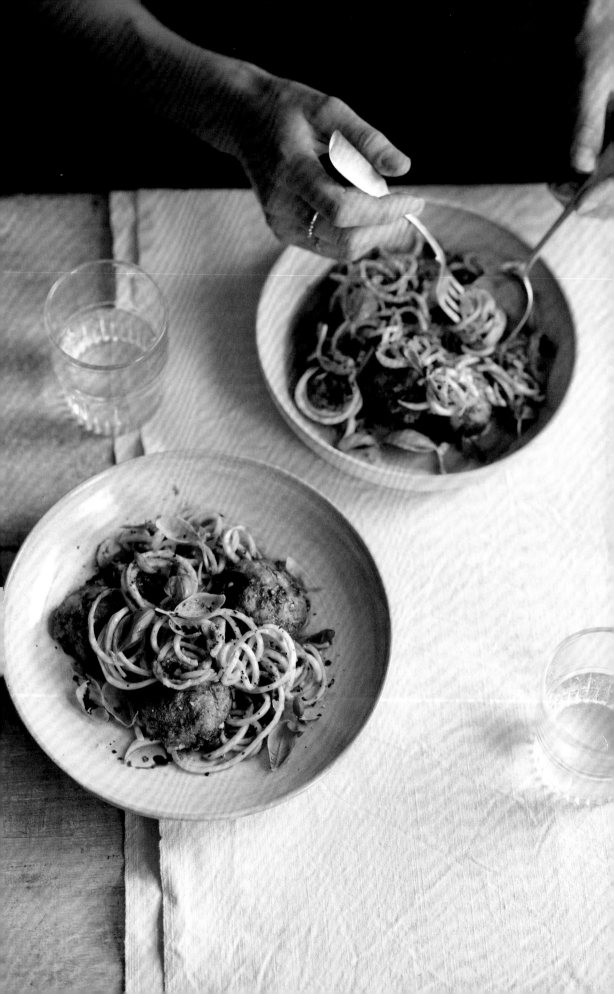

Index

A

almonds 11
   broccoli bread 126
   cauliflower pizza 144
   fennel and chocolate cake 56
   fennel and date balls 54
   pumpkin, cherry and almond pie 174
   rhubarb and peach crumble 60
apples: carrot muffins 200
   spiced fennel, Puy lentil and apple salad 50
artichokes see globe artichokes; Jerusalem artichokes
Asian-style broth 110
asparagus 30–9
   asparagus and mushroom breakfast stack 32
   asparagus and shallot tart 38
   asparagus and spinach soup 34
   asparagus and sweet potato frittata 32
   asparagus and wild rice salad 36
aubergines 240–51
   aubergine and artichoke caponata 244
   aubergine, artichoke and garden pesto salad 246
   aubergine fritter burgers 250
   baked aubergine with preserved lemon yoghurt 242
   Indian-style aubergine stacks 245
   marrow and aubergine masala 284
   roasted vegetable tabbouleh 274
   spiced aubergine fritters 248
   tomato and aubergine curry 146
avocados: artichoke heart and pomegranate salad 42
   avocado dressing 254
   avocado salad 226
   avocado salsa 136
   cucumber and avocado gazpacho 78
   cucumber and red pepper nori rolls 80
   cucumber, avocado and coconut smoothie 82
   green spring salad 114
   Mum's rice salad 78
   oyster mushrooms and avocado on toast 234
   radish, avocado and tofu 'voké' bowl 72
   spiced root vegetable rosti 210
   spiced stir-fried Brussels sprouts with tofu 122
   stuffed sweet potatoes 184
   sweet potato, black rice and chilli tortillas 180
   vegetable-fried rice with avocado 230

B

bananas: carrot muffins 200
   ice cream 56
   rhubarb banana bread with compote 64
   rhubarb granita and banana ice cream sundae 62
barley: carrot, broccoli stalk and barley soup 19
basil 9
   pea and cashew pesto 28
   pesto 238
beans see borlotti beans; butter beans etc

beetroot 208–17
   beetroot and coconut curry 216
   beetroot and shallot fritters 214
   beetroot crêpes with tarragon mushrooms 212
   beetroot slaw 236
   candy beetroot and blood orange salad 213
   herb-roasted root vegetables 188
   pea and cashew pesto with quinoa and pickled beetroot 28
   spiced root vegetable rosti 210
the best barbecue slaw 116
black beans: cauliflower tortillas 136
   pepper and black bean salad 254
   pumpkin feijoada 168
bok choy see pak choi
borlotti beans: artichoke and borlotti bean salad 44
bread: asparagus and mushroom breakfast stack 32
   broad bean bruschetta 14
   broccoli bread with artichoke spread 126
   flatbreads topped with spinach and egg 86
   panzanella 262
   see also toast
broad beans 12–19
   asparagus and wild rice salad 36
   broad bean and broccoli hummus 19
   broad bean and buckwheat salad 18
   broad bean and herb frittata 16
   broad bean bruschetta 14
   pea and broad bean pasta 24
broccoli 124–33
   broad bean and broccoli hummus 19
   broccoli and coconut soup 129
   broccoli and red lentil stew 132
   broccoli bread with artichoke spread and radishes 126
   broccoli carpaccio with hoisin sauce 130
   butternut squash and sweet potato gnocchi with broccoli 164
   carrot, broccoli stalk and barley soup 197
   green spring salad 114
   leek and broccoli bake 222
   roasted broccoli with chilli 128
   super green salad 130
broth, Asian-style 110
bruschetta, broad bean 14
Brussels sprouts 118–23
   Brussels sprout and coconut dal 122
   Brussels sprouts, peanut and pumpkin seed salad 120
   spiced stir-fried Brussels sprouts with tofu 122
   sprouts and spelt rigatoni with tomato-cashew sauce 120
buckwheat 10
   broad bean and buckwheat salad 18
   onion and buckwheat patties 226
   red onion and blood orange salad with buckwheat 230

roasted carrots, buckwheat and pecan salad 196
roasted vegetable tabbouleh 274
burgers: aubergine fritter burgers 250
mushroom burger 236
butter beans: flatbreads topped with spinach and egg 86
marrow and bean stew 286
Portobello mushroom, tomato and bean bake 238
spinach and butter bean dip 74
butternut squash 154–65
butternut squash and rosemary soup 156
butternut squash and sweet potato gnocchi 164
butternut squash tacos 160
creamy butternut squash curry 163
roasted butternut squash with tahini and tamari
seeds 158
za'atar-roasted butternut squash 162

C

cabbage 112–17
the best barbecue slaw 116
green spring salad 114
roasted cabbage and lentils 114
super green salad 130
see also pak choi
cacao powder: fennel and chocolate cake 56
fennel and date balls 54
cakes: courgette loaf cake 280
fennel and chocolate cake 56
rhubarb banana bread 64
candy beetroot and blood orange salad 213
capers: leek, black lentil and caper salad 222
leeks, peas and capers on sourdough toast 220
caponata, aubergine and artichoke 244
caramel: porridge with pumpkin and salted caramel 172
caraway seeds, artichoke fritters with 44
cardamom 10
carpaccio, broccoli 130
carrots 191–201
carrot, broccoli stalk and barley soup 197
carrot cassoulet 198
carrot, fennel and celery salad 194
carrot muffins 200
crudités with dips 74
heritage carrot and black rice salad 194
honey-roasted parsnips and carrots 206
roasted carrots, buckwheat and pecan salad 196
spiced root vegetable rosti 210
cashew nuts 11
Brussels sprout and coconut dal 122
butternut squash tacos 160
kale and chilli salad with cashews 94
pea and cashew pesto 28
pesto 238
stuffed sweet potatoes 184
sweet potato massaman curry 178
tarragon pesto 36
tomato-cashew sauce 120
cassoulet, carrot 198
cauliflower 134–47
broccoli and red lentil stew 132
cauli cous cous and cranberries 140
cauliflower frittata 138
cauliflower fritters with sweet and sour sauce 141
cauliflower pizza with lemon-infused tomatoes 144

cauliflower steak with warm green lentil salad 142
cauliflower tortillas 136
crudités with dips 74
leek and broccoli bake 222
smooth pepper soup 257
stuffed Romano peppers 258
tomato and aubergine curry with cauliflower rice 146
the ultimate vegetable curry 278
celery: carrot, fennel and celery salad 194
ceps: Asian-style broth 110
cherries: pumpkin, cherry and almond pie 174
chickpea flour: kale pakoras 92
chickpeas: broad bean and broccoli hummus 19
golden sweetcorn patties 293
Jerusalem artichoke polpette 190
kale, giant chickpea and celery stew 94
onion and buckwheat patties 226
red pepper and chickpea dip 74
sweetcorn polpette 294
chillies: chilli sambal 96
kale and chilli salad 94
kale pakoras 92
pea and broad bean pasta 24
roasted broccoli with chilli 128
smoky pepper and sweet potato chilli 256
som tam salad 264
spiced okra curry 152
sweet potato chilli 182
chives 9
chocolate: fennel and chocolate cake 56
fennel and date balls 54
chowder, sweetcorn and kohlrabi 290
chutney 245
cinnamon 10
cloves 10
coconut milk: beetroot and coconut curry 216
broccoli and coconut soup 129
Brussels sprout and coconut dal 122
creamy butternut squash curry 163
Malaysian laksa and courgetti 276
mushroom curry 238
porridge with pumpkin and salted caramel 172
sweet potato massaman curry 178
sweetcorn and kohlrabi chowder 290
coconut water: cucumber, avocado and coconut
smoothie 82
coconut yoghurt see yoghurt
coriander 9
corn on the cob: grilled corn on the cob with herb
dressing 290
raw mushroom and sweetcorn salad 234
the ultimate vegetable curry 278
see also sweetcorn
courgettes 272–81
artichoke heart and pomegranate salad 42
courgette loaf cake 280
cucumber, fennel, spinach and courgette juice 82
leek and broccoli bake 222
Malaysian laksa and courgetti 276
pak choi and satay noodles 108
roasted vegetable tabbouleh 274
stuffed courgettes with tapenade 276
sweetcorn polpette 294
the ultimate vegetable curry 278

warm salad with roasted radishes and courgettes 70
see also marrow
cous cous, cauli 140
cranberries, cauli cous cous and 140
crêpes, beetroot 212
crudités with dips 74
crumble, rhubarb and peach 60
cucumber 76–83
broad bean bruschetta 14
coconut tzatziki 248
cucumber and avocado gazpacho 78
cucumber and red pepper nori rolls 80
cucumber, avocado and coconut smoothie 82
cucumber dip 92
cucumber, fennel, spinach and courgette juice 82
Mum's rice salad 78
radish and quinoa salad 68
the ultimate chopped salad 88
cumin 10
curry: beetroot and coconut curry 216
creamy butternut squash curry 163
marrow and aubergine masala 284
mushroom curry 238
spiced okra curry 152
sweet potato massaman curry 178
tomato and aubergine curry 146
tomato curry 269
the ultimate vegetable curry 278

D
dairy alternatives 11
dal: Brussels sprout and coconut dal 122
okra and dal 150
dates: fennel and date balls 54
hoisin sauce 130
porridge with pumpkin and salted caramel 172
dill 9
dips: broad bean and broccoli hummus 19
coconut raita 284
crudités with dips 74
cucumber dip 92
red lentils and cherry tomatoes 270
red pepper and chickpea dip 74
spinach and butter bean dip 74
drinks: cucumber, avocado and coconut smoothie 82
cucumber, fennel, spinach and courgette juice 82

E
edamame beans: green spring salad 114
super green salad 130
Ed's tomato sauce and pasta 266
eggs 11
asparagus and mushroom breakfast stack 32
asparagus and sweet potato frittata 32
broad bean and herb frittata 16
cauliflower frittata 138
flatbreads topped with spinach and egg 86
kale and pea omelette 96
okra and egg-fried rice 152
parsnip rosti with fried egg 204
pea, leek and tarragon omelette 22
pepper and black bean salad 254
spiced root vegetable rosti with poached egg 210
vegetable-fried rice with avocado and a fried egg 230

F
fava beans see broad beans
feijoada, pumpkin 168
fennel 48–57
carrot, fennel and celery salad 194
cucumber, fennel, spinach and courgette juice 82
fennel and chocolate cake 56
fennel and date balls 54
honey and tamari-roasted fennel salad 52
spiced fennel, Puy lentil and apple salad 50
spiced okra curry 152
tomato and aubergine curry 146
fennel seeds 10
flatbreads topped with spinach and egg 86
flour 11
frittata: asparagus and sweet potato frittata 32
broad bean and herb frittata 16
cauliflower frittata 138
fritters: artichoke fritters with caraway 44
aubergine fritter burgers 250
beetroot and shallot fritters 214
cauliflower fritters 141
spiced aubergine fritters 248

G
gazpacho, cucumber and avocado 78
ginger: onion and ginger jam 228
super green salad with tahini and ginger 130
globe artichokes 40–7
artichoke and borlotti bean salad 44
artichoke fritters with caraway 44
artichoke heart and pomegranate salad 42
aubergine and artichoke caponata 244
aubergine, artichoke and garden pesto salad 246
broccoli bread with artichoke spread and radishes 126
Italian vignole 46
gnocchi, butternut squash and sweet potato 164
golden sweetcorn patties 293
grains 10
granita, rhubarb 62
green beans: green spring salad 114
marrow and bean stew 286
som tam salad 264
watercress and roasted tomato salad 102
green spring salad 114

H
haricot beans: carrot cassoulet 198
hazelnuts: broad bean and buckwheat salad 18
herb dressing 290
herb-roasted root vegetables 188
herbs 9–10
heritage carrot and black rice salad 194
hoisin sauce, broccoli carpaccio with 130
honey: fennel and chocolate cake 56
honey and tamari-roasted fennel salad 52
honey-roasted parsnips and carrots 206
hummus, broad bean and broccoli 19

I
ice cream 56
rhubarb granita and banana ice cream sundae 62
icing 280

Indian-style aubergine stacks 245
ingredients 9–11
Italian vignole 46

J
Jerusalem artichokes 184–91
    herb-roasted root vegetables 188
    Jerusalem artichoke and shallot soup 188
    Jerusalem artichoke polpette 190

K
kale 90–7
    the best barbecue slaw 116
    Italian vignole 46
    kale and chilli salad 94
    kale and pea omelette 96
    kale, giant chickpea and celery stew 94
    kale pakoras 92
kitchari, spinach 88
kohlrabi: sweetcorn and kohlrabi chowder 290
Korean-style pak choi and tofu 106

L
ladies' fingers see okra
laksa, Malaysian 276
leeks 218–23
    leek and broccoli bake 222
    leek, black lentil and caper salad 222
    leeks, peas and capers on sourdough toast 220
    pea, leek and tarragon omelette 22
lemon: baked aubergine with preserved lemon yoghurt
    242
    broccoli and red lentil stew with preserved lemons
        132
    pea and broad bean pasta with lemon 24
lentils: broccoli and red lentil stew 132
    Brussels sprout and coconut dal 122
    heritage carrot and black rice salad 194
    leek, black lentil and caper salad 222
    okra and dal 150
    red lentils and cherry tomatoes 270
    roasted cabbage and lentils 114
    spiced fennel, Puy lentil and apple salad 50
    spinach kitchari 88
    stuffed marrow 286
    warm green lentil salad 142
lettuce: artichoke heart and pomegranate salad 42
    smoky pepper and sweet potato chilli 256
limes: avocado dressing 254
    som tam salad 264
    za'atar-roasted butternut squash with lime yoghurt
        162
lychees: sweet and sour sauce 141

M
macaroni: Mac and Tom 268
Malaysian laksa and courgetti 276
mangoes: the best barbecue slaw 116
    charred sweetcorn and mango salad 292
marrow 282–7
    marrow and aubergine masala 284
    marrow and bean stew 286
    stuffed marrow 286
    see also courgettes

masala, marrow and aubergine 284
massaman curry, sweet potato 178
mayonnaise, vegan 194
'meatballs' see polpette
mint 10
muffins, carrot 200
Mum's rice salad 78
mung beans: Indian-style aubergine stacks 245
mushrooms 232–9
    Asian-style broth 110
    asparagus and mushroom breakfast stack 32
    beetroot crêpes with creamy tarragon mushrooms
        212
    leek and broccoli bake 222
    mushroom burger with salsa verde 236
    mushroom curry 238
    oyster mushrooms and avocado on toast 234
    Portobello mushroom, tomato and bean bake 238
    raw mushroom and sweetcorn salad 234
    smoky pepper and sweet potato chilli 256
    the ultimate chopped salad 88

N
noodles, pak choi and satay 108
nori rolls, cucumber and red pepper 80
nuts 11
    see also almonds, hazelnuts etc

O
oats: asparagus and shallot tart 38
    carrot muffins 200
    pastry 174
    porridge with pumpkin and salted caramel 172
    quinoa porridge 62
    rhubarb and peach crumble 60
okra 148–53
    okra and dal 150
    okra and egg-fried rice 152
    spiced okra curry 152
olives: tapenade 276
omelettes: kale and pea omelette 96
    pea, leek and tarragon omelette 22
onions 224–31
    onion and buckwheat patties 226
    onion and ginger jam 228
    pickled onions 136, 158, 228, 250
    red onion and blood orange salad 230
    stuffed marrow 286
    three-onion 'voké' bowl 228
    tomato and onion salad 262
    vegetable-fried rice 230
oranges: candy beetroot and blood orange salad 213
    red onion and blood orange salad 230
oyster mushrooms and avocado on toast 234

P
padrón peppers, Spanish-style 254
pak choi 104–11
    Asian-style broth with pak choi, ceps and quinoa 110
    Korean-style pak choi and tofu 106
    pak choi and satay noodles 108
pakoras, kale 92
panzanella 262
papaya: som tam salad 264

parsley 9
    aubergine, artichoke and garden pesto salad 246
parsnips 202–7
    herb-roasted root vegetables 188
    honey-roasted parsnips and carrots 206
    parsnip rémoulade 206
    parsnip rosti with fried egg 204
pasta: Ed's tomato sauce and pasta 266
    Mac and Tom 268
    pea and broad bean pasta with lemon 24
    sprouts and spelt rigatoni with tomato-cashew
        sauce 120
pastry 100, 174
patties: golden sweetcorn patties 293
    onion and buckwheat patties 226
peaches: rhubarb banana bread with compote 64
    rhubarb and peach crumble 60
peanut butter: pak choi and satay noodles 108
    satay sauce 80
peanuts: Brussels sprouts, peanut and pumpkin seed
    salad 120
    som tam salad 264
pearl barley: carrot, broccoli stalk and barley soup 19
peas 20–9
    aubergine, artichoke and garden pesto salad 246
    Italian vignole 46
    kale and pea omelette 96
    leeks, peas and capers on sourdough toast 220
    pea and broad bean pasta 24
    pea and cashew pesto 28
    pea, leek and tarragon omelette 22
    pea soup with black rice 26
    watercress quiche 100
    see also sugarsnap peas
pecans 11
    courgette loaf cake 280
    roasted carrots, buckwheat and pecan salad 196
pepper 11
peppers 252–9
    beetroot and coconut curry 216
    butternut squash and rosemary soup 156
    carrot cassoulet 198
    creamy butternut squash curry 163
    cucumber and red pepper nori rolls 80
    leek and broccoli bake 222
    Mum's rice salad 78
    mushroom curry 238
    pepper and black bean salad 254
    pumpkin feijoada 168
    red pepper and chickpea dip 74
    smoky pepper and sweet potato chilli 256
    smooth pepper soup 257
    Spanish-style padrón peppers 254
    stuffed Romano peppers 258
    sweet and sour sauce 141
    sweet potato chilli 182
    the ultimate vegetable curry 278
pesto 238
    aubergine, artichoke and garden pesto salad
        246
    pea and cashew pesto 28
    tarragon pesto 36
pickles: pickled onions 136, 158, 228, 250
    pickled radishes 72, 74

pistachios: honey-roasted parsnips and carrots 206
    pea soup with black rice 26
    roasted pumpkin and black rice 170
pizza, cauliflower 144
polpette: Jerusalem artichoke polpette 190
    sweetcorn polpette 294
pomegranate seeds: artichoke heart and pomegranate
    salad 42
porridge: porridge with pumpkin and salted caramel 172
    quinoa porridge 62
Portobello mushroom, tomato and bean bake 238
potatoes: asparagus and spinach soup 34
    broad bean and herb frittata 16
    spiced root vegetable rosti 210
pumpkin 166–75
    porridge with pumpkin and salted caramel 172
    pumpkin, cherry and almond pie 174
    pumpkin feijoada 168
    roasted pumpkin and black rice 170
pumpkin seeds 11
    Brussels sprouts, peanut and pumpkin seed salad
        120
    butternut squash tacos 160
    roasted butternut squash with tahini and tamari
        seeds 158
    watercress risotto with pumpkin seeds 102

Q
quiche, watercress 100
quinoa 10
    Asian-style broth with quinoa 110
    Brussels sprouts, peanut and pumpkin seed salad
        120
    cucumber and red pepper nori rolls 80
    pea and cashew pesto with quinoa 28
    quinoa porridge with rhubarb and berry compote 62
    radish and quinoa salad 68
    radish, avocado and tofu 'voké' bowl 72
    stuffed courgettes with tapenade 276

R
radishes 66–75
    the best barbecue slaw 116
    broccoli bread with artichoke spread and radishes
        126
    crudités with dips 74
    Mum's rice salad 78
    pickled radishes 72, 74
    radish and quinoa salad 68
    radish, avocado and tofu 'voké' bowl 72
    three-onion 'voké' bowl 228
    warm salad with roasted radishes and courgettes 70
raita, coconut 284
ranch dressing 88, 136
raspberries: quinoa porridge with rhubarb and berry
    compote 62
red cabbage: the best barbecue slaw 116
red pepper and chickpea dip 74
rémoulade, parsnip 206
rhubarb 58–65
    quinoa porridge with rhubarb and berry compote 62
    rhubarb and peach crumble 60
    rhubarb banana bread with compote 64
    rhubarb granita and banana ice cream sundae 62

rice 10
  asparagus and wild rice salad 36
  beetroot and coconut curry 216
  heritage carrot and black rice salad 194
  marrow and aubergine masala 284
  marrow and bean stew 286
  Mum's rice salad 78
  mushroom curry 238
  okra and egg-fried rice 152
  pea soup with black rice 26
  pumpkin feijoada 168
  roasted pumpkin and black rice 170
  spiced stir-fried Brussels sprouts with tofu 122
  spinach kitchari 88
  stuffed Romano peppers 258
  sweet potato, black rice and chilli tortillas 180
  sweet potato chilli 182
  three-onion 'voké' bowl 228
  tomato curry 269
  vegetable-fried rice with avocado 230
  watercress risotto with pumpkin seeds 102
  see also wild rice
rigatoni: sprouts and spelt rigatoni 120
risotto, watercress 102
rocket: heritage carrot and black rice salad 194
  leek, black lentil and caper salad 222
root vegetables: herb-roasted root vegetables 188
  spiced root vegetable rosti 210
  see also carrots, parsnips etc
rosemary 10
  butternut squash and rosemary soup 156
rosti: parsnip rosti 204
  spiced root vegetable rosti 210

S
salads: artichoke and borlotti bean salad 44
  artichoke heart and pomegranate salad 42
  asparagus and wild rice salad 36
  aubergine, artichoke and garden pesto salad 246
  avocado salad 226
  the best barbecue slaw 116
  broad bean and buckwheat salad 18
  Brussels sprouts, peanut and pumpkin seed salad
    120
  candy beetroot and blood orange salad 213
  carrot, fennel and celery salad 194
  charred sweetcorn and mango salad 292
  green spring salad 114
  heritage carrot and black rice salad 194
  honey and tamari-roasted fennel salad 52
  kale and chilli salad with cashews 94
  leek, black lentil and caper salad 222
  Mum's rice salad 78
  panzanella 262
  pepper and black bean salad 254
  radish and quinoa salad 68
  raw mushroom and sweetcorn salad 234
  red onion and blood orange salad 230
  roasted carrots, buckwheat and pecan salad 196
  roasted vegetable tabbouleh 274
  som tam salad 264
  spiced fennel, Puy lentil and apple salad 50
  super green salad 130
  tomato and onion salad 262

the ultimate chopped salad 88
  warm green lentil salad 142
  warm salad with roasted radishes and courgettes 70
  watercress and roasted tomato salad 102
  salsas 250
  avocado salsa 136
  salsa verde 236
salt 11
  porridge with pumpkin and salted caramel 172
sambal, chilli 96
satay sauce 80, 108
seeds 11
  see also pumpkin seeds; sunflower seeds
shallots: asparagus and shallot tart 38
  beetroot and shallot fritters 214
  Jerusalem artichoke and shallot soup 188
shoyu sauce 72
slaws: beetroot slaw 236
  the best barbecue slaw 116
smoky pepper and sweet potato chilli 256
smooth pepper soup 257
smoothie: cucumber, avocado and coconut 82
som tam salad 264
soups: Asian-style broth with pak choi, ceps and quinoa
    110
  asparagus and spinach soup 34
  broccoli and coconut soup 129
  butternut squash and rosemary soup 156
  carrot, broccoli stalk and barley soup 197
  cucumber and avocado gazpacho 78
  Jerusalem artichoke and shallot soup 188
  Malaysian laksa and courgetti 276
  pea soup with black rice 26
  smooth pepper soup 257
  sweetcorn and kohlrabi chowder 290
soya yoghurt see yoghurt
Spanish-style padrón peppers 254
spelt rigatoni, sprouts and 120
spices 10
spinach 84–9
  asparagus and spinach soup 34
  cucumber, fennel, spinach and courgette juice 82
  flatbreads topped with spinach and egg 86
  pea and cashew pesto with quinoa and pickled
    beetroot 28
  pea soup with black rice 26
  salad 198
  spinach and butter bean dip 74
  spinach kitchari 88
  the ultimate chopped salad 88
  watercress quiche 100
  watercress risotto 102
spring greens: butternut squash tacos 160
sprouts see Brussels sprouts
squash see butternut squash
'steak' seasoning 132
stews: broccoli and red lentil stew 132
  carrot cassoulet 198
  kale, giant chickpea and celery stew 94
  marrow and bean stew 286
  pumpkin feijoada 168
  see also curry
stock, vegetable 11
sugarsnap peas: green spring salad 114

leek, black lentil and caper salad 222
pak choi and satay noodles 108
super green salad 130
sundae, rhubarb granita and banana ice cream 62
sunflower seeds 11
roasted butternut squash with tahini and tamari seeds 158
tarragon pesto 36
watercress risotto 102
super green salad 130
swede: carrot cassoulet 198
sweet and sour sauce, cauliflower fritters with 141
sweet potatoes 176–85
asparagus and sweet potato frittata 32
butternut squash and sweet potato gnocchi 164
smoky pepper and sweet potato chilli 256
stuffed sweet potatoes 184
sweet potato, black rice and chilli tortillas 180
sweet potato chilli 182
sweet potato massaman curry 178
sweet potato wedges 183
sweetcorn 288–95
avocado salad 226
beetroot slaw 236
charred sweetcorn and mango salad 292
golden sweetcorn patties 293
raw mushroom and sweetcorn salad 234
sweetcorn and kohlrabi chowder 290
sweetcorn polpette 294
the ultimate chopped salad 88
see also corn on the cob

T
tabbouleh, roasted vegetable 274
tacos, butternut squash 160
tahini: broad bean and broccoli hummus 19
roasted butternut squash with tahini and tamari seeds 158
super green salad with tahini and ginger 130
tamari: cucumber and red pepper nori rolls 80
hoisin sauce 130
honey and tamari-roasted fennel salad 52
roasted butternut squash with tahini and tamari seeds 158
shoyu sauce 72
tapenade, stuffed courgettes with 276
tarragon: creamy tarragon mushrooms 212
pea, leek and tarragon omelette 22
tarragon pesto 36
tarts: asparagus and shallot tart 38
pumpkin, cherry and almond pie 174
watercress quiche 100
three-onion 'voké' bowl 228
thyme 10
toast: leeks, peas and capers on sourdough toast 220
oyster mushrooms and avocado on toast 234
tofu: Korean-style pak choi and tofu 106
radish, avocado and tofu 'voké' bowl 72
spiced stir-fried Brussels sprouts with tofu 122
tomatoes 260–71
artichoke and borlotti bean salad 44
asparagus and mushroom breakfast stack 32
aubergine and artichoke caponata 244
cauliflower pizza with lemon-infused tomatoes 144

Ed's tomato sauce and pasta 266
Jerusalem artichoke polpette with tomato sauce 190
Mac and Tom 268
marrow and bean stew 286
mushroom curry 238
panzanella 262
Portobello mushroom, tomato and bean bake 238
red lentils and cherry tomatoes 270
smoky pepper and sweet potato chilli 256
smooth pepper soup with sun-dried tomatoes 257
som tam salad 264
spiced okra curry 152
sprouts and spelt rigatoni with tomato-cashew sauce 120
sweet potato chilli 182
tomato and aubergine curry 146
tomato and onion salad 262
tomato curry 269
tomato sauce 144, 294
watercress and roasted tomato salad 102
tortillas: cauliflower tortillas 136
sweet potato, black rice and chilli tortillas 180
turmeric 10
tzatziki, coconut 248, 250

U
the ultimate chopped salad 88
the ultimate vegetable curry 278

V
vegan mayo 194
vegetable-fried rice 230
vegetable stock 11
vignole, Italian 46
'voké' bowls: radish, avocado and tofu 72
three-onion 228

W
watercress 98–103
salad 198
watercress and roasted tomato salad 102
watercress quiche 100
watercress risotto 102
white beans: warm salad with roasted radishes and courgettes 70
wild rice: asparagus and wild rice salad 36
broccoli and red lentil stew 132
Mum's rice salad 78

Y
yoghurt: baked aubergine with preserved lemon yoghurt 242
coconut raita 284
coconut tzatziki 248, 250
icing 280
ranch dressing 136
vegan mayo 194

Z
za'atar 162
za'atar-roasted butternut squash 162

Acknowledgements

A huge thank you to the amazing team who helped bring my recipes to life. To the brilliant Issy Crocker, who always manages to capture something magical in each photograph. To the very clever Emily Ezekiel, whose golden touch makes every dish look devourable. To the delightful Kitty Coles, who helped prepare the recipes, and to Steph McLeod, whose cool calmness brought tranquillity to all our shoot days.

To the whole team at Bloomsbury, Xa Shaw Stewart and Lisa Pendreigh for their continued support, guidance and marvellous editing, as well as Richard Atkinson.

To the amazing Norma MacMillan, who was able to untangle my words and make every one sing.

To Pete Dawson and Alice Kennedy-Owen at Grade for the beautiful design.

To my agent Dorie, who is always so positive and supportive of everything that I want to do.

To my entire team at Detox Kitchen for their commitment and passion, which makes running a company impossibly enjoyable.

To all of our customers and friends, who have supported, believed and eaten with us since we launched in 2012. None of this would be possible without you and I am so thankful for everyone who continues to come back for more.

And finally, to my family. My mum, whose unfaltering support and kindness has meant that I can strive for my dreams. My dad, who continues to inspire every dish that I cook. For my little people, Fin and Eva, you make each day happier and cooking for you makes everything way more fun. And finally my husband, whose patience, kindness and understanding during the writing of this book made it all that little bit more magical.

This book is dedicated to my husband Ed

BLOOMSBURY PUBLISHING
Bloomsbury Publishing Plc
50 Bedford Square, London, WC1B 3DP, UK

BLOOMSBURY, BLOOMSBURY PUBLISHING and the Diana logo are trademarks
of Bloomsbury Publishing Plc

First published in Great Britain 2018

The information contained in this book is provided by way of general guidance in relation
to the specific subject matters addressed herein, but it is not a substitute for specialist
dietary advice. It should not be relied on for medical, health-care, pharmaceutical or
other professional advice on specific dietary or health needs. This book is sold with the
understanding that the author and publisher are not engaged in rendering medical,
health or any other kind of personal or professional services. The reader should consult
a competent medical or health professional before adopting any of the suggestions in
this book or drawing inferences from it

The author and publisher specifically disclaim, as far as the law allows, any responsibility
from any liability, loss or risk (personal or otherwise) which is incurred as a consequence,
directly or indirectly, of the use and applications of any of the contents of this book

If you are on medication of any description, please consult your doctor or health
professional before embarking on any fast or diet

A catalogue record for this book is available from the British Library

Library of Congress Cataloguing-in-Publication data has been applied for

ISBN: 978-1-4088-8446-1

10 9 8 7 6 5 4 3 2 1

Project Editor: Norma MacMillan
Designer: Peter Dawson, Alice Kennedy-Owen / GradeDesign.com
Photographer: Issy Croker
Food and Prop Stylist: Emily Ezekiel
Indexer: Hilary Bird

Printed and bound in China by C&C Offset Printing Co., Ltd

Bloomsbury Publishing Plc makes every effort to ensure that the papers used in the
manufacture of our books are natural, recyclable products made from wood grown
in well-managed forests. Our manufacturing processes conform to the environmental
regulations of the country of origin.

To find out more about our authors and books visit
www.bloomsbury.com and sign up for our newsletters